D0641953

The Engaged Workforce

The Engaged Workforce

Proven Strategies
to Build a Positive
Health Care Workplace

Jo Manion, PhD

Health Forum, Inc.
An American Hospital Association Company
CHICAGO

AHA
press

This publication is designed to provide accurate and authoritative information in regard to the subject matter covered. It is sold with the understanding that neither the authors nor the publisher are engaged in rendering legal, accounting, or other professional service. If legal advice or other expert assistance is required, the services of a competent professional should be sought.

The views expressed in this publication are strictly those of the authors and do not necessarily represent official positions of the American Hospital Association.

Portions of this book were published in earlier form in *Create a Positive Health Care Workplace!* by Jo Manion, PhD (Chicago: Health Forum, Inc., 2005).

Portions of chapter 8 are reprinted from *Polarity Management* by Barry Johnson, copyright © 1992, 1996. Reprinted by permission of the publisher, HRD Press, Amherst, MA, (800) 822-2801, www.hrdpress.com.

⛩ is a service mark of the American Hospital Association used under license by AHA Press.

Copyright © 2009 by Health Forum, Inc., an American Hospital Association company. All rights reserved. No part of this publication may be reproduced, stored in a retrieval system, or transmitted, in any form or by any means, electronic, mechanical, photocopying, recording or otherwise, without the prior written permission of the publisher.

Printed in the United States of America—04/09

Cover design by Cheri Kusek

ISBN: 978-1-55648-359-2   Item Number: 088709

Discounts on bulk quantities of books published by AHA Press are available to professional associations, special marketers, educators, trainers, and others. For details and discount information, contact AHA Services, Inc., P.O. Box 933283, Atlanta, GA 31193-3283 (Phone: 1-800-242-2626; E-mail: AHA-orders@pbd.com).

Library of Congress Cataloging-in-Publication Data

Manion, Jo.
    The engaged workforce : proven strategies to build a positive health care workplace / Jo Manion.
        p. ; cm.
    Includes bibliographical references and index.
    ISBN 978-1-55648-359-2 (alk. paper)
  1. Health services administration. 2. Personnel management. 3. Medical personnel . I. Health Forum (Organization) II. Title.
    [DNLM: 1. Health Services Administration. 2. Organizational Culture. 3. Personnel Management. W 84.1 M2782e 2009]
    RA971.M34676 2009
    362.1068'3—dc22   2008054089

This book is dedicated to:

My husband, Craig, my constant source of love, support, and encouragement.

The many health care leaders who are trying, every single day, to make their departments and organizations positive, healthy places to work in the face of the many challenges in today's business environment.

Contents

List of Figures and Tables

About the Author and Contributors

Jo Manion, PhD, RN, NEA-BC, FAAN, is a speaker, accomplished author, and senior management consultant who offers practical and creative approaches to organizational and professional issues. Since the early 1990s, she has worked with organizations and individuals engaged in creating effective cultural change, developing leadership capacity, and transforming organizational structures. Her focus is on creating positive workplace environments with high-impact retention strategies.

As a widely published author, she has written books on organizational innovation and intrapreneurship, creation of team-based health care organizations, and leadership. The second edition of *From Management to Leadership: Practical Strategies for Health Care Leaders* was released in 2005. She also co-authored *Nature's Wisdom in the Workplace: Managing Energy in Today's Healthcare Organization*.

She has published dozens of articles and book chapters on current issues in health care and is a frequent contributor to *H&HN OnLine*. Dr. Manion is a fellow in the American Academy of Nursing. After growing up in the Midwest, she earned her undergraduate and graduate degrees from Marycrest College and the University of Iowa. In addition, she has a master's degree and a doctorate in human and organizational development from the Fielding Graduate Institute in Santa Barbara, California. She makes her home with her husband and their two dogs in the Orlando, Florida, area.

Sharon H. Cox, MSN, RN, is principal consultant and sole proprietor of Cox & Associates, a health care consulting and training company in Brentwood, Tennessee. As a registered nurse and nurse manager, she worked for twenty years in both clinical and administrative positions in academic health centers. She has also worked for more than twenty years in consulting and staff development for health care organizations in the United States and Canada. Cox is a member of the editorial board of *Nursing Management* magazine and co-author of *Core Skills for Nurse Managers* (published by HCPro in 2004). She is primary author of *Nature's Wisdom in the Workplace: Managing Energy in Today's Healthcare Organization*. She holds a master of science degree in nursing from the Medical College of Georgia in Augusta.

Mary G. Jenkins, MA, is an organization development consultant, lecturer, and author specializing in strategic planning and system design. She has worked with a wide range of clients in business, education, government and health care including Shell Oil, Saturn Corporation, the U.S. Government Accountability Office, and the State of Michigan. Jenkins is co-author of *Abolishing Performance Appraisals: Why They Backfire and What to Do Instead,* and she is a contributor to *Managing Human Resources in the 21st Century: From Core Concepts to Strategic Choice* (published by South-Western College Publishing in 1999). She holds a master's degree in labor and industrial relations from Michigan State University in East Lansing.

Preface

WORKFORCE SHORTAGES, both current and impending, are reported to top the list of the health care executive's concerns in this and future decades. Creating a positive workplace culture is a key factor in attracting good people to an organization as well as in retaining them. The composition of the workforce is changing significantly from years past. "Our economy is rapidly changing from a money economy to a satisfaction economy" (Seligman 2002, p. 165). Seligman is referring to the increasingly accepted recognition that beyond a certain safety net, money no longer is the primary motivator for most employees. Although this is especially true in times when jobs are abundant, the trend over the past twenty years has moved in the direction of employees being more motivated to remain with a job because of the work experience rather than the monetary rewards of working. Thus, the organization with a strongly positive work environment has the competitive edge in attracting and retaining high-quality employees.

A few years ago, it was common in health care organizations to claim that the manager is the chief retention officer in his or her department. This book recognizes and emphasizes that maintaining a vibrant workforce is a responsibility shared by both managers and employees. Having strong, savvy leaders who understand and embrace their role in both recruiting and retaining employees is crucial. However, it is not enough. As the illustration on the this page shows, a positive work environment is possible only through the active participation of all key stakeholders working in partnership.

Three Factors Important in Creating a Positive Workplace

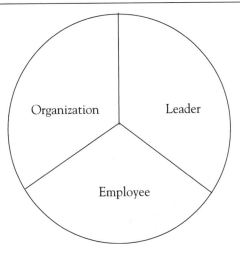

In fact, a primary working premise of this book is that the possibility of a positive work environment only exists when there is an active and dynamic state of interdependence among the organization, its leaders and managers, and its employees. And that healthy state of interdependence is characterized by positive adult-to-adult relationships among all members of the organization, with employees and leaders alike owning the responsibility for their own performance, knowledge and skill development, career progression, and morale.

To say that the manager is the chief retention officer for the department implies that he or she is primarily or even solely responsible for creating a culture of engagement that retains high-performing employees. Although an individual leader may achieve a high level of success independent of a supportive organization or participating employees, the sustainability of such success is short term at best. In the same way, an individual employee may not be able to influence an entire organization, and yet to ignore the possibility of an individual's influence is to fly in the face of both experience and historical events. However, when all three aspects of the system are working in concert, remarkable and sustainable results can be attained. A positive and supportive organizational culture coupled with effective leaders and engaged employees is the absolute best-case scenario. Indeed, it could be argued that the presence of any one of these factors alone increases the likelihood that the other two will develop.

With that said, this book has been written primarily from the perspective of the leader's role with the belief that much of what is offered here is also completely applicable to the individual employee. Some interpretation and application may have to be done by the reader; however, by and large, the concepts are appropriate for any employee. Although in some cases the application of a particular concept under discussion is made

Influence and Interdependence of the Organization, Leader, and Employee

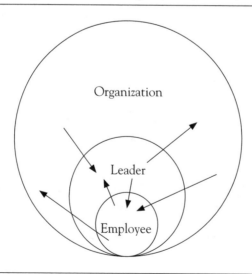

directly to the organizational level, this book is not primarily focused on the organizational scale as much as it is on the individual scale. Clearly, to create and support positive workplaces, an overhaul of culture in health care organizations must occur. Although this approach is apparent in many places throughout the book, this work is not intended to be a true organizational development book in that context. Questions at the end of each chapter offer conversation points from the perspective of the organization, the leader/manager, and the individual employee. And while these conversation points can lead to lively, engaged dialogue for those involved, the principles in this book will be applied only with strong and effective leadership skill.

For all of the emphasis on, and importance of, retention and the current focus on the quality of the employee's experience of the workplace, a body of evidence-based practice is finally emerging that can be evaluated to determine which strategies are most effective. In the past, the literature reported almost any intervention that someone thought was a good idea. The net was cast broadly in the hope of success, rather than offering targeted interventions that were demonstrated to be effective. This book in its earlier form was an attempt to provide a more focused view of strategies that are based on the evidence provided through research. Although the emphasis is on an evidence-based approach, the suggestions and strategies offered are immanently practical and applicable in any health care setting. This second edition continues the same focus.

Part I

The first section of the book contains four chapters and represents the foundation upon which the initiatives and interventions in the remainder of the book are based. Chapter 1 focuses on introductory material; it asks and attempts to answer the question, "Where should we put our energies: recruitment or retention?" It explores the high cost of turnover in its many aspects, with a special emphasis on the hidden cost of losing good people. Additional information on recruitment processes are included here.

Chapter 2 explores the reasons people work. A historical review of work and its importance for the human experience is presented. Drawing from the psychological, sociological, and organizational development literature and research, this chapter summarizes briefly what is known about the intrinsic motivators, that is, those internal forces that cause an individual to do what he or she does. For some readers, this brief description will be a review of familiar concepts that serves as a reminder of that knowledge. For others, it is the organizational context of this chapter that will be helpful, and for yet others, the information presented may be new. The value of this chapter is that it serves as a guidepost in evaluating the workplace. Although intrinsic motivators are those forces within the individual that compel action, an effective leader understands these concepts and uses leadership interventions to create an environment that increases the likelihood that these forces will be acted upon. Additional new content on the drivers behind human behavior are included in this second edition.

Chapter 3 presents a summary of what is known about organizational commitment. This chapter is included because of the recognition that although the intrinsic motivators are what get a person to work, what keeps the individual there is yet another important aspect to understand. Although the intrinsic motivators are closely linked to a person's organizational commitment, these concepts are separated into two chapters for ease of presentation and assimilation. Again, understanding the lessons of evidence-based practice about employee commitment is a fundamental step in evaluating any work environment. Chapters 2 and 3 give the manager and the individual employee the ability to assess their workplace and target their interventions rather than using the shotgun approach (trying everything in the hope that something will hit the target).

The fourth chapter is considered foundational because it sets the stage for moving forward into the second part of the book. The goal of a positive work environment is to ensure that the people who are there are happy. This chapter offers a brief review of the remarkable field of positive psychology, highlighting the recent research findings that shed light on the creation of a positive work environment. The business case for happiness at work is examined, and the results of a study of health care workers who report experiencing joy through their work are shared. The chapter concludes with a discussion of the techniques that have been documented and demonstrated to induce lasting happiness in people. Practical strategies for increasing happiness levels in work groups are offered.

Part II

The second section focuses specifically on strategies that have been found to be related to a positive work environment. Chapter 5 begins this section by reviewing the results of a research study conducted in order to understand more fully what first-line health care managers actually do to create a culture of retention in their organizations. The examples and stories from the research participants offer vivid and rich suggestions for those interested in creating a culture of retention. The findings suggest a variety of organizational ramifications and specific direction for the leaders to whom these managers directly report. A self-assessment instrument has been added to this edition so the reader can compare his or her own work environment to the research findings. The chapters that follow in the rest of the book are based on these findings.

Chapters 6 and 7 present strategies that directly flow from this study and from what is known about the intrinsic motivators and organizational commitment. Creating healthy working relationships and nurturing a sense of community within the workplace are well-documented strategies with long-lasting impact. For managers and employees who are naturally talented in the area of relationships, these chapters serve as a review and checkpoint. For those who experience some difficulty with relationships or who are interested in improving their relationships in the workplace, these chapters are essential. Although the chapters emphasize the basics of a healthy working relationship, work from the field of emotional intelligence is also explored. Emotional competencies of both individuals and work teams or work groups are examined. Chapter 7 addresses the relationships within groups of people. Important concepts of team are presented, and the developmental process of community creation is reviewed. Specific strategies that can be used to enhance the formation of a vibrant, healthy sense of community are addressed.

Getting results is the focus of the next two chapters. Chapter 8 presents strategies for getting results, including actual techniques such as problem solving, appreciative inquiry, and polarity management. Models of shared decision making used in health care organizations today are also briefly examined. General principles, rather than a specific, cookie-cutter approach, are offered.

Chapter 9 discusses the basic principles for creating an innovative work environment. In too many health care organizations today, people with good ideas are meeting almost insurmountable resistance. Too often even the finest employee gives up when it comes to getting a good idea heard and implemented. A positive work environment is considered to be one that is responsive, dynamic, and continuously improving. Yet many structural and philosophical barriers impede getting good ideas implemented. This chapter offers suggestions on how such barriers can be addressed.

The final chapter on specific strategies is chapter 10, "Influencing Performance." Exemplary managers and high-performing employees simply do not tolerate poor performance from others, nor do they settle for "work-arounds." Instead, they deal with performance issues, each in their own way. The concept of positive discipline is presented as well as other basic techniques for dealing with shortfalls in performance. Difficult behaviors such as those resulting from workplace incivility and pervasive negativity and personality disorders are briefly addressed.

Part III

The third section contains material related to challenging and difficult situations. The content is based on requests and questions from readers of *Create a Positive Health Care Workplace!* over the past four years. Chapter 11 addresses specific environmental challenges. Included is an examination of challenges to creating a positive workplace in a union environment, as well as in long-term care facilities and academic institutions.

Chapter 12 focuses on the issue of complexity in the health care workplace as it relates to generational differences. Although the issues related to having four generations active in the workforce have been apparent for several years, the increasing demands placed on managers and organizations to deal with heightened diversity makes this a topic worth exploring. Both the differences between members of the various generational cohorts and the universality of human experience are addressed. Practical and immediately applicable strategies are offered. The remainder of this chapter focuses on efforts to retain the older worker. Members of the Baby Boom generation are reaching retirement age and precipitating a rapidly approaching collision of demographics. This issue is not just local but also global for the health care workforce. And it is certainly not a concern just for health care but also for the economy of all nations.

In Conclusion

Each chapter concludes with a brief summary and a list of questions suggesting ramifications for the organization, the manager, and the employee. Considering these ramifications is challenging because they require thoughtful reflection and honesty with oneself. A lot of spin takes place in today's health care organizations. When the organization knows what people are looking for, it can relatively easily design an advertising campaign that attracts individuals. Meeting the promises implied in the advertisement is something else. Organizations that are good at spin may do well in the short run because they are able to attract new employees. However, keeping those employees is quite another story.

This book is written for health care organizations and professionals who are serious about undertaking the challenging work of creating or maintaining a positive work culture and environment. As Fred Lee (2004) points out, this is the difference between marketing and selling. The basic principle of selling is to convince people that they want what the organization has. The concept of marketing is to have what people want. This book takes the approach that the healthiest, most long-term successful organizations will be those that strive to create a positive workplace that people want.

Acknowledgments

As in any work of this magnitude, it is impossible to acknowledge everyone who had an impact on my ideas and work. There are, however, several noteworthy contributions by others that I would like to acknowledge.

First, I would like to acknowledge those colleagues who shared their experiences and ideas through interviews on various topics. Their contributions have made this edition richer and a more in-depth work. Second, I would like to acknowledge the contributions of my research participants. I have learned so much from them. They gave of their time and ideas unstintingly and helped me not only to learn but also to recapture my own enthusiasm and excitement for the work that we do. They are certainly the joyful part of any research project!

Third, I would like to extend my thanks to all of the teachers who have imparted their knowledge, given me guidance, or provided me with opportunities over the years, including those who have served a formal teaching role in my life as well as the many authors who have shared their knowledge with me. Others gave me learning opportunities either through my work or through writing for publication. All of these experiences have blessed me with a richness of perspective and understanding that I might not otherwise have had. Thanks to you all.

And, finally, I would like to thank Christopher Hund, project editor for AHA Press. His insight, perspective, and persistence have all helped this book develop. Thanks for your attention to detail!

The Engaged Workforce

I

Foundations for Understanding Engagement in the Workplace

THE FIRST PART of this book introduces the key concepts behind the creation of positive workplaces and explores the challenge of recruiting and retaining a vibrant health care workforce. Part I also presents key concepts that will help increase understanding of the complex issues surrounding intrinsic motivation and the meaning and purpose of work. In addition, the first four chapters of this book review the historical literature on the subject of work as well as recent research in psychology and organizational development.

Specifically, chapter 1 discusses health care workforce issues with a focus on the challenges of recruitment and retention. Chapter 2 explores the meaning of work, and chapter 3 examines commitment as both a personal issue and an organizational challenge. Chapter 4, the last chapter in part I, introduces the idea of finding happiness and joy through work and in health care workplaces. Chapter 4 also explores the new field of positive psychology and offers specific interventions to help employees find happiness in their work and workplaces.

1

Considering Workforce Issues

Jo Manion

Never before have organizations paid more attention to talent. . . .
Keeping it. Stealing it. Developing it. Engaging it.
Talent is no longer just a numbers game; it's about survival.
—Beverly Kaye and Sharon Jordan-Evans

Today, building and maintaining a vibrant workforce are inextricably linked to, and embedded in, the strategic focus of virtually every health care organization. No health care organization can achieve its strategic imperatives without the full partnership of engaged, talented, and skilled employees. And with workforce shortages already evident today and certain in the future, simply attaining a high-performing workforce itself has become a strategic imperative.

As the challenges faced by today's organizations mount—and they are formidable—they can only be met with highly engaged and effective employees working hand in hand with organizational leaders. Trends and challenges today include such issues as transparency, increased consumer direction and participation, digitization and the electronic medical record, increased use of hospitalists and new roles such as the clinical nurse leader and the doctor of nursing practice, anticipated reimbursement changes, decreasing budgets, and impending chaos in the insurance market. Even the settings for providing care are shifting like sand in a windstorm. Medical tourism, stand-alone emergency departments, and retail site clinics staffed by nurse practitioners are a few examples. New practice models include physician practices based on e-mail and text messaging and remote patient monitoring devices that are Internet based (Larkin 2008). Increasing regulation such as nurse staffing ratio laws and new Medicare payment rules that preclude "never events" from being reimbursed all add layers of complexity to an already almost impossibly complex system. These may be just the tip of the iceberg as nanotechnology and advances in genetic enhancements occur and with new entrants like Google getting into the field of maintaining personal health records.

In recent years, escalating shortages of health care workers have received the attention of every professional association, regulatory agency, health care consulting practice, and major health care system. Report after report has outlined the extent of shortages among clinical professionals as well as support staff. Although shortages vary by geographical area, state after state reports high vacancy rates that represent unfilled positions that are likely to remain difficult, if not impossible, to fill. Topics related to workforce shortages fill the agendas of professional meetings and are the subject of seminars all around the country. All of these activities attest to the level of anxiety and concern that health care leaders and executives are currently experiencing.

Unfortunately, a potentially dangerous side effect accompanies this ongoing emphasis on the health care workforce challenge: It is easy to become habituated to this bad news. At some point, organizational leaders may stop listening because they are certain that they have heard all of the bad news before. It is interesting to speculate on the day in the not-too-distant future when today's high turnover and vacancy rate crisis becomes the norm. Chronic workforce shortages seem to be the future if only because of colliding demographics as Baby Boomers, a large portion of the current workforce, reach retirement age.

To believe that the workforce shortage issue can be solved once and for all is probably shortsighted to the point of being delusional. At one recent hospital association annual meeting, a conversation was overheard during which one hospital executive proudly told another, "We've got the nursing shortage licked. We don't have any open vacancies. The shortage is over for us." The hospital executive in question really should have gone back and looked carefully at his demographics before congratulating himself. Of course, sometimes this type of questionable self-assurance is an attempt to find some measure of comfort in what has become an environment fraught with seemingly continual and often insurmountable challenges. In 2007, chief executive officers (CEOs) were surveyed, and 65 percent identified shortage of registered nurses (RNs) and talent competition as a top priority. Employee retention was ranked as a priority by 57 percent (Colosi 2007).

The health care sector is not alone in facing workforce challenges. McKinsey & Company conducted a yearlong study involving seventy-seven companies and almost six thousand managers and executives. The conclusion: "The most important corporate resource over the next 20 years will be talent: smart, sophisticated people who are technologically literate, globally astute, and organizationally agile" (Fishman 1998, p. 104). In the McKinsey & Company review of the changing workforce, it is clear that the supply of qualified workers is decreasing at the same time workforce demands are increasing. "The search for the best and brightest will become a constant, costly battle, a fight with no final victory. Not only will [organizations] have to devise more imaginative hiring practices, they will also have to work harder to keep their best people" (Fishman 1998, p. 104).

An extensive review of the health care research literature on workforce shortages is not included here for two reasons. First, anyone reading this book has probably read the same studies and reports and already knows their content and conclusions. Reference to pertinent findings are made to support chapter content. Second, while some people might have found such a review fascinating and exciting reading, it is doubtful that such people are the ones who would read this book. Spending energy rereading and synthesizing what must surely be self-evident to most people seems futile. Instead, several major observations are summarized here as they pertain to workforce issues and several ideas about the concept of retention are offered.

Basic Conclusions

Here are the conclusions from the extensive literature on workforce shortages that have ramifications for meeting the challenge of workforce development and maintenance:

1. At various times, critical shortages of key health care workers have occurred. The shortages will likely continue to plague health care delivery and even worsen in the future. In the recent past, shortages have been quantitatively documented in most health care professional groups, including nurses, pharmacists, imaging technicians, physical and occupational therapists, laboratory specialists, social workers, and information technology specialists and managers (AHA 2007). The degree of the shortages varies by location and is often cyclical in nature. The impending loss of Baby Boomers from the workforce is likely to significantly affect health care organizations in many ways that are unrecognized at this time. Chapter 12 explores in more detail the issue of retaining the older worker.

   Awareness is increasing that this issue is more than a local, regional, or even national one. It has emerged as a global issue.

   The current worldwide shortage of health care workers is estimated to be more than 4 million. In the industrialized world, the World Health Organization (WHO) projects that the need for health care workers will increase by 20 percent over the next 20 years, due to the demands of the aging populations. Maintaining present levels of care will require an extra 8.5 million health care workers by 2025. By 2010—the United States itself will not have enough health care workers to meet demands. (Pittman and Svensson 2008, para. 3)

   Far more serious shortages are being seen in developing countries. National health care issues and inequities in health care systems have stimulated the migration of workers from developing countries to those who have the resources to pay. This situation creates a serious ethical dilemma and increased difficulties for the home country struggling with the need to retain workers and continue to invest in their education.

2. Creating a positive work environment is important regardless of the existence of workforce shortages, and yet doing so is much more difficult in the face of shortages. Inadequate staffing levels affect employees adversely and fuel more turnover. Recruiting during times of high vacancy is more difficult, workload is heavier for current employees,

resignations increase, and the cycle continues. A positive work environment directly affects the quality and level of service, the number of errors, the productivity of employees, and the financial well-being of the organization (AHA 2007; Williams et al. 2007; Stanton 2004; Needleman et al. 2002; Aiken et al. 2002).

During times of workforce shortages, a positive work environment becomes a competitive edge that makes an organization even stronger and more viable. Parsons, Cornett, and Golightly-Jenkins (2006) identify seven elements of a healthy workplace. Gilbert (2007) would add the last bullet. These are:

- Excellence in patient care/customer service
- Effective and efficient clinical processes and systems
- Effective and efficient business processes and systems
- Ongoing professional development
- Effective and efficient staffing systems
- Established organizational and team behavioral norms
- Workable, safe, and welcoming physical environment
- Ethical wisdom at every level in the organization

The assertion that a positive workplace is a crucial strategic initiative is validated by the number of national and international initiatives and efforts seeking to create healthier workplaces. These include but are not limited to the Good Work initiative based at The University of Pennsylvania; the Robert Wood Johnson Foundation grants for its program Transforming Care at the Bedside; the emphasis on healthy practice environments internationally; and the increased interest in obtaining recognized designations of excellence such as Magnet status, Employer of Choice designation, or the Malcolm Baldrige National Quality Award. Even the Joint Commission has published a white paper on the nursing shortage that identifies creating a culture of retention as the first strategy for addressing what it calls "the evolving nursing crisis" (Joint Commission 2002).

3. Many reasons for the shortages have been suggested, and several have been very well documented. However, the decreasing size of the generational cohorts means that fewer people are available for recruiting. In addition, the declining attractiveness of health care as a career opportunity is significant. The problem is multifaceted and complex.

4. Not only common sense but also a wealth of research support the contention that a positive workplace increases satisfaction levels on the part of employees. When employees are dissatisfied, they are more likely to be looking for their next job. In one study, 69.4 percent of respondents who reported low levels of trust and commitment in their workplace indicated that they were likely or very likely to leave their current employer (Gregory et al. 2007).

5. Not all health care organizations experience workforce shortages in the same way. Many recognize that the only substantial difference

between them and their competitors is the skills, knowledge, commitment, and abilities of the people who work in the organization. These organizations act accordingly and treat their employees well. Unfortunately, just as many organizations follow a philosophy that regards employees as easily replaceable units who should consider themselves lucky just to have a job. As Stanford University professor Jeffrey Pfeffer said, "Loyalty isn't dead . . . but toxic [organizations] are driving people away. There isn't a scarcity of talent—but there is a growing unwillingness to work for a toxic organization" (Webber 1998, p. 154). Pfeffer went on to say that organizations short on talent probably deserve to be. Sounds a bit harsh, but perhaps he has a point.

6. All the principles shared in this book are based on the underlying assumption that strong leadership exists in the organization. None of the strategies suggested here are quick fixes. The first step in any organization is ensuring that leaders are prepared for the challenges they face and supported with resources and continuing development opportunities.

The Cost of Turnover

Turnover is an issue even during times when employees are plentiful and every position in the organization is filled. Turnover occurs when an employee leaves his or her position and must be replaced. It is always an expensive proposition for an organization, although some turnover is to be expected and is even desirable. People who have not been with the organization since the beginning of recorded history can help others see things from a new perspective. Turnover provides the opportunity to welcome new people who bring fresh and unique ideas to the organization. This opportunity assumes, however, that others are willing to listen to them.

Occasionally, the loss of a particular employee or manager may even be a cause for celebration. Everyone has worked with disruptive, toxic, or simply unproductive people in his or her career. Take the case of Agnes. Agnes creates disruption and chaos wherever she goes. She is difficult to work with and is a constant source of complaint. Either Agnes is complaining about something or someone or her co-workers are complaining about Agnes. When a co-worker looks at the next day's schedule and sees that Agnes is scheduled, panic sets in. The knowledge that Agnes will have to be dealt with the next day is enough to sink anyone into a bad mood for the rest of the day. In fact, it is enough to cause the co-worker to consider calling in sick rather than face a day working with her. When Agnes finally blows up and resigns in a fit of pique, everyone breathes a sigh of relief. Her manager grabs the resignation letter, immediately copies it, and personally delivers it to the human resources department before Agnes can change her mind. Losing employees like Agnes is a positive kind of turnover.

Undesirable turnover is the loss of people who will be highly missed by members of the work group. Such employees are highly productive, and they often contribute constructive ideas. These are the skilled, temperate people who work well with others. They are at work when scheduled and often volunteer to cover for others when needed. When these people resign, everyone is sorry to see them go. Understanding the ways in which turnover is expensive may encourage everyone involved to work diligently to avoid unnecessary turnover.

Financial Cost

The first cost of turnover—the financial cost—is obvious. The financial loss that results from the resignation of a single employee has been estimated to range from 150 to 250 percent of the employee's annual salary. The range is wide simply because a multitude of factors must be considered. The most obvious factors include the actual cost of advertising the vacancy and the hours spent reviewing applications and conducting interviews. In addition, the cost of replacement help in the form of expensive temporary employees to cover the position until a new person can be hired must be considered as well as the cost of new employee training and orientation. Regardless of the thoroughness with which costs are captured, even conservative estimates of financial costs are significant for an organization.

A study conducted by the Voluntary Hospitals of America is illuminating (Gelinas and Bohlen 2002). As part of the study, several member hospitals were evaluated carefully on the basis of their actual vacancy rates. For example, in one organization, replacement costs were projected to be 22 percent of total payroll base compensation. The average replacement cost per skilled employee was estimated to be almost $29,000. When these estimates were applied to the organization's actual number of turnovers, it was determined that reducing turnover from 31 percent to 25 percent would result in a cost savings of more than $800,000 per year. If the turnover rate could be reduced even further, to 20 percent, savings would total more than $1.4 million per year. This type of case study can be done in any organization by using actual turnover data.

At least three important points should be considered in examining the financial cost of employee turnover. First, a common reaction to proposals for spending money on retention efforts is the refrain, "We don't have the money." The truth is that reducing turnover could yield a significant amount of found money that could be used to fund improved retention efforts. One such study clearly demonstrates this concept. The University of Michigan Health System implemented a preparation program for 400 staff preceptors that emphasized education, coaching, and skill development in preparation for its support of new hires. The initial program resulted in a decrease in its vacancy rate of 68 percent over a two-year period of time. Turnover rates decreased by 27 percent over a three-year period. Additionally, the satisfaction levels and retention rates of the new hires also increased (Baggot et al. 2005). Funding of residency programs for new graduate professionals has also been demonstrated to be a solid investment for the future, saving money in the long run (Thrall 2007).

Another retention strategy illustrates the point that short-term financial considerations may cost more in the long run. A critical care director in one acute care hospital was faced with high nurse vacancy rates and excessive costs of per diem and temporary agency nurses. He developed a plan that included over-hiring one RN per critical care unit and demonstrated startling results. Not only did staff satisfaction levels improve but also vacancy rates fell from almost 18 percent to under 5 percent and control of the budgeted salary expense improved. "Instead of facing an unfavorable variance of $1,440,000, the year resulted in an unfavorable variance of $220,000, translating to a 650% improvement" (Cutruzzula and Cipriano 2007, p. 32).

Second, managers and executives ought to have a clear idea of just how much turnover is costing the organization. Otherwise, resources may not be used wisely. For example, in one department over several years, the manager worked hard to keep a key night-shift position filled. New employees who began optimistically lasted, on average, less than three months before they resigned. The permanent employees on the night shift had been there for years. Their expectations were quite high, and they purposely created difficult situations for the new people in order to test their abilities. The old-timers were just plain toxic. They complained bitterly about nobody wanting to work with them on the graveyard shift, but they failed to see that they were a large part of the reason why no one stayed. Finally, after years of replacing new employees for this shift, the manager pulled together the cost information and sat down with these long-tenured employees and showed them the facts. She said, in essence, "You are costing this department too much. I can't afford to keep you. If you are unable to accept the next new employee and help him or her assimilate into the department, I am going to have to let you go. I just cannot afford you." They got the message.

In too many organizations today, health care managers do not have accurate or timely information about turnover costs in their department. Very few have specific quantitative data about factors important to retention, such as employee and physician satisfaction levels, the length of recruitment time for open positions, or even basic information such as the overall vacancy rate.

The final point in considering the financial cost of turnover is that it is important to test assumptions held. There are many misperceptions about turnover. For example, it is obvious that the more highly paid professionals in the organization represent a higher cost of turnover in terms of cost per employee. For this reason, organizations focus on shortages of professionals such as registered nurses, licensed pharmacists, and skilled therapists and technicians. However, employees who make a lower wage may actually represent a larger turnover cost to the organization because of the sheer number of turnovers in these positions. For example, in a long-term care facility, nursing assistants deliver 80 to 90 percent of the direct patient care. Not only are there higher numbers of these workers but the annual turnover rate among these employees is reported to be as high as 99 percent (Riggs and Rantz 2001). Therefore, the total turnover cost for certified nurse assistants can be much higher than that for registered nurses in long-term care facilities. In acute care organizations, turnover among entry-level environmental service and dietary workers can represent a tremendous cost because hospitals employ large numbers of these workers and they tend to turn over more frequently.

Damage to the Brand

Another cost of turnover, damage to the brand, is often hidden, and many people in health care have not even considered this serious issue. *Damage to the brand* is a business term that refers to the negative impact that a single product can have on a whole line of products when the product fails to meet the customers' expectations.

At a state hospital association meeting, John Houck (2003) reported on the results of a nursing retention study. He introduced damage to the brand as a concept that can have significant ramifications for health care organizations. In his study, Houck reported finding that more than 30 percent of the nurses who left hospitals during the period of time studied did not take new hospital positions. Instead, they chose positions in another area of health care or opted out of health care altogether. Houck talked about his previous business experience in the clothing industry, and he pointed out that when a new clothing design or product is released, sales figures are closely tracked. Retailers are interested not just in how many of the items are purchased but also in how many people repurchase the same item. According to Houck, a repurchase rate of 30 percent represents a significant problem. Products with low rates of repurchase are quickly pulled from the shelves because the sale of unsatisfactory new products can damage sales for the entire brand.

What Houck was referring to is the thinking that goes on in the head of the consumer. For instance, a person may try a new style of Levis®. If they do not fit right or look good or if no one notices them the first time they are worn, most people do not say, "Gee, I didn't make a very good buying decision here." Instead, they say something like, "Boy, Levis just aren't what they used to be. I guess I had better start looking around at some other brands and maybe try something different next time."

The concept of damage to the brand has significant ramifications for the health care sector. Take the example of Sally, a young registered nurse who recently graduated from college. In her first work experience, fresh out of school, she was assigned to work in the telemetry department of an acute care hospital. She was just three months out of nursing school, and she was assigned to work as the night charge nurse with only one other registered nurse, who was also a recent graduate. Was it any wonder that she began thinking about quitting and becoming a florist? She did not say to herself, "This hospital is using new graduates inappropriately." Instead, she said, "Nursing isn't for me. This is too hard. This isn't what I thought it would be." If no one is available to help this new graduate process her negative experience, this situation can signal the beginning of the end for this career.

Everyone tends to generalize on the basis of limited experience and condemn the entire "brand" of experiences rather than just the single negative experience. In Sally's case, the brand is hospital nursing or even nursing as a whole. Employees' experiences determine the judgments and decisions they make about the organization, the profession, the specialty, and so on. Health care organizations can no longer afford to recruit good people and then provide a negative work experience. Every time this happens, far more is lost than one promising employee. In a study by Aon Consulting in partnership with the American Society of Healthcare Human Resources Administration, Runy (2003) reports that 64 percent of the health care workers studied think about leaving or have begun to make plans to leave their health care careers.

Loss of Experience, Knowledge, and Connections

The third cost of turnover, loss of experience, knowledge, and connections, is not easily quantifiable. When a valued employee leaves an organization, the departure represents far more than a financial loss to the organization. Also lost is experience with and knowledge of the organization that can take the organization months and even years to replace. People who have been with an organization have learned the ropes—both the formal and the informal ways to get things done. They know who to talk to about a problem, and they know how to navigate the ins and outs of a complex work situation. They have learned from their mistakes in order to gain this hard-won, tacit knowledge.

Experienced employees who have tenure in the organization also have formed relationships and connections both within their immediate work group and within the larger system. These relationships often help them to accomplish needed results. When such connections and relationships are severed, re-establishing them takes a significant amount of time. When turnover occurs frequently, those employees who remain in the organization often become more cynical and less inclined to form new attachments to the replacement employees.

One organization provides a clear example of this type of cost. A series of retreats for employees was held in the women's services department. The department was experiencing very high turnover rates, approaching 40 percent annually. During the retreat, several long-term employees made the comment that a pact had been established among the more seasoned, tenured employees. They had become tired of continually orienting new people and trying to get to know them only to have them resign within their first few months on the job. The long-term employees had decided that they were not going to talk to any of the new employees until they had been there for at least six months. It was just too exhausting for them to try to form a new relationship before they were certain that the new person was likely to stay. Furthermore, the long-term employees felt demoralized, so they had decided to stop having going-away parties for departing employees. The effect of the pact on the new employees was evident in their comments: "No one talks to us." "Sally just had her last day, and she's been here for 20 years . . . and no one even brought in doughnuts." Their natural conclusion: "No one cares about each other here."

When employees come and go frequently, building connections and satisfying, productive relationships becomes exhausting. In another organization, the CEO was concerned about the relationship between a senior vice president and the employees in his departments, who were experiencing problems related to trust and openness. This vice president was the fifth to whom these people had reported within the past five years. Employees naturally were hesitant to trust and extend themselves in relationship to this person. Forming relationships takes a lot of energy and a willingness to extend one's self. Continually reforming and re-establishing similar relationships over and over again begins to feel like a no-win situation for most people, and eventually even the most optimistic person becomes unwilling to make the investment.

Another major, indirect cost of turnover is the impact on patient safety. "According to the Joint Commission on the Accreditation of Healthcare Organizations (JCAHO), inadequate orientation and training of nurses is a factor in 58% of serious errors" (Baggot et al. 2005, p. 139). Furthermore, inadequate staffing levels were a factor in 24 percent of 1,609 sentinel events over a five-year period. The patient safety literature covers this issue thoroughly.

Impact on Remaining Employees

The final hidden cost of turnover is the sense of rejection that those who remain in the organization often experience. Especially when the individual leaving is a valued, strong colleague or leader, the individual's choice to leave can feel like a personal rejection. The person has chosen to take another opportunity and is basically saying, "I can do better elsewhere." If this happens too many times, even the most steadfast employee may begin to question his or her own commitment to stay. As one senior-level executive said in an interview: "I want to work in a system people want to come to, not a place where they are leaving." He was referring to the exodus of good people he had watched over the years, which he found personally very demoralizing.

This felt rejection can also influence how managers respond to the employees who resign. When a valued employee's resignation is perceived as a personal rejection, managers and co-workers alike feel hurt and even betrayed, especially when they have worked hard to help the person develop his or her skills and abilities over time. In some cases, the manager may have worked hard to create opportunities and meet the person's needs, and it can be difficult for the manager to rise above his or her personal disappointment and concern about finding a replacement. Unfortunately, how the manager responds may determine whether the employee will consider returning to the organization in the future.

During the past several years, it has become evident that many people are disappointed in the reality of their new job after they have left an organization for a better opportunity. Savvy recruiters and managers stay in touch with employees who have left and make it clear that they will be welcomed back if they want to return. Some organizations have even reinstated full benefits at the level they were at the time of resignation when employees return within a certain period. Managers and work groups have found a variety of ways to keep in touch with people. Some managers actually include former employees on their holiday greeting card lists, or they telephone them periodically to simply say hello. In other cases, being invited to alumni events that highlight the kinds of things that are going on in the department or organization serves to keep former employees informed of changes. Including them in holiday parties or department get-togethers is another way to encourage a continued sense of connection. Increased attention is being given to the recruitment of former employees as a viable strategy.

The alternative for the manager to letting people know he or she is still interested and cares about them as a potential colleague is to allow former employees to believe that the manager and the organization no longer care about them. Such feelings can create ill will in the community and make recruiting high-quality people more difficult.

Consider this true-life example. A young pharmacist named Tom interviewed at two organizations. One was a small community hospital, and the other was a large tertiary medical center. Tom chose the smaller organization because of the work he would be doing. When he told the recruiter at the large medical center of his choice, the recruiter became very angry with him. She simply could not believe that he would choose the smaller organization. Within about two months, Tom realized that he had made a mistake. He was not doing the work he had been promised but instead had been assigned a different job. He was very disappointed. When he was encouraged by a colleague to recontact the recruiter from the larger organization, he refused, saying, "You just don't know how angry she was. I couldn't possibly call her back." This young man, with his doctorate in pharmacology, is unlikely to ever consider the larger organization again because the recruiter reacted to his decision in a very negative way based on her own personal disappointment.

In a study that examined nurses' perceptions of factors prompting them to leave their job, several nurses referred to being treated poorly by their managers when they resigned. In these cases, the managers' negative actions or comments remained vivid in the memories of the study participants. For example:

- "No manager from my department said good-bye to me. They never acknowledged it was my last day after 18 years of employment. I left thinking I made the best decision I could."
- "I remember the day I told my manager I was quitting. She asked me what was I going to do and when I told her, she replied, 'When or if you do come back, you'll work nights and every weekend.'" (Cline, Reilly, and Moore 2003, p. 52)

Re-recruiting good former employees has tremendous advantages. When highly skilled individuals leave for other opportunities but years later remember the support they felt during the resignation process, they are more likely to consider returning to the organization. Such employees are often better for their time away, because they have gained new perspectives and different experiences. In this way, returning employees may even be considerably more valuable than when they left. Even when they are not interested in returning to the organization, they may refer other colleagues to it.

Current employees play a significant role in recruiting former employees as well. Co-workers often keep in touch with their former colleagues. The more positively they continue to speak of their workplace, the more likely the former employees are to consider returning at some point in the future. Employees can also let their departing colleagues know when new positions open up, and thus they can serve as a trusted bridge between the former workplace and the former employees.

A recent survey by Korn/Ferry International found that 64 percent of 4,000 respondents said they would consider returning to a previous employer (Vestal 2006). Often referred to as *boomerang* or *rebound employees*, their return must be given careful consideration. In addition to the many advantages already enumerated, however, some unintended negative effects may arise. Was the individual a high-performing employee? Why did the individual leave? Was it for more experience? Was it dislike of the previous job? And, if so, has that job changed significantly or at all? Will the person be rehired at a higher level of pay than former co-workers are now making? Will this become a source of contention in the department?

Re-recruiting former employees actually starts at their resignation. The leader's ability to be open and communicate personal disappointment at the loss of a valued employee means the door is open for the separating employee to return some day.

Psychological Resignation

"Resignation is not just a behavioral act; it is also a state of being" (Manion 2000, p. 25). Probably the most dangerous form of turnover is that which occurs when the individual leaves emotionally and psychologically and yet remains physically. A person does not have to resign officially for turnover to occur. Managers sometimes deceive themselves when they look at low vacancy rates and conclude that they do not have a turnover problem. However, most managers and work groups understand psychological resignation because they have experienced it themselves.

Employees who resign psychologically are often referred to as *on-the-job retired*. When employees are not fully engaged but have instead psychologically retired from their jobs, their level of productivity plunges. They come to work late or not at all, and the other members of the team must carry heavier workloads to meet the team's goals. Having even 10 or 20 percent of the employees in a work group working below speed creates tremendous morale problems for the rest of the employees.

Thus, turnover may not be adequately addressed just by filling vacant positions. Recruitment efforts need to emphasize finding high-quality employees who are likely to remain committed and engaged in their work and full participants in the workplace. Good managers and savvy employees understand that they must continually re-recruit talented applicants and encourage optimal performance among all employees. In other words, keeping talented and dedicated employees is just as important as recruiting new ones.

The Metrics

Currently, several forms of measuring workforce effectiveness are available, including approaches from productivity measures to employee satisfaction rates. However, adding recruitment and labor management metrics are also important. Evaluating recruitment effectiveness can be accomplished by examining the percentage of open positions filled, time taken to fill each position, quality of hires, labor supplier dependability, and percentage of job offers accepted (Lauter 2007).

It is also important to carefully examine the employee turnover information for the organization. Are experienced employees or inexperienced employees leaving? Are they being replaced with experienced or inexperienced people (Jones 2005)? What is the tenure of the employee? In a recent study, a survey was mailed to a random sample of newly licensed registered nurses in 35 states. Of those who responded, about 13 percent had changed jobs after the first year, and 37 percent reported that they felt ready to change jobs. This accounts for 50 percent of this sample (Kovner et al. 2007). The organization never regains its return on investment from the resource-intensive orientation period of these new graduates if they move on to their second job so quickly.

Experience is not the only consideration. Overall turnover rate in the facility may hide some important facts. Where is the turnover the highest? Is it in departments such as housekeeping or dietary? Is it in the laboratory, nursing, or pharmacy? Another piece of information that is often missing is whether the organization is losing its high or low performers. Applying this concept is resisted by many managers. However, sorting employees into high, middle, and low performers and then tracking turnover would provide more complete information about the organization's turnover picture.

Managers are often held accountable for the turnover in their departments. However, all turnover is not the same, and acknowledgment of this fact ought to be taken into account. For instance, is a staff position vacated because the employee is promoted to a higher position in the organization? This type of turnover should be commended rather than counted against a manager. Is the turnover expected? For example, perhaps an employee joined the department in an entry-level position to help him or her through the course of an education program and graduation has occurred. In this case, the position was always intended to be a time-limited one. Is the position vacated because the availability of a long-awaited internal transfer became available? When managers feel penalized for turnover regardless of these considerations, it creates a hostile and punitive work environment.

Recruitment versus Retention

Recruitment and retention are closely linked. Making sure that all recruitment practices work well will yield little if the new recruits leave within a few months of joining the organization or department. In fact, finding good people and convincing them to give the organization a try but then having them move on within a relatively short period of time simply increases the level of cynicism and demoralization within the entire health care system. And it also takes a great deal of energy and effort that ultimately makes everyone involved feel nonproductive. It is important, then, to measure the outcomes of recruiting and staffing strategies for effectiveness. These measures include standards such as applicant flow, interview-to-offer time, average experience of hired candidates, time-to-fill and cost per hired employee, and bottom-line savings against the cost of temporary employees (Colosi 2007).

Of course, recruitment efforts need to be top-notch in a competitive labor market. And many organizations have stepped up their efforts in this area and have enjoyed increased success. However, these efforts do not mean that all is well throughout the entire community. Kalisch (2003) conducted an extensive study of recruitment processes and systems in 122 acute care hospitals throughout the United States. The findings were appalling, especially considering the competitive nature of the talent pool in health care. Example after example of just plain poor practices was found. It is worth examining Kalisch's results here, at least briefly.

Kalisch identified a total of thirty markets. Ten qualified nurses participated in the study and played the role of potential employees. The nurses were coached extensively on a standard procedure for applying and interviewing at the hospitals. One of the ten nurses applied to, and interviewed with, each of the 122 hospitals in the study.

The study results showed that problems within the recruitment process were widespread and began with the pre-interview contacts. The pre-interview problems ranged from no response to letters and inquiries to cases of extensive telephone tag. The overall quality of the letters and brochures provided by the hospitals was rated as fair to poor. Such communication problems create issues because applicants base their decisions on whether to interview at a given organization primarily on the quality, nature, and timeliness of letters, telephone contacts, e-mails, and brochures and other printed materials.

The interview experiences of the nurses also left a lot to be desired. The problems began with the directions to the facility, the parking experience, the physical appearance of the facility, and the helpfulness of the information desk personnel. Additional problems concerned the welcomes received by the applicants as well as waiting times, testing requirements, interview lengths, and interview environments. A few examples are described here to indicate the degree of problems encountered.

"In 55 percent of the interviews, the recruiter was expecting the candidate but no interviews had been set up with the managers of the units being considered. . . . [For example,] one critical care applicant flew from one end of the country to the other to interview in a well known medical center only to have no one available for the interview" (Kalisch 2003, p. 472). In another instance, "Even though I had a prearranged interview, when I got there, the secretary didn't know who I was. She paged the recruiter once but refused to do it again or to call anyone else to see me. This was despite me telling her I was from 2500 miles away!" (Kalisch 2003, p. 472). Another applicant was told by a nurse manager that she had no time to interview her and the applicant would need to wait for the assistant manager. She waited sixty-five minutes.

Other applicants reported receiving a similar reception. They were often left to wait in an area where they were able to see or hear the person with whom they were supposed to interview. "I sat there 20 minutes waiting and watching the recruiter sip coffee. There was no apology offered for being late." Another said, "I could hear her on the phone talking about last Saturday's date and this was 25 minutes after my interview was to start" (Kalisch 2003, p. 473). And unfortunately, these were not the only problems. At some organizations, the candidates' applications and resumes were misplaced, interviews were shortened to as little as five minutes, interview environments were negative, and postinterview follow-up was lacking. Shockingly, 91 percent of the organizations provided no interview follow-up at all.

Kalisch's study offers insight into potential problem areas, and the results of her study should jolt any manager or executive into realizing that the assumption that the organization's recruiting practices are effective is risky and dangerous. Evaluation of the organization's recruitment efforts is necessary. The process can start by asking new hires about their experience during the recruitment process and devising a way of following up with the candidates who did not select the organization to find out what they experienced when they contacted the recruiter.

Fortunately, problems in the recruitment process can be fixed when they are recognized and the importance of their impact is appreciated. The National Association for Health Care Recruitment (NAHCR) is a very positive source for this kind of information. (The organization's Web site address is www.nahcr.com.) The NAHCR provides workshops for recruiters as well as other helpful resources such as handbooks and toolkits. The NAHCR also offers a credentialing exam for recruiters.

Exemplary recruiting practices in organizations often include the redesign of the recruitment function to more broadly involve the recruiters. The recruiter is responsible not only for the successful hiring of staff but also for satisfaction ratings from managers, the recruits, and other external contacts. Adequate numbers of recruiters for the level of vacancies in the organization are also necessary. "Industry standards indicated the need for one recruiter for every 35–45 open positions" (Ellerbe, Ostermeier, and Shelley 2006, p. 39). The role can be more active, soliciting leads and following up from job fairs and conferences rather than passively awaiting applications to process.

Many organizations today have figured out that simply getting the new recruit to his or her home department is only the first step. More attention is being paid to the initial experience of the employee to ensure that it is positive and anchors the individual in the culture and everyday life of the department. Turnover rates of new hires is high during the first year; reports indicate a range of 30–35 percent (Baggot et al. 2005; Bowles and Candela 2005). By the end of the hire's second year, turnover has been reported at an astounding 57 percent (Bowles and Candela 2005).

Bowles and Candela conducted a study to determine RNs' perceptions of their first nursing experience, and if they left the position, why. "The vast majority of recent RN graduates believed that the working environment was stressful and not conducive to providing safe patient care" (2005, p. 133). Of the study participants, 54 percent reported the work atmosphere as negative, 42 percent said patient supplies were not available in the department, and 62 percent reported that administration did not listen to staff concerns. Staffing levels were inadequate, said 79 percent, resulting in less time to spend with patients. There were also positive findings. Most believed the staff worked together as a team, co-workers were helpful to them, managers were supportive, and continuing education was encouraged.

"Hiring top talent is only the first step. Health care organizations need to ensure that they open their arms to new hires, help them settle into the job and provide support at every step" (Lauter 2006, p. 1). Significant money is spent on identifying and courting new hires, but once the deal is made, efforts to engage and retain these vital employees must be ongoing. Although the rest of this book addresses this issue at length, included here are some suggestions for immersing that new hire immediately.

Sending a personalized note or letter to the new employee's home welcoming him or her to the organization and department is a positive way to greet the person before he or she physically arrives. One manager has everyone in the department sign the letter personally. Providing reading material ahead of time or items of interest gets the newcomer in the loop early. Greeting him or her with a roster of the entire work group or team that includes names and a bit of information about each co-worker gives the new hire a head start on getting to know everyone.

Orientation programs that acquaint the individual quickly with the organization and its people are also helpful. Having work space and related items and issues ready for the person when he or she arrives shows a spirit of interest and welcome. Assigning mentors or preceptors who help the person assimilate into his or her new role provides support and an early contact. Remaining in communication with the individual throughout the first year to determine experiences and issues can help increase engagement and demonstrate continued interest in and value of the person. Often a recruiter continues to be part of this process through the first year. Managers and executives who are vested in talent management processes ensure they have an active role in welcoming new employees.

Summary

This chapter explores employee turnover as a key challenge in today's health care organizations. The costs of turnover are considered, with emphasis given to the hidden costs such as potential damage to the brand; the feeling of rejection and lowered morale experienced among managers and co-workers; and the organization's loss of experience, knowledge, and connections. The concept of turnover extends to individuals who may not physically leave but separate psychologically. Finally, a challenge is offered to evaluate carefully the organization's recruitment practices to ensure efforts to attract high-quality candidates are maximized. Once the impact of current and future workforce shortages has been considered fully, it is possible to go to the next challenge: creating a more positive workplace for employees.

Conversation Points

Organizational Perspective

1. Does the organization provide managers with accurate, department-specific workforce data on a timely basis? Do the data include vacancy and turnover rates and the average length of time a position is open before it is filled?
2. Are new employees tracked to determine their length of employment so that problem areas can be illuminated? Are there any "revolving door" departments, shifts, or positions?
3. How are managers being held accountable for their turnover levels? What are some of the valid reasons for turnover?
4. How much does turnover cost the organization financially on an annual basis?
5. Is your human resources department adequately resourced for recruitment efforts? Has an assessment of the recruitment process been performed? Do you know where the problems are? What is the success rate on a long-term basis?
6. Do managers and recruiters have a process for matching a potential employee's strengths with the open position? Is job fit an important issue that is considered? Are managers skilled in behavioral questioning?

Leader Perspective

1. Do you have accurate, timely data on turnover, cost of turnover, and vacant positions for your department? Do you know how long it takes you to replace employees?

2. When an employee resigns, do you meet with the person to determine the issues and reasons? Do you graciously let the individual know you are disappointed and that he or she would be welcomed back in the future (if this is the case)?

3. How do you make new employees feel welcome and encourage their assimilation into the work group? Do you have regular points of contact with new employees to assess their progress?

4. How strong is the orientation program in your department? Do you meet regularly with new employees to determine how they are doing?

5. Are there any problems in your recruiting and interviewing processes that need to be fixed?

6. Have you clearly identified the skills and strengths needed for each of the positions for which you typically interview candidates? Do you use behavioral questioning to determine fit and suitability of a potential applicant?

7. Do you take steps to stay in touch with former employees? Do you take any action to recruit former employees for open positions?

8. Have you been tolerating any employees who have resigned psychologically rather than dealing with their lack of performance?

9. How are current employees included in the interview process?

Employee Perspective

1. Do you know what the recruitment process is in your department?

2. How actively do you or your co-workers participate in interviewing or meeting with potential applicants?

3. How do you support and encourage new employees?

4. Do you participate in the orientation of new employees?

5. Do you keep in touch with departing co-workers and continue to talk positively about the workplace? Do you have any role in helping to bring former employees back to the organization?

2

Understanding Why People Work

Jo Manion

*To have a firm persuasion in our work—to feel that what we do
is right for ourselves and good for the world at exactly the same time—
is one of the great triumphs of human existence.*
—David Whyte

WHEN MANAGERS are asked about why people work, 89 percent of them answer, "for the money" (Kaye and Jordan-Evans 2002). Whether these managers were giving a quick, flippant answer to an age-old question or whether they truly believe that the people they work with are working primarily for the money may never be known. What is known, however, is that when managers believe that employees work mostly for the extrinsic rewards they receive (the salary and benefits), this belief influences them in a variety of ways. Because managers have little or no significant influence on what employees in the organization are paid, this belief can inadvertently absolve the managers of any responsibility for substantially influencing the attitudes and behavior of their employees. In other words, such managers develop a mind-set based on the premise that "it's not my problem if people here aren't motivated." Starting from this negative viewpoint leads supervisors and managers to take little positive action to influence the employees with whom they work.

On the other hand, when people in management positions are encouraged to think more deeply about the reasons why people work, they quickly come to see that the answer to the question, "Why do people work?" is considerably more complex than it first appears. A full investigation of the meaning of work in the lives of people reveals a multitude of reasons why people work. And, in fact, when employees are working in a particular organization only because of the money, the chances are significant that they are going to be less committed and productive than their counterparts who have deeper reasons for working. In short, research has clearly documented that money is not the primary reason why people work (Kovner et al. 2006; Atchison 2003). It is a satisfier, not a motivator.

The first step to creating a positive workplace is to build on a full understanding of the reasons why people work. An appreciation of the complexities and subtleties of this issue informs leaders and employees who are trying to create a positive work environment. In fact, it is virtually impossible to create such an environment unless factors well beyond the satisfiers and extrinsic motivators are considered. This chapter explores the question of why people work and examines the research in the area of intrinsic motivation.

Meaning of Work

Why do people work? What is the meaning of work in our lives? Throughout the centuries, these questions have been considered by the great thinkers of the time. The answers they offered were influenced by various theological and philosophical perspectives, as well as by the societal issues and social structures of the day.

A variety of historical viewpoints are held as to why humans work. Contemporary perspectives are represented in the publications of Meilaender (2000), Naylor (1996), Erikson and Vallas (1990), Applebaum (1992), and Amott and Matthaei (1991).

Work Is an Essential Element of Life

Meilaender and a group of scholars interested in the ethics of everyday life met over a five-year period under the auspices of the Institute of Religion and Public Life at the University of Notre Dame. Meilaender notes that the group read, wrote, conversed, argued, and continually sought ways for deepening their own understanding of the "meaning of human life as ordinarily lived" (Meilaender 2000, p. v). This work led to the publication of several anthologies covering various aspects of everyday life. The anthology entitled *Working: Its Meaning and Its Limits*, edited by Meilaender (2000), provides an in-depth examination and historical perspective on work and the meaning it has held for humans over the centuries. (See figure 2-1.)

Meilaender presents four main categories that capture the meaning of work over the centuries. The four categories include work as co-creation, work as necessary for leisure, work as dignified but irksome, and work as vocation. The anthology includes a variety of readings, essays, biblical passages, stories, and poems that illustrate each of the major categories. The readings and other written materials add richness and depth to this work and serve to illustrate the four categories.

Figure 2-1.   The Meaning of Work as Categorized in the Literature

---

Work is an essential element of life
   Work as co-creation
   Work as necessary for leisure
   Work as dignified but irksome
   Work as vocation

Work is a way to fulfill individual, emotional, and psychological needs
   Need for self-identity and self-esteem
   Need to contribute to society
   Need for independence from the control of others
   Need for social relationships
   Need for achievement, competence, and accomplishment

Work as Co-creation

Work can be understood as co-creation. The first book of Genesis in the Old Testament of the Bible is used to illustrate a mandate to participate with God in the care of His creation. Meilaender quotes an excerpt from Dorothy Sayer's essay, "Why Work?" which describes this sentiment well (Meilaender 2000, p. 43):

> Work should be looked upon not as a necessary drudgery to be undergone for the purpose of making money, but as a way of life in which the nature of man should find its proper exercise and delight and so fulfill itself to the glory of God. That it should, in fact, be thought of as a creative activity undertaken for the love of the work itself; and that man, made in God's image, should make things, as God makes them, for the sake of doing well a thing that is worth doing.

Thus, from a Judeo-Christian perspective, work is not something that a person does to live, but instead it is the thing one lives to do. And it should embody the full expression of an individual's faculties, "the thing in which he finds spiritual, mental, and bodily satisfaction, and the medium in which he offers himself to God" (Meilaender 2000, p. 43). In both the Hebrew and Christian ideology, God is portrayed as a worker, laboring six days to make the world and stopping on the seventh to rest (Applebaum 1992).

A citation attributed to Walter R. Courtenay reinforces this notion of work as an act of co-creation with God. "God gave man work, not to burden him, but to bless him, and useful work, willingly, cheerfully, effectively done, has always been the finest expression of the human spirit" (Naylor, Willimon, and Osterberg 1996, p. 36).

Regardless of one's religious beliefs, this concept of work as co-creation is compelling because it seems to correspond to the desire many people express for work that is meaningful and productive. In the literature relevant to the meaning of work in our lives, many of the articles and books are about meaningful work rather than about the meaning of work. It is helpful to differentiate between these two closely interrelated concepts. The relationship exists in that for many people the reason for work relates to their need to have an impact on the world. Meaningful work, work that makes a difference to others, is one source of meaning for them.

Although meaningful work may be one reason or motive for working, it is not the only one. Work has other meanings for humans as well. These other meanings are explored in the following pages.

Work as Necessary for Leisure

The idea that work is necessary for leisure has its roots in classical thinking. For many of the great Greek philosophers, work was important simply because it makes leisure possible. Not only does work make leisure possible but it is through the presence of work that we are able to clearly distinguish work from leisure. Today, leisure is thought of as freedom from work, most commonly amusement or time off that refreshes a person before a return to work. For Aristotle, in contrast, leisure was the pursuit of silence and contemplation.

The contemplative life was thought to be superior; in fact, contemplation was considered the highest form of existence. The contemporary concept of leisure is very different. For most people who experience weekends, holidays, and vacations as leisure, nothing could be farther from the contemplative life than leisure. Indeed, many return to work every Monday looking for a respite from the hectic pace that today's leisure entails.

Work as Dignified but Irksome

The third category of thought about work as presented by Meilaender and his colleagues (2000) also has its basis in biblical teachings. The concept of work as dignified but irksome is first apparent in the book of Genesis. Man, who has fallen into sin, is now condemned to toil for the bread he eats. And his toil is made even more difficult by a recalcitrant earth that brings forth only thistles and thorns. Simply observing ordinary human experience throughout history tells us that work is often burdensome. Over the centuries, humans have enslaved other humans to provide a source of labor. The peasants and serfs of early centuries and the wage earners of early factories certainly were exploited for their labor. The work histories of many groups employed in the secondary labor markets (composed of part-time, seasonal, or temporary employees) are replete with examples of exploitation, physical and psychological abuse, and working conditions that were not just unhealthy but sometimes actually incompatible with life. Even today in the Japanese culture, the word *karoushi* refers to a sudden death from overwork (Tubbs 1993).

At times, this category of thought also described work as a duty and an obligation. However, de Man (1929) found in his research that the Christian theology of the obligatory nature of work is a strong influence only in an indirect and unconscious way. It is not something verbalized in the workers' reports he analyzed. Quite apart from the theological aspects, de Man did find that, although every kind of working activity contains elements that make it a delight, it also contains elements that make it a torment. He reviewed examples of the words used in various languages that relate work to difficulties and turmoil. According to de Man, these examples were:

> not merely a legacy from the days when the social subordination of the worker made work degrading. Just as in the legend of the Fall, work is a symbol for punishment, so it lies in the nature of things that all work is felt to be coercive. Even the worker who is free in the social sense, the peasant or the handicraftsman, feels this compulsion, were it only because, while he is at work, his activities are dominated and determined by the aim of his work, by the idea of a willed or necessary creation. Work inevitably signifies subordination of the worker to remoter aims, felt to be necessary, and therefore involving a renunciation of the freedoms and the enjoyments of the present for the sake of a future advantage. (de Man 1929, p. 67)

Such dignified yet irksome elements fall at opposing ends of the spectrum, but they can be seen in every piece of work. When the aim of work is one chosen voluntarily by the worker, work is seen as a sacrifice. When the aim is one imposed on the worker from an external source, work is more likely felt as punishment. Thus, according to de Man, every worker is both creator and slave. "Freedom of creation and compulsion of performance, ruling and being ruled, command and obedience, functioning as a subject and functioning as an object—these are the poles of a tension which is immanent in the very nature of work" (de Man 1929, p. 67).

Work as Vocation

Work as a vocation, the last category identified by Meilaender (2000), was articulated most clearly during the Protestant Reformation. This category is related to the belief that work is a calling or vocation. People came to think that God's blessing sanctified their work and gave significance to it. Thus, no matter how menial their work might be, anyone could glorify God by doing his or her work joyfully and with dignity. Clearly, the idea of experiencing joy through work is a major construct in religious teachings and remains a contemporary message as well.

The idea of work as a calling is a powerful affirmation of daily life. Thinking of work as a vocation emphasizes that "work is a social activity contributing in some way to the good of all" (Meilaender 2000, p. 12). Applebaum points out that with Martin Luther and John Calvin were the beginnings of the modern-day work ethic, starting with "the concept of calling as a Christian duty, and the admonition to be successful in commercial enterprise, something which was looked down upon in the ancient and medieval world" (Applebaum 1992, p. 582). Interestingly, this new Protestant work ethic took two different directions. On the one hand, it promoted hard work and business enterprise while stressing thrift and business success. On the other hand, it stressed the need for respect of the working man, common ownership of land, and the redistribution of goods and services so that none would suffer. The first direction seems to support capitalism, whereas the second seems to support socialism.

The idea of work as vocation is often thought of in today's contemporary world as social obligation. Dick Richards examines the need of humans to bring passion and commitment to work and to create workplaces that not only honor but also support these qualities. He addresses the meaning of work in terms of a sense of social obligation: "All work creates something. Artfulness demands that we engage with the process of the work and with its product. The meaning of the work resides in the meaning of what we create. . . . We have a chance to work artfully when we believe that our work makes the world a better place" (Richards 1995a, pp. 35–36).

Work Is a Way to Fulfill Individual, Emotional, and Psychological Needs

Although Meilaender's work has provided a useful overview, there is another category of thought related to why people work. In the contemporary world, for at least part of the population, the meaning of work revolves around the desire to satisfy inherent human needs and motivations. "Work, if it has great significance for our lives, tends to be symbolic, having value for us because it helps to fulfill some human need other than work" (Naylor 1996, p. 46). This idea is a common theme in contemporary discussions and examinations of the meaning of work.

In 1994, Brian Dumaine wrote an article titled "Why Do We Work?" for *Fortune* magazine. In it he notes that if people are asked why they work, many say it is to make money. Yet, he asks, if that is entirely true, how does this motivation account for people continuing to work after winning the lottery or after having made enough money to retire? He notes that when Robert Weiss, a research professor at the University of Massachusetts, "asked people in a survey whether they'd work if they had inherited enough to live comfortably, roughly eight out of ten people said yes" (Dumaine 1994, p. 196).

More and more people today, especially among the Baby Boomers, "are looking to their work to satisfy some deeply individualistic, emotional and psychological need" (Dumaine 1994, p. 196). This is a recurring theme in the literature. In today's world, work is probably the most important single factor in status and self-respect for the individual, according to Applebaum (1992), who has studied the concept of work in ancient, medieval, and modern times. "The kind of work one performs, one's occupation, and one's employer are all indicators of the type of power and income which one can command and, with that, the type of consumption goods one can command" (Applebaum 1992, p. 286).

The idea that work fills personal, emotional, and psychological needs is supported by the findings of de Man (1929), who in 1926 read seventy-eight autobiographical reports from workers in Germany. Although one might think these participants are worlds apart from people living today, many of the themes and motivations identified are similar to the thinking today. The following needs are often fulfilled by contemporary work: a sense of self-identity and self-esteem; a capacity to contribute to wider society; a need for independence from the control of others; a need for social relationships; and a sense of achievement, competence, and intellectual accomplishment.

Self-Identity and Self-Esteem

A recurrent theme in the literature is the importance of work in forming individual self-identity. When de Man (1929) published his *Joy of Work*, he reported many examples and excerpts from workers' autobiographies that illustrated this point:

> A smith (case 49), a man endowed with vigorous artistic impulses, says: "How much I had identified myself with the work I turned out, became clear to me whenever I had to hand it over. I felt that it really contained a part of my personality, and I was often on the verge of throwing up my job at the factory and of returning to handicraft." (de Man 1929, p. 38)

De Man went on to note that there was a wide tendency to associate a high valuation of one's occupation with a high valuation of one's self.

> This is no less true today, and many people define themselves by the job or position held or the professional status enjoyed. Personal identity is closely tied up with work. The danger, of course, is when the job or work ends. In

today's tumultuous business environment characterized by downsizing and layoffs, mergers and acquisitions, identifying oneself too closely with the organization can be quite risky.

In *Working*, Studs Terkel (1972) quotes an unemployed, forty-five-year-old construction worker expressing his frustration and discouragement: "Right now I can't really describe myself because . . . I'm unemployed. . . . So you see, I can't say who I am right now. . . . I guess a man's something else besides his work, isn't he? But what? I just don't know" (Terkel 1972, p. 44).

E.P. McKenna found this out the hard way. While she was writing *When Work Doesn't Work Anymore: Women Work and Identity*, her high-achieving, executive husband discovered that his job had been restructured off the organizational chart. "With a tap of the delete key much of who he was and much of what he cared for was wiped away. . . . I knew . . . that it was going to take a while for him to sort out the man and the work. It had been a long time since he'd had to" (McKenna 1997, p. 224).

Self-esteem is closely related to self-identity. It refers to the value the person places on self. Many authors identify the positive effects work has on an individual's self-esteem (Amott and Matthaei 1991; Applebaum 1992; Aptheker 1989; Bookman and Morgen 1988; de Man 1929; DeChick 1988; Erikson and Vallas 1990; Gould, Weiner, and Levin 1997; Greiff 1999; Grossman 1990; Hesse-Biber and Carter 2000; Josselson 1996; McKenna 1997; Naylor 1996; Schuster 1990; Seiling 1997; Spencer 1982). Significant evidence shows that working increases a woman's sense of well-being (Hesse-Biber and Carter 2000), and why should it be any different for men? Warren Bennis, a well-known leadership scholar, notes that "work really defines who you are. So much of a person's self-esteem is measured by success at work" (Dumaine 1994, para. 9).

In his book *Joy: 20 Years Later*, Schutz's (1989) description of joy closely relates to his own self-esteem. Although Schutz's work is based on personal experience rather than on systematic research, the connection with joy and self-esteem is worth noting here:

> Joy is the feeling that comes from the fulfillment of my potential. Fulfillment brings to me the feeling that I can cope with my environment; the sense of confidence in myself as a significant, competent, lovable person who is capable of handling situations as they arise, able to use fully my own capacities, and free to express my feelings. Joy requires a vital, alive body, self-contentment, productive and satisfying relations with others, and a successful relation to society. (Schutz 1989, p. 11)

Contribution to Society

The desire to make a difference, to be part of something bigger than oneself, and to contribute to the wider society has been identified by many investigators as a driving factor in finding meaning in the workplace today. This idea is related to Meilaender's (2000) concept of work as co-creation. Based on his research, Terez (1999) reports that virtually all people have a driving desire to make a difference. "Believing your work can make a real difference in the world has motivated many people over the years" (Dumaine 1994, para. 17). This theme is found in several of the studies examining workers' experiences of joy (Worthington 1994; DiSciullo 1997). "[A] therapist . . . experiences joy in seeing her clients growing and developing skills to handle their life better" (DiSciullo 1997).

Independence from the Control of Others

Independence from the control of others is related to increased competence as well as to earning capacity based on the work (Hesse-Biber and Carter 2000; McKenna 1997). Especially for women, who in prior times were completely dependent on their husband or father for their income and financial assets, the ability to earn produces a powerful sense of independence. Independence also increases an individual's sense of personal satisfaction.

Independence, however, also has a shadow side. As Durning (1993, para. 15) notes:

> Members of the consumer class enjoy a degree of personal independence unprecedented in human history, [and] yet hand in hand comes a decline in our attachments to each other. Informal visits between neighbors and friends, family conversation, and time spent at family meals have all diminished in the United States since mid-century.

In fact, affluence has "broken the bonds of mutual assistance that adversity once forged" (Durning 1993, para. 14).

Social Relationships

Work is a key source of social relationships. Schuster (1990) studied gifted women at the University of California Los Angeles. The women came from a range of socioeconomic backgrounds. In her interviews with the women, Schuster sought to determine what characterized the essence of work for them, what aspects of their careers gave meaning and value to their lives. According to Schuster (1990, p. 204):

> For nearly all the gifted women—regardless of their technical competence, their creative ability, the nature of their work, their income, or their level of "success"—the issue of interactive communication stood out as the most salient characteristic of their work lives. In nearly three-quarters of the interviews, the gifted women described themselves, their achievements, and their sense of professional well-being in terms of relationships.

This observation is supported by the work of several other authors in the same volume. The experience of a woman's relationships in the workplace is central to the meaning that her work has in her life (Grossman 1990). Although there is evidence that women are more relationally oriented than men (Gilligan 1982; Miller 1976), the importance of relationships in the workplace does not seem to be a gender-specific issue. The value of work relationships is further emphasized by Applebaum (1992), who notes that work remains a major arena for social interaction. Even when people do not find satisfaction in their work, they often enjoy the social contacts they make at work.

Achievement, Competence, and Accomplishment

For many people, the value of their work lies in the sense of achievement and accomplishment that accompanies it. Dumaine (1994, p. 204) points out that work is a source of feedback and recognition related to this achievement: "Psychologists say few of us have the inner resources to live without constant and meaningful praise." And, in fact, several participants in DiSciullo's (1997) research identified feedback from their work as a source of joy. McKenna (1997) interviewed many women who focused their expectations for fulfillment and recognition largely on their careers. Greiff (1999) suggests that, for many, work represents the single most important source of accomplishment and intellectual satisfaction. A sense of capability and competence is also critical, and it is closely related to intellectual stimulation.

Historical Changes in the Meaning of Work

Ample evidence supports the idea that the meaning of work has undergone significant change since the advent of the Industrial Revolution in the mid-nineteenth century. As the United States, along with other industrializing countries, moved away from the predominantly agricultural societies of earlier centuries, the meaning of work was significantly altered. Similarly, the societal changes that began in the mid-twentieth century with the application of modern computer and communications technologies will continue to affect what work means for the foreseeable future.

Emergence of Industrialization and Capitalism

Throughout history, the context and location of work have varied. In the early days, work took place in the home and the community. With the decline of the agrarian age and the beginning of the Industrial Age, for the first time in history work moved into large factories and buildings where people came together to do their work. This remarkable change had many ramifications for society, all of which have been documented elsewhere. With the rise of capitalism and the formation of early bureaucracies, the voices and concerns of Karl Marx and Max Weber became prominent.

Marx believed that work is of prime and absolute importance to humans. "Man's essential activity is his work" (Applebaum 1992, p. 584). Marx argued that work went beyond irksome; that is, workers in an industrial society become alienated from their work because capitalism, in particular, dehumanizes the workers' relationship to their work. As workers become objects of work and an instrumental part of work processes, feelings of alienation become inevitable.

This viewpoint was contradicted by de Man (1929), who found that "'mechanised work' and 'work at the machine' are not the same thing. Among those who experience the highest joy in work . . . most of them are among the far more numerous machine workers, who, feeling themselves to be masters and overseers of the machines, have not the same reason to dread repetitive work" (de Man 1929, p. 112). In his study of German workers, de Man found that although the majority of those he studied were Marxian socialists, their personal experience was quite different from Marxian theory. In fact, for many workers, he found that working in industrial settings and learning the skills needed to master the machinery resulted in increased self-esteem and pride.

Introduction of Scientific Management

As the Industrial Age progressed and the continuing impact of mechanization became evident, so did another major change: the introduction of scientific management techniques. The writings of Frederick W. Taylor, a mechanical engineer, emphasized the importance of productivity and efficiency and were widely applied in business and industrial settings during the early twentieth century. Taylor's principles of scientific management included the following:

- Specialization of work into narrow jobs
- Precise and minute specification of jobs
- Constant repetition of tasks by the same workers
- Lack of a need for any judgment or discretion on the part of workers

With the advent of Taylor's scientific management methods and the institution of assembly-line organization of work, the de-skilling of workers began. As work functions were reduced to simple, repetitive, and monotonous tasks, much of the joy of work (as least in the industrial sector) disappeared. Therefore, although Marxian theory seemed to have been contradicted by de Man's work, an explanation for the discrepancy is apparent. De Man was reporting on the early effects of mechanization, when workers' lives were made easier by the machinery and workers gained a sense of mastery that increased their self-esteem. However, as the machines became more sophisticated and easier to operate, monotony set in. Many studies and writings of the day reported widespread dissatisfaction with work in industrial society. Soon work was seen as an "instrumental activity, as a means for acquiring income for subsistence and consumption, and that there [was] little or no satisfaction or meaning to be found in the workplace" (Applebaum 1992, p. 586).

Application of Bureaucratic Organizational Structures

Not only has capitalism and the continual pursuit of material goods affected the meaning of work, but changes in the structure of the organizations in which work is carried out has also had an impact. In the late nineteenth century, industrialized organizations were characterized by despotic management practices based on nepotism, political favoritism, and institutionalized corruption (Nadler and Tushman 1997). The bureaucratic model was developed as a reaction to the subjugation and cruel treatment of workers and the subjective decision making that characterized the managerial practices of the early Industrial Revolution (Bennis 1966).

The notion of bureaucracy as an organizational structure was first articulated by Max Weber, a German sociologist, around the beginning of the twentieth century. At the time, the bureaucracy was considered a radical idea and represented a remarkable advance over the traditional management practices of the time. Precursor structures were based on the arbitrary application of patrimonial authority. Weber believed that a modern bureaucracy "formulated on rational legal precepts was capable of sweeping other forms of organization before it" (Clegg 1990, p. 35).

Weber's bureaucracy was a management design based on formalized procedures, clear chains of command in the management hierarchy, and staffing decisions based on merit and technical expertise. The basic precepts of this design include:

- Division of labor based on functional specialization
- Well-defined hierarchies of authority
- Systems of rules that dictate the rights and duties of employees
- Established procedures for dealing with specific work situations
- Interpersonal relationships characterized by impersonality
- Promotion and selection practices based on technical competence

Meaning of Work in Contemporary Society

The simultaneous convergence of these three factors—capitalism, scientific management, and bureaucratic organizational structure—heavily influenced the way the meaning of work is perceived today. The contributions of Weber and Taylor combined to result in the emergence of a new organizational structure, the machine bureaucracy. This new structure perfectly fed the goals of capitalism. Productivity gains were enormous, and this structure became the dominant design of both industry and large corporations. It has been so prevalent that most managers have "grown up" with this model firmly and completely embedded in their approach to organizational design. Health care workers have been heavily socialized in the model of the professional bureaucracy, which has many of the same characteristics as the machine bureaucracy. The only difference is that the professional bureaucracy is based on a professional model rather than a business model. Over time, however, Weber became extremely concerned about the dehumanizing aspects of the bureaucracy and its impact on the creativity and free expression of the humans who worked within it.

The bureaucracy is still the predominant structure in many sectors of society (health care, education, finance, manufacturing, and government, for example). Morgan (1998) has traced the proliferation of multinational conglomerates, and he suggests that they are at least one example of the impact of an accelerated pace of mergers resulting in megacompanies that will significantly affect our lives in the future.

Clearly, bureaucratic structure has an impact on the meaning derived from work. The negative impact of increasingly massive and complex bureaucracies on the average worker is a common and repetitive theme in the contemporary business literature (Waterman 1992; Tushman and O'Reilly 1999; Stacey 1992; Snow, Lipnack, and Stamps 1999; Silberstang 1995; Seiling 1997; Ryan and Oestreich 1991; Reina and Reina 1999; Pinchot and Pinchot 1994; Morgan 1998; Hock 1999; Hirschhorn 1997; Helgesen 1995; Gowing, Kraft, and Quick 1998; Gould, Weiner, and Levin 1997; Denhardt 1981; Bowles 1991, 1997; Bennis 1970).

In addition, the attitude that work is only performed for money is still prevalent today and has become a significant issue in health care. McKenna is one of the most eloquent contemporary authors to discuss this subject. In the mid-1990s, she surveyed and interviewed almost 1,200 women about their work. Many reported a strong sense of dissatisfaction when they discovered they had basically created a level of consumption expectation that required continual feeding. One individual noted: "We quickly found that going to work also meant having to work. Quite apart from whether we wanted to or not—and most of us did—it just was a shock how quickly choice became necessity" (McKenna 1997, p. 27). In other words, the women's additional income raised the standard of living obtainable and soon became an expectation and "need" rather than a choice that provided discretionary funds. Another participant in McKenna's study noted that her dissatisfaction began when she realized that she and her husband both needed to work simply to maintain their standard of living. For many Americans, especially those who exist in one of the labor markets other than the upper tier of the primary segment, work is mostly about making a living, although the real living goes on after work hours.

One of McKenna's participants was articulate in describing the impact of increasing bureaucracy on her work life. As a woman in the publishing field, she had a long career marked by increasing success. However, as the years passed, the organization for which she worked became larger and larger through mergers and acquisitions. Jane told this story:

> When I was twenty-two, I worked for the editor-in-chief, who, in turn, worked for the head of the company. Twenty-two years later I was a vice president and editor-in-chief of a seventy-nine-million-dollar division. I worked for a president and publisher who, in turn, worked for a group president who worked for a CEO for the group who worked for a corporate executive vice president who worked for. . . . You get the picture.
>
> [For Jane it signaled the end of the community and therefore the end of communal purpose.] The work became increasingly purposeless. I didn't want to move on to the next level. I liked what I did and was happy doing what I was doing, but I just didn't want to be doing it in an increasingly meaningless way. I couldn't devote enough attention. . . . I really felt I wasn't doing it any better, I was just doing it thinner. I was more spread out. (McKenna 1997, p. 33)

Will this trend continue into the coming age of knowledge? Will knowledge workers (those who possess and develop highly specialized technical knowledge) experience less satisfaction when computer programs begin taking over decision making, the synthesis of data, and the all-important process of converting data into useful information?

Creation of a Positive Workplace

Throughout time a great deal of thought has been devoted to the question of why people work. The readings were reviewed in this chapter in an attempt to provoke a deeper level of thinking on the part of leaders in contemporary health care organizations. When the deeper, more compelling reasons people work are understood, they can be considered in terms of their influence in the organization. "Getting people to do their best work, even in trying circumstances, is one of managers' most enduring and slippery challenges" (Nohria, Groysberg, and Lee 2008, p. 78). Understanding human motivation is crucial.

Four Basic Drives

Motivation is what makes a person behave in a particular way. It is the underlying energy that compels action in a particular direction. There are at least two major ways of approaching this issue. The first involves recent research that identified human drives. Work done by Nohria, Groysberg, and Lee (2008) involves a review and synthesis of cross-disciplinary research in the fields of neuroscience, biology, and evolutionary science in addition to two recent research studies these authors conducted, which surveyed 385 employees from two global businesses and employees from 300 Fortune 500 companies. In these two studies, the definition of motivation focused on four commonly measured workplace indicators of motivation: engagement, satisfaction, commitment, and intention to quit. These two studies found that four drives underlie human motivation. Nohria, Groysberg, and Lee (2008, p. 80) propose that "the four drives are hardwired into our brains, and the degree to which they are satisfied directly affects our emotions and, by extension, our behaviors." The four drives are:

1. The drive to acquire. People are driven to acquire, not just physical things, like money, food, clothing, and housing, but also intangibles, such as social status, and experiences.
2. The drive to bond. "Many animals bond with their parents, kinship groups, or tribe, but only humans extend that connection to larger collectives such as organizations, associations, and nations" (p. 80). When this drive is met, the results are positive emotional experiences, and when they are not, loneliness and isolation can be common. The researchers believe this explains why employees feel a sense of belonging to the organization as a whole as well as their part

of the organization. It also explains the tremendous loss of morale when the organization betrays them and explains why it is so difficult for workers to break out of their silo (their particular part of the organization). The bond, or attachment, is usually strongest to their closest colleagues.

3. The drive to comprehend. People are invigorated by working out answers to problems, and they attempt to make sense and explain the world they inhabit and what is happening in it. "Employees are motivated by jobs that challenge them and enable them to grow and learn, and they are demoralized by those that seem to be monotonous or to lead to a dead end" (p. 81).

4. The drive to defend. This drive has to do with a need to defend and protect one's property and accomplishments, family and friends, and ideas and beliefs against external threats. When significant fear and resentment exists in the workplace, this drive is perhaps being thwarted. This drive has to do with aggressive and defensive behavior, but also the need to create organizations with a clear mission and goals, good intentions, and a sense of justice.

Nohria, Graysberg, and Lee (2008, p. 80) believe that an organization's ability to meet these four fundamental drives explains "on average, about 60% of employees' variance on motivational indicators." Each of the four drives may have a different impact on the strength of the motivational indicators. For example, the drive to bond had the greatest impact on commitment, which is clearly supported by the organizational development literature on affective commitment as presented in chapter 3. They suggest that a way for an organization to improve the overall motivation of employees is to focus on all four of these drives. The absence of one can affect the ability of the organization to meet the other drives.

The Intrinsic Motivators

The second major area to examine is the literature that explores intrinsic motivation. Intrinsic motivators are those forces within an individual that cause the person to act. Intrinsic motivators are of primary importance to leaders in organizations because the motivators exist independent of the leaders' actions. In other words, when an employee is intrinsically motivated to do what needs to be done, the leader's presence is of secondary importance. People who are intrinsically motivated know what needs to be done and want to do it. Such people are going to do the right thing whether the manager is standing there or not. When leaders understand the intrinsic motivators that drive employee performance, they can reinforce these powerful factors by their leadership actions, thus increasing the impact in the workplace.

Thomas, in *Intrinsic Motivation at Work: Building Energy and Commitment* (2000), offers a solid conceptual framework for understanding the intrinsic motivators. He also offers a compelling case for their contribution and importance in today's work world. "The new work role is more psychologically demanding in terms of its complexity and judgment, and requires a much deeper level of commitment. While economic rewards were pretty good for buying compliance, gaining commitment is a far different matter" (Thomas 2000, p. 5). He clearly believes that external motivators (such as money and benefits) are no longer enough to compel workers to act. When intrinsic motivators are present, individuals are more likely to feel energized and vitally connected to their work. Much of the work on intrinsic motivation is further substantiated by recent work in the field of positive psychology, which is discussed in chapter 4.

Thomas (2000) developed a model for creating a work environment that engages employees and taps into their creative potential. His work is based on the premise that a positive workplace leads to increased positive energy and commitment on the part of employee-colleagues. Thomas's work is worth noting here because he bases his conclusions on an extensive review of the psychological, sociological, and organizational development literature.

Based on his research and experience, Thomas identifies four factors that people find intrinsically motivating. These include meaningful work, choices in carrying out that work, a sense of competence, and the ability to make progress toward reaching desired outcomes. Based on further research and reading, the model has an additional factor likely to be an intrinsic motivator, the presence of healthy relationships.

Under this framework, leadership interventions become clear. Managers need to inspire and focus employees on the meaning of their work, create choices for the workers, coach for continual development and competence, and ensure that progress occurs and can be measured. In addition, managers have a responsibility to focus on the quality of relationships in the workplace. (See figure 2-2.)

Application of Intrinsic Motivators at the Organizational Level

The following subsections examine each of the five intrinsic motivators with special emphasis on their application in today's health care organizations.

Focus on the Meaningfulness of the Work

"People have a desire to be engaged in meaningful work—to be doing something they experience as worthwhile and fulfilling" (Thomas 2000, p. 12). For many people, work is composed of tasks that serve a particular end or accomplish a specific purpose. When a person is clear about what the purpose is, he or she can make intelligent decisions about the work. Rather than seeing work as a necessary evil or something that costs in a substantial way, the individual can see the work itself as meaningful and rewarding. Schwartz (2007, p. 68) says that "People tap into the energy of the human spirit when their everyday work and activities are consistent with what they value most and with what gives them a sense of meaning and purpose. If the work they're doing really matters to them, they typically feel more positive energy, focus better, and demonstrate greater perseverance."

Figure 2-2.   Leadership Strategies Based on the Fulfillment of Intrinsic Motivators

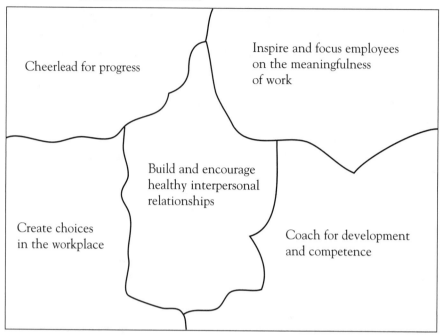

For example, a woman whose second career was nursing was interviewed for a research project and asked about her experience of joy through her work. At the time of the study, the nurse was employed in the outpatient recovery area of a diagnostic center. Over the course of the interview, she casually mentioned that after four years as a nurse, she was nearing the salary level she had reached in her manufacturing job before she entered nursing school. When asked about the higher-paying job in manufacturing, the nurse indicated that she would never return to manufacturing even though the money was better. She was committed to her work as a nurse because she believed she made a difference for every patient she helped. In her words, our world "can live without chrome bumpers for our cars," but it could not survive without someone to care for the sick and injured (Manion 2002a). To her, the meaningfulness of her work far outweighed any financial considerations.

Reed (2007, p. 52) proposes that employees must be connected with their passion for caring and service as one key condition for employee discretionary effort to manifest itself: "Most employees chose a health care career because of an *innate desire to make a difference in the world and in the lives of other people*" (emphasis in original). When the mission, vision, and goals of the work group, the department, and the organization are in alignment with each other, this impact is even more pronounced. Because, by its very nature, health care encompasses some of the most meaningful work known to humankind—the care of the sick and vulnerable—it is easy to conclude that health care work is inherently meaningful. Leaders and managers may be tempted to think that no specific action need be taken to enhance the meaning of health care work for their employees. Such an assumption, however, would be counterproductive for several reasons.

First, many individuals who work in health care organizations perform such a narrow part of the organization's work that they may not see how their work is connected to the well-being of patients. Examples of such workers include the messenger who delivers patient mail, the maintenance worker who paints the walls, the housekeeper who empties the trash, and the collection clerk who handles patient accounts in the business office. Managers can help all types of employees understand the contributions they make to patient care and the importance of their work. In addition, health care workers who work directly with patients can share their stories with those who work behind the front lines as a means of inspiring others.

At Medtronic, a medical device manufacturer in Minneapolis, the annual holiday gathering for employees is a prime example of the power of sharing stories. This program is broadcast to 30,000 employees worldwide and features the stories of patients who have benefited from the company's products. "Our people end up feeling personally involved in our company's mission to restore people to full life. They can see the end result of their work. Many of them are profoundly moved by the patients' stories" (Johnson 2005, p. 3), says Paul Erdahl, vice president of executive leadership and development. By "putting a human face on its mission," the company is an industry leader in achieving high employee retention rates.

Second, leaders along with employees must be continually alert to events or situations that indicate that the organization is not living up to its stated mission and values. When organizational decisions and behaviors contradict what employees believe to be the mission of the organization, the resulting dissonance can severely affect the employees' sense of meaning. (This subject is considered more fully in chapter 3.)

Finally, especially in today's organizations, managers must continually seek to reduce the amount of unnecessary work that creeps into jobs. Few health care workers chose their field because they wanted to spend half of their time documenting and recording what they did. Increased regulation in health care has resulted in an increased focus on paperwork and compliance with arbitrarily established rules, often at the cost of time spent in the delivery of the actual service in the department (AHA 2001). Add to this dissatisfaction the amount of duplicative work, and it is apparent that the point is rapidly being reached where health care workers are beginning to believe that meaningless requirements have replaced the meaningful work in their jobs.

Create Choices

Choice is a second intrinsic motivator. A sense of choice related to tasks or responsibilities creates the feeling that a person's views, ideas, and insights are important. Choice also involves the feeling of ownership and personal responsibility for the outcomes of one's behaviors or decisions. "Choice takes on extra importance when we are committed to a meaningful purpose. Then a sense of choice means being able to do what makes sense to you to accomplish the purpose" (Thomas 2000, p. 65).

A manager in today's workplace may have little control over the individual's initial choice to be there, in other words, whether the person must work or not. However, as explored in chapter 3, on organizational commitment, choice is crucial for ensuring that people feel engaged and committed to their work. A freely made choice to work or to be employed in a particular organization is instrumental to employees' feelings of commitment. Beyond this effort, however, leaders and managers have a great deal of control over this intrinsic motivator.

Shared decision making, empowerment, and delegation are common ways to increase each employee's ability to make choices in his or her work. Giving people the authority to make decisions that fall within their scope of responsibility and trusting them to do so are important leadership behaviors. Creating a climate characterized by a nonblaming, positive response to mistakes is another way to encourage employees to make decisions and show initiative.

Johnson (2005, p. 3) says that organizations must let employees know that they can exercise choice: "Jobs that provide variety and the freedom to make decisions and mistakes engender extensive loyalty." When people are allowed the opportunity to take ownership and be responsible for projects, they have the chance to develop new skills and show what they can do.

Coach for Competence

"You have a sense of competence on a task when you feel that you are performing your work activities well—when your performance of those activities is meeting or exceeding your own standards" (Thomas 2000, p. 77). Most people are more likely to enjoy work at which they are good. Seligman (2002) defines authentic happiness as occurring when a person knows his or her signature strengths and then crafts a life that uses these strengths in all aspects of life, including work. In other words, a person is more likely to be happy when he or she is engaged in work that taps into key abilities and is a reflection of competence. This is the core idea of the third intrinsic motivator.

The potential ramifications of personal competence in health care work are enormous. The role of the leader as coach is to help followers increase their level of competence, whether technical or interpersonal. Providing opportunities and learning resources, emphasizing individual growth, and ensuring an organizational philosophy of continuous learning are all important.

Selecting the right person for the right work and helping individuals modify work that does not use their competencies or signature strengths are also crucial. According to Buckingham and Coffman (1999, p. 148), "casting is everything. . . . If you want to turn talent into performance, you have to position each person so that you are paying her to do what she is naturally wired to do. You have to cast her in the right role." This is reinforced in chapter 10 in the section on job fit.

This message is reinforced by Jim Collins's research into why some organizations are able to make the leap from being good performers to exceptional performers while others are not. "The executives who ignited the transformations from good to great did not first figure out where to drive the bus and then get people to take it there. No, they first got the right people on the bus (and the wrong people off the bus) and then figured out where to drive it" (Collins 2001, p. 41). Furthermore, in determining who the right people are, exceptional organizations place greater emphasis on character attributes than on specific experience or education (Collins 2001; Manion 2004b). It is not that specific skills or knowledge are unimportant. Exceptional leaders know that skills and knowledge are teachable whereas character traits are ingrained.

Crafting work that fits an individual is another aspect of the manager's role. Loehr and Schwartz (2003) describe their extensive experience in coaching sports athletes as well as corporate athletes (their term for performers in the work world). They share example after example of individuals who came to them for coaching because they were exhausted and nearly depleted of energy. These people had lost a sense of connection and competence in their work. Sorting through what they are extremely good at is a key aspect of redefining the work so that it engages a person's full capabilities (Loehr and Schwartz 2003; Seligman 2002). Using a strengths-based approach to coaching employees is heavily emphasized today in the management literature (Buckingham and Coffman 1999; Buckingham and Clifton 2001; Henry and Henry 2007). A case study illustrating this approach can be found at the end of chapter 4.

Another potential role of the leader is to create work environments that are more likely to lead to optimal experience or flow on the part of employees. Csikszentmihalyi (1990, 1997, 2003) has done extensive research on the concept of flow. He defines flow as an optimal experience that is the unintended side benefit of engaging in activities during which an individual is stretched to the limits by challenges that are worthwhile. It includes both a sense of mastery and a sense of involvement or participation in an event. "Flow is the state in which people are so involved in an activity that nothing else seems to matter; the experience itself is so enjoyable that people will do it even at great cost, for the sheer sake of doing it" (Csikszentmihalyi 1990, p. 4). Competence is an important element of this concept, because flow requires a person to stretch but not exceed one's abilities. When a task does not challenge, boredom or apathy rather than flow is the result. But when the challenge exceeds the ability to master it, frustration is the outcome.

Flow is also described as engagement. In fact, when a person is in flow, engagement is so deep that time passes without notice. A quick examination of most health care workplaces reveals multiple barriers to the experience of flow. Endless interruptions; the need to be in constant contact with the rest of the world, as evidenced by the preponderance of beepers and cell phones; and the never-ending bombardment of overhead announcements, environmental noise, and e-mails are just a few examples of interruptions that break or prevent flow.

An important payoff when employees work with a sense of their own competence is that it leads to the emotion of pride. In an interview about his latest book, *Why Pride Matters More Than Money*, Katzenbach (2003) said that "it's more important for people to be proud of what they are doing every day than it is for them to be proud of reaching a major goal. That's why it's crucial to celebrate the 'steps' as much as the 'landings.' The best pride builders are masters at spotting and recognizing the small achievements that will instill pride in their people" (quoted in Byrne 2003, p. 66). Feeling pride is not to be mistaken for acting prideful in the sense of arrogance. Pride represents the positive emotion that accompanies personal accomplishment.

Recognize and Celebrate Progress

Another strong intrinsic motivator is a sense of progress. A feeling of having made progress occurs when a person feels like activities have had the impact intended, when work is achieving its purpose. Little is more discouraging than the feeling that nothing has changed as a result of intense effort and hard work. When progress is seen, one experiences a sense of momentum and enthusiasm, and the energy to continue the work becomes available.

An ancient Greek legend portrays the exquisite torture of a being for whom meaningful work is an inherent part of his nature. According to the legend, as punishment for an offense against the gods, Sisyphus is doomed to push a large boulder up to the top of a hill and then stand aside and let the boulder roll back down to the bottom of the hill. Then his work begins again as he pushes the same boulder to the top of the same hill over and over again for all of eternity.

The research on what brings people joy in their work clearly indicates that seeing results and making progress are essential for most people (de Man 1929; Manion 2002a, 2003). The ramifications for health care leaders are multifold. Barriers to progress within the system need to be analyzed and removed. For too many years the same problems have been tolerated in health care systems. Implementing an effective process improvement approach is not just the latest consulting fad or organizational culture change; it is crucial if employees and managers alike are going to have the tools to make both incremental and substantial changes in the system. The responsibility for true process improvement must be shared by both employees and managers. (Chapter 8 explores approaches for getting results and making progress.)

Systems for measuring progress are also critical to support this motivator. Without such systems, managers and employees find it difficult to track progress and recognize results. Such accountability systems are notoriously weak in health care organizations. For example, even with the current emphasis and focus on the leader's responsibility in recruitment and retention, few health care managers have access to department-specific measures of vacancy and turnover rates or survey results of satisfaction among patients, employees, and physicians. Yet department managers are being held accountable for outcomes in areas where measurements are inadequate or so outdated as to be useless.

A final consideration for leaders is how they can recognize and reward progress. Progress that is not recognized goes by unacknowledged. For example, a hospital in the Southeast was positioning itself to become part of a larger health care system. In order to appear as financially viable as possible, each segment of the system was asked to make a substantial contribution in the form of reducing its operating expenses. In the organization's large home health agency, the managers were expected to reduce their operating expenses by $1.5 million over the next year. These managers were exceptional leaders who worked closely with their employees in order to achieve this result. The employees were instrumental in designing and implementing a workforce reduction that was well received. In only nine months, a reduction of $1.2 million was achieved.

Subsequently, the two managers were called to a meeting with the system's chief executive officer and chief financial officer to report on their progress. For an hour, the executives badgered, questioned, and basically harangued the two department managers looking for a way to make the remaining $300,000 in cuts. No mention was made of the progress they had achieved, nor were any commendations offered for the exemplary way the initial results had been obtained. Imagine the level of interest and motivation that these two managers felt when they left the meeting. Both left the organization within six months.

The studies on happiness also support Thomas's (2000) conclusion regarding meaning and progress. "Happiness grows less from the passive experience of desirable circumstances than from involvement in valued activities and *progress toward one's goals*" (Myers and Diener 1995, emphasis added). These conclusions and recommendations reinforce directly the idea that work has meaning because it creates opportunities for achievement and competence.

Celebrating and recognizing progress is not as easy as it sounds. Many leaders have natural reservations about celebrating too early, and some may believe that there is not enough time during the busy day to celebrate. However, people pay attention to what is emphasized, and celebrations let people know what the organization considers really important.

Establish and Support Healthy Relationships

People clearly are more highly motivated to perform in a particular way when they have positive, healthy relationships with others in the workplace. Employees are not likely to go the extra mile for co-workers whom they actively dislike or for whom they feel no respect. When people enjoy healthy, positive relationships with others in the workplace it leads to stronger commitment to the organization and affects the quality of care provided. Co-worker friendliness and cooperation are important reasons health care workers stay with their jobs (Strachota et al. 2003;

Kangas, Kee, and McKee-Waddle 1999). It has become conventional wisdom that the relationship between employees and their manager is one of the most crucial in determining employees' commitment to stay with the organization.

Research in positive psychology also supports this assertion. (Healthy working relationships are examined more fully in chapter 6.) At this point, it is enough to point out that the establishment of positive relationships and a sense of connection to the people in the work environment increase the level of intrinsic motivation experienced by an individual.

Application of Intrinsic Motivators at the Individual Level

Understanding and applying the key intrinsic motivators are essential for every leader who wants to influence individual behavior. Understanding this model is also helpful for individual employees because it can help one make better choices about one's work (Manion 2008). Most people work in some form of gainful employment throughout the decades of their adult lives. For some, work is just a job, a way to earn money in order to do other things or meet personal needs. Many people see their work as a career, and throughout the years they continue to accumulate skills and achievements as a result of that work. Seeking promotions and new work opportunities is part of the process. When that upward progress is halted, the enjoyment of work is often lost and careers end. Yet for others, their work is more of a calling, work that is done for other reasons. Such people would do the work and enjoy it even in the absence of more traditional extrinsic rewards such as financial benefits or the recognition and adulation of others.

At times throughout a person's years in the work world, he or she comes to crossroads that raise the question of whether to stay with a particular job or move on. Understanding the five intrinsic motivators (mentioned above) provides an approach for considering and thinking about the decision (Manion 2002b).

As shown in figure 2-3, specific questions can be asked and explored to help decide whether the current work situation continues to meet personal needs. Sorting these questions by the intrinsic motivators may help individuals focus on key issues. The answers to the questions range along a continuum, as shown in figure 2-4. Plotting one's location on the continuum can provide a picture of what the current situation is like. It then becomes easier to determine whether a clear pattern or a mix of high and low responses emerges. When a person sees where he or she lands on the continuum, the following questions can be asked:

- Is there anything I want to do about the ratings that are low?
- Can I influence these lower ratings in any way?
- Which actions are within my scope of authority and responsibility?
- Which of these are of the highest priority for me?

Figure 2-3. **Using Intrinsic Motivators to Answer the Question, Should I Stay or Should I Go?**

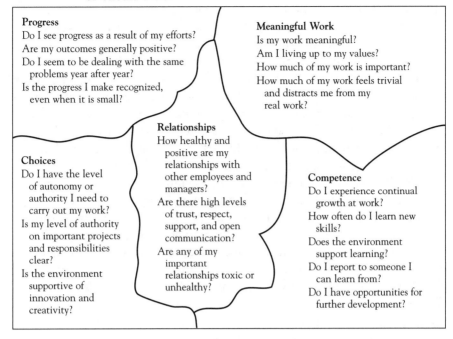

Progress
Do I see progress as a result of my efforts?
Are my outcomes generally positive?
Do I seem to be dealing with the same problems year after year?
Is the progress I make recognized, even when it is small?

Meaningful Work
Is my work meaningful?
Am I living up to my values?
How much of my work is important?
How much of my work feels trivial and distracts me from my real work?

Relationships
How healthy and positive are my relationships with other employees and managers?
Are there high levels of trust, respect, support, and open communication?
Are any of my important relationships toxic or unhealthy?

Choices
Do I have the level of autonomy or authority I need to carry out my work?
Is my level of authority on important projects and responsibilities clear?
Is the environment supportive of innovation and creativity?

Competence
Do I experience continual growth at work?
How often do I learn new skills?
Does the environment support learning?
Do I report to someone I can learn from?
Do I have opportunities for further development?

Figure 2-4. **Self-Assessment of Current Job in Terms of Intrinsic Motivators**

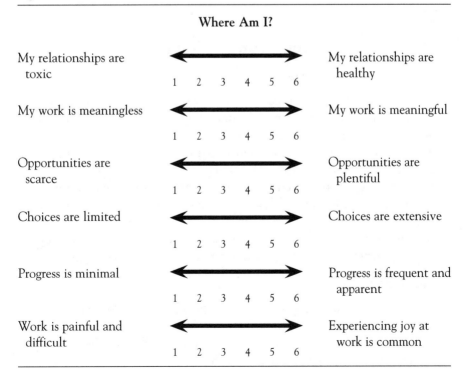

Where Am I?

My relationships are toxic   ⟷   My relationships are healthy
1   2   3   4   5   6

My work is meaningless   ⟷   My work is meaningful
1   2   3   4   5   6

Opportunities are scarce   ⟷   Opportunities are plentiful
1   2   3   4   5   6

Choices are limited   ⟷   Choices are extensive
1   2   3   4   5   6

Progress is minimal   ⟷   Progress is frequent and apparent
1   2   3   4   5   6

Work is painful and difficult   ⟷   Experiencing joy at work is common
1   2   3   4   5   6

Summary

The understanding of work has undergone change over the centuries. Throughout history, the meaning of work as proposed by the thinkers of the time has revolved around work as co-creation, work as necessary for leisure, work as dignified but irksome, and work as a calling. Today, one of the predominant ways the meaning of work is viewed is related to meeting the highly individual, emotional, and psychological needs of each employee. Many of the answers to the question about why people work are clearly interrelated, and any given individual is likely to identify several factors as motivating. The reasons for working manifest differently in each individual, and they are likely to change according to life stage, circumstances, and sociocultural perspective.

Clearly, organizational leaders as well as employees who understand the meaning of work in an individual's life are more likely to use this knowledge to build a strong, supportive work environment. And when the workplace fails to support any of the five intrinsic motivators (the need for meaningful work, choice and autonomy, competency, progress, and healthy working relationships) and these motivators are missing, it is likely that what is left to influence employee behavior are only the financial rewards of working. To the degree that jobs are interchangeable, if a person can easily replace this job with another that is similar, financial rewards are not very satisfying. Atchison (2003) notes that a common mistake of health care leaders is to try a quick-fix approach for improving employee morale and motivation rather than focusing on the deeper issues. If the organization is not a good place to work, money in the form of salaries and perks is not going to solve the underlying problems.

Conversation Points

Organizational Perspective

1. In what ways does the organization have initiatives that support the intrinsic motivators (meaningful work, competence, progress, autonomy, and healthy relationships)?
2. Are the organization's actions and stated beliefs about people and their motivation consistent with each other?
3. Does the organizational culture build on the intrinsic motivators? For example, are stories shared about meeting the mission that inspire others and increase the sense of pride employees feel? Are organizational structures in place to enhance employee competence, such as a strong educational department, career counseling services, and succession planning?

Leader Perspective

1. Examine your own beliefs about why people work. Do you have any employees for whom you think the primary motivator is money? Is there anything you can do to influence this situation? How can you build on the intrinsic motivators in your department?

2. What is the level of autonomy you expect of employees in your department? Do you transfer ever-increasing responsibility to employees?
3. Do you ask your employees about their individual challenges? Do you know what their aspirations and hopes are?
4. Do employees in your department feel a sense of pride and meaningfulness about their work?
5. How actively do you coach employees?
6. What is the quality of relationships among employees in your department and between your department and others in the organization?
7. Is visible progress being made on the problems in your department, or are you dealing with the same problems over and over again?

Employee Perspective

1. What is the meaning of work in your life? Beyond the obvious (it pays the bills), what is the deeper meaning of work in your life?
2. Do you spend more time at work doing tasks influenced by external demands rather than by a strong, clear sense of your own purpose?
3. Have you ever worked in a job where you felt like the work was meaningless? Did this make it difficult to go to work? What was the impact on your feelings about the job?
4. Do you feel like you have an appropriate level of decision-making authority for you to do your work well? What could you do if you feel like it is inadequate?
5. Is personal competence a motivator for you? Is it important that you are highly skilled and capable in your work? Think of times you did not feel competent or capable in your work. How did this affect your motivation for going to work?
6. How do you help others in the workplace increase their competency levels? Are you involved in coaching your co-workers?
7. How do you see progress in your workplace as a result of your efforts?

3

Building Organizational Commitment

Jo Manion

*Commitment is the will of the mind to finish what the heart has begun
long after the emotion in which that promise was made has passed.*
—J. Maxwell

WHAT KEEPS people at work once they get there? Understanding the intrinsic motivators and drivers helps a manager to recognize the factors that are important to employees. Ensuring that individuals are able to fulfill these intrinsic needs in the workplace increases the likelihood of employee commitment to the organization. Organizational commitment is another area to explore in understanding how to create positive workplaces. In previous decades, most organizations followed a traditional command-and-control approach to management in which employees were expected to do as they were directed without question. At best, compliance was the outcome. Compliance, however, often is not enough in today's complex and challenging work environment (Thomas 2000). The very nature of the relationship between the organization and employees has undergone a tremendous shift. Not only do workers today not expect to work for the same organization for decades, they do not want to. "The lifetime-employment contract was never the way to build employee loyalty . . . emphasizing a company's purpose . . . also engenders loyalty, especially when employees see the connection between their values and the company's mission" (Johnson 2005, p. 3).

Today, the role of leadership requires building a workforce among whom commitment is strong. For this reason, the concept of commitment is explored thoroughly in this chapter. The more understanding and knowledge a leader has about how commitments are made and what can be done to influence the process, the more likely it is that targeted approaches are used for creating a positive work environment. Commitment goes both ways: Organizations and leaders must create environments that evidence commitment to employees. However, employees also owe the organization a certain loyalty whereby they experience good intentions and positive engagement in their work (Spitzer 2007).

This chapter is adapted from Jo Manion, Strengthening Organizational Commitment, *The Health Care Manager* 23(2): 167–76. Copyright © 2004 and used by permission of Lippincott Williams & Wilkins.

Leadership is more than influencing others to follow a specific direction; it is creating a desire in the followers to do so (Manion 2005). "It is relatively easy to lead people where they want to go; the transformational leader must lead people to where they *need to be* to meet the demands of the future" (Wolf, Triolo, and Ponte 2008, p. 202). Although it is difficult or even impossible to teach people how to build commitment through reading and classroom work, a thorough understanding of the concept reveals several specific steps that can be taken by leaders to increase the level of employee commitment.

Peter Senge (1990, p. 10) describes the importance of commitment shared by leaders and followers when he writes about leading learning organizations: "We have seen no examples where significant progress has been made without leadership from local line managers, and many examples where sincerely committed CEOs have failed to generate any significant momentum." In other words, no leader accomplishes a major change or program initiative alone; such change requires a vital partnership with followers, all working in concert to carry out the plan.

In this chapter, liberal use of the term *leader* is used in recognition of the fact that both managers and employees function in leadership roles. Leadership roles are often assumed in organizations without the benefit of managerial authority. In fact, a key way that employee-leaders influence people without the benefit of legitimate authority is through the approaches discussed in this chapter.

Compliance versus Commitment

In the past, when formal managers were considered the primary source of leadership in the organization and the command-and-control methodology was still acceptable, compliance seemed fairly easy to attain. Employees were simply told what to do, and they were expected to acquiesce regardless of their own opinions or ideas. Basically, compliance means conformance. People do what they have been directed or asked to do. There may be very little personal involvement. In contrast, commitment is a personal pledge to a position or an issue. It requires giving oneself in trust to the issue or solution. In other words, compliance is a matter of the mind, but commitment is a matter of the heart.

Two factors in today's environment make mere compliance inadequate. The first is the nature of the workforce. A clear majority of today's health care workers are mature and experienced professionals, and they feel more involved in their work than ever. Second, the changes occurring in health care delivery are no longer mere tweaks in the system; they are fundamental, complex alterations to the very way service is delivered. For this deep level of change to be successful, more than mere compliance is required from the individuals who are expected to implement the changes.

Understanding the underpinnings of personal and organizational commitment is crucial for the leaders working in today's health care business environment. Accelerating change, developing organizational challenges and crises, increasing workforce shortages, and mounting environmental pressures make the need for committed and fully engaged employees more critical than ever.

Commitment Defined

Commitment is the act of pledging or engaging oneself. To commit is defined as binding or obligating oneself as in committing to a promise, a certain cause or course of action, or another person.

Concept of Commitment

A review of the classic literature on organizational development sheds further light on the concept. Brickman and his colleagues studied commitment extensively and report that it is "a force that stabilizes individual behavior under circumstances where the individual would otherwise be tempted to change that behavior. . . . Commitment is whatever it is that makes a person engage or continue in a course of action when difficulties or positive alternatives influence the person to abandon the effort" (Brickman, Wortman, and Sorrentino 1987, p. 2).

Commitment is seen in the workplace daily when people remain at work despite unpleasant or rapidly deteriorating conditions. Most employees can remember days when everything seemed to go wrong and they would rather have been somewhere, anywhere, else. It is commitment that keeps the person at work.

Commitment contains a directional element (Trigg 1973). An individual can never just be committed; one must be committed to something or someone. Commitments are not free floating; they are attached to a person or a thing. Also implied in commitment is a strong evaluative element; people must believe in the truth and inherent value of that to which they commit themselves. Commitment indicates a belief that an organization or a job is a good one and that it is worth supporting and important in some way. People do not commit to organizations that they believe are trivial, deceitful, or potentially corrupt. They make a judgment about an organization or job in light of their values.

Every individual has certain beliefs, and commitment involves a personal dedication to the actions implied by those beliefs. Therefore, commitment is more than belief; it is a belief strong enough to actually compel action. To illustrate this observation, consider the example of membership in a professional association. Members of the profession obviously evidence differing levels of commitment to their professional association. One professional may believe that the association advances the profession, which is of value, but she may choose not to join and support the association. In this case, no action would be taken and thus no commitment would be exercised, even though the association's value is recognized. Another professional may join the association and pay dues, but he may not participate on committees and task forces or attend local membership meetings. A third professional may choose to become an active member of the association by participating and contributing in numerous ways. This member would demonstrate a higher level of commitment than the member who merely paid his dues.

The essence of commitment is in the "relationship between the 'want to' and 'have to.' . . . Commitment involves three elements: a positive element, a negative element, and a bond between the two" (Brickman, Wortman, and Sorrentino 1987, p. 6). Therefore, commitment is a distinctive and compelling psychological process. The connection between the two elements, not merely their joint presence, is critical for commitment. Furthermore, the nature of this connection and bonding determines the nature of the commitment. Negative elements exist in even the most absorbing commitments, for example, the spouse who nurses her partner through a devastating and lengthy terminal illness; the manager who spends inordinate amounts of time at work, often at the expense of his personal relationships; or the highly skilled surgeon who made heavy sacrifices to learn her skills and puts herself at risk on a daily basis in the exercise of those skills. Similarly, a positive element can be present in even the most alienated commitment. "People who stay with a job or marriage after the life has gone out of it may no longer have the reason that initially drew them, but they still have reasons, they still have something of value that they do not wish to lose. . . . Thus the pension the person derives from the job, or the reputation and security from the marriage, become more valuable" (Brickman, Wortman, and Sorrentino 1987, p. 7). In other words, the investment made in the commitment has become more important than the original reason for the commitment.

> People experience commitment in at least two different ways. If the negative element is salient, persistence is the manifestation. If the positive element is stronger, enthusiasm is manifest. Persistence characterizes behavior that people continue to enact despite their sense that it calls for them to make sacrifices and resist temptations—they may have to work hard and resist the pleasure of quitting. Enthusiasm characterizes behavior that people enact without ambivalence about what the behavior costs, out of a sense that the behavior itself is meaningful. Persistence in commitment reflects the call of duty; enthusiasm goes beyond the call of duty. (Brickman, Wortman, and Sorrentino 1987, p. 10)

The manifestation of commitment is an important consideration for leaders in the workplace. Employees who seem to have lost their enthusiasm may not leave the organization, but their unhappiness may mean that the negative aspects of their job have overtaken the positive. Logically, when persistence is all that is keeping the employee in the job, it seems likely that the individual is closer to the next step, severing the commitment. And remember, as pointed out in chapter 1, termination occurs when the employee either "walks with the feet" and physically leaves a job or an organization or "walks with the heart" and emotionally leaves. Both forms of resignation result in the loss of commitment or engagement.

Interestingly, adversity plays an important role in the formation of commitment (Lydon and Zanna 1990). Without the negative element or adversity and the existence of alternatives that must be sacrificed, a true choice has not been made. Adversity can serve as a catalyst in the development of commitment. It can strengthen and affirm a commitment. For example, researchers have found that romantic love develops more strongly in the face of opposition.

Process of Commitment

Brickman, Wortman, and Sorrentino (1987) describe five stages in the process of commitment. Recognizing these stages may help in understanding the process of commitment and the issues related to each stage. Briefly described here, these stages also give insight into the making, as well as the breaking, of commitments.

Stage 1: Exploration

In stage 1, the level of commitment can be described as exploratory. During this stage, the potential activity or relationship is explored with concern only for what positive elements exist that might make further exploration worthwhile. Commitments at this stage can be considered a pre-commitment in that they often involve a positive orientation toward the potential object of commitment and significant reflection has not yet occurred. Stage 1 commitment can be characterized as positive and somewhat superficial. For example, recall the early stages of a job search or the exploration of a possible promotion.

Stage 2: Testing

Stage 2 can best be described as a testing phase. By this point in the process, some negative events have been encountered, and a need has arisen to assess one's willingness and ability to accommodate these events. The individual may have been involved in testing the environment, for example, to determine the willingness of a manager or co-workers to make concessions and contribute in some meaningful way to the employment relationship. The person may test himself or herself to determine presence of the ability to solve a problem or accomplish a task or activity. This stage also involves a search for information, but the focus is on the negative and troubling aspects rather than on the positive attributes inherent in the first stage. The focus at this point is external, and the crisis involves encountering unfamiliar and perhaps unexpected events. In other words, in stage 2, the honeymoon is over. The new job or organization has failed to meet expectations in some way.

Stage 3: Passion

Passionate describes stage 3. This stage is characterized by the first major synthesis of positive and negative elements as well as recognition of the entire process as a commitment. Commitments at this stage are fiercely positive (with an almost complete denial of negative features), and the person is highly self-conscious (Brickman, Wortman, and Sorrentino 1987). The individual at this stage of commitment development is sometimes experienced by self and others as fanatical, with compliance to behavioral actions that are rigid and without regard to their cost. It is almost as though the individual needs a more rigid, positive view in order to remain committed once a more realistic view of the negative elements in the situation appears.

Stage 4: Familiarity

Stage 4 can be characterized as quiet. This stage emerges more slowly as the energy needed to maintain the passion of stage 3 fades along with the ambiguity of the previous stage. The crisis of stage 4 occurs when the object of the commitment is attained and energy must be refocused on sustaining the commitment. Familiarity and comfort, characteristic of this stage, can undermine the effort required to sustain the commitment. As Maxwell (2003, p. 8) says, "Commitment is the will of the mind to finish what the heart has begun long after the emotion in which the promise was made has passed."

The orientation of this stage is intrinsic, with any threat coming from inside the person. The crisis comes in the form of boredom. When this stage is reached in a work commitment, many people begin looking for new opportunities or new ways to experience the job's challenge again.

Stage 5: Integration

Stage 5 commitment can be described as integral. This level of commitment represents a higher level of integration of both positive and negative elements. Stage 5 integration is more flexible and complex than earlier bonding. The structure supports awareness of both the positive and the negative elements, allowing the entire commitment to flow in and out of consciousness. During stage 5, "individuals have the capacity to treat their commitments in a cognitively simple or mindless way, simply acting out of habit or following a well-known script" (Brickman, Wortman, and Sorrentino 1987, p. 179).

Organizational Commitment

Recognizing the five stages of commitment increases understanding of how commitment is established and what the process of commitment looks like. The stages establish clarity about expected reactions, and this clarity can be reassuring for people who may feel confused by the dynamics of the process.

Perhaps one of the most important reasons to understand the stages of commitment formation is that understanding increases appreciation for the process. As a process, commitment is dynamic rather than static, and its characteristics change as it becomes deeper and more strongly affirmed.

Understanding the process of commitment also helps a leader see helpful interventions at different stages. For example, at stage 4 (familiarity), the manager can play an important role by working with the employee to find new opportunities to explore or challenges to undertake. It is also beneficial for an employee to understand the process of commitment because it may encourage him or her to seek additional responsibilities and opportunities in the current position rather than leaving because the work has become boring. Finding win-win solutions based on an understanding of the dynamics of commitment becomes more likely.

Commitment has been studied in numerous contexts, but the focus here is on commitment in the work setting. Organizational commitment can be defined in many ways, with the simplest definition being that organizational commitment is an employee's expressed "intent to stay." Wiener (1982) points out that behaviors resulting in organizational commitment possess the following characteristics: (1) the behaviors reflect some personal sacrifice made for the sake of the organization, (2) the behaviors show persistence, and (3) the behaviors indicate a personal preoccupation with the organization, such as devoting a great deal of personal time to organization-related activities. These characteristics vary in degree depending on the strength of each individual's level of commitment to the organization.

Other elements of organizational commitment include (Kanter 1972; Makin, Cooper, and Cox 1996):

- A strong belief in, and acceptance of, the organization's goals
- A willingness to exert effort on behalf of the organization
- A strong desire to maintain membership of the organization
- Group cohesiveness

Group cohesiveness is the "ability of people to 'stick together,' to develop the mutual attraction and collective strength to withstand threats to the group's existence" (Kanter 1972, p. 67). Job satisfaction as an expression of organizational commitment is clearly linked to the employee's intent to stay with an organization (Kleinman 2004).

Types of Organizational Commitment

Extensive research has revealed three specific types of organizational commitment: continuance, affective, and normative. Understanding these different types of commitment enables leaders to have a more significant degree of influence on the level of commitment experienced by employees.

Continuance Commitment

Continuance commitment is based on the employee's recognition that benefits as well as sacrifices are inherent in aligning with the system as well as sacrifices. Continuance commitment is based on a cognitive process. The balance between sacrifices and rewards must tip in the direction of rewards for an employee to remain in the system. For example, the person stays with the organization because the financial rewards are too great to leave, vacation accrual is at a high level, or the person does not want to lose the respect and relationships established. In other words, it costs too much to leave.

Early research on commitment focused on "side bets" (Becker 1960). In the organizational context of employment, the term *side bet* is used quite loosely but can refer to anything of value that the individual has invested—including money, ego, time, and effort—that would be lost or deemed worthless if the employee were to leave the organization. Such investments include contributions to nonvested pension plans, organization-specific skills or status, and any specific organizational benefits that could not be duplicated elsewhere. Thus, it is the threat of a loss that binds the person to the organization.

Employees committed to the organization primarily for financial reasons such as pay and benefits are not as likely to feel commitment to the values of the organization (Mayer and Schoorman 1998; McNeese-Smith 2001; McNeese-Smith and Crook 2003). In fact, they may actually become a liability to the organization because such employees experience higher levels of job dissatisfaction and deliver lower levels of job performance compared with employees who are committed to the organization's values (Meyer et al. 1989).

Affective Commitment

Affective commitment occurs as a result of events that increase the employees' level of emotional connection to their work group and lead to enhanced group cohesiveness (Kanter 1972; Iverson and Buttigieg 1999). Over the years, research has found that lower rates of turnover have been related to strong emotional and affiliative ties with the work group. Employee friendliness and cooperation are reasons health care workers stay with their jobs (Strachota et al. 2003; Kangas, Kee, and McKee-Waddle 1999). When the commitment to relationships within the workplace is strong, emotional ties bind members to each other as well as to the community they form (Barney 2002).

In today's world, a sense of community within the workplace has become increasingly important for many people as it may be the only source of community in which they participate. Chapter 7 explores the concept of community in the workplace more thoroughly.

Affective commitment is based on the strength of positive feelings that increase the emotional bond. It also explains why turnover costs more than money. Turnover ruptures relationships and threatens the cohesiveness of the work group (Barney 2002; Manion 2000).

Normative Commitment

The third form of organizational commitment is based on the recognition by the person that his or her personal values and beliefs fit with those of the organization. "Commitment to uphold norms, obey the authority of the group, and support its values, involves primarily a person's evaluative orientations. When demands made by the system are evaluated as right, moral, just, or expressing one's own values, obedience to these demands is regarded as appropriate" (Makin, Cooper, and Cox 1996, p. 69). When normative commitment exists, employees and work groups are less likely to deviate from rules and challenge authority. Normative commitment is also referred to as moral commitment.

Normative commitment explains at least partially why congruence between an organization's (or a leader's) stated values and its actions is so critical. A break in moral commitment occurs when employees perceive that the organization or one of its leaders is acting in ways inconsistent with the organization's stated beliefs or in ways significantly different from the employees' values. Everyone has seen the effects of such inconsistencies at one time or another. For example, one middle-size community hospital in the Midwest stated clearly that its most important value was providing high-quality patient care. Yet the hospital's employees openly and disdainfully argued that the true value held by the organization was high-quality physician care. Employees pointed to numerous and highly visible examples of instances when hospital executives failed to put patients first, giving physicians what they wanted instead of giving patients what they needed. For this organization, "Patients first" started as a catchy phrase meant to exemplify the organization's values but eventually became a roadblock to building employee commitment.

Employee Commitment to the Organization

Although the three different types of commitment may lead to stronger organizational support and affiliation, the nature of each of these links to employees is quite different. "Employees with a strong affective commitment remain with the organization because they want to, whereas those with strong continuance commitment remain because they need to" (Meyer et al. 1989, p. 152). As a result, the daily performance and behavior of these two types of employees are different. Those who value and want to remain part of the organization are likely to exert considerable effort on behalf of the organization, but those who feel compelled to stay to avoid financial or other costs may do little more than the minimum required to retain their employment.

Unfortunately, the results of multiple studies reveal that many health care workers are not highly committed to their job or to the organizations for which they work (Seligman 2002; AHA 2003). Fifty-two percent of health care workers admit to having a low level of commitment to the job they perform and the institutions for which they work (AHA 2003).

In today's health care organizations, it is relatively easy to find many employees who have "stayed, but left" or who "psychologically resigned" a long time ago. Such employees can be easily identified by co-workers because they rarely behave in a manner that exhibits strong affective commitment. In fact, studies have shown that job performance and promotability are negatively related to continuance commitment (Meyer and Allen 1984). More recent research has found that affective and normative commitment lead to positive organizational outcomes (such as lower absenteeism and intention to leave as well as a higher acceptance of change), but continuance commitment leads to greater inflexibility. In terms of rewards and benefits, merely introducing higher wages increases the person's "perception of low alternatives but has no effect on improving the alignment of employee goals with the organization" (Iverson and Buttigieg 1999, p. 327).

Leadership Interventions

When leaders understand the essential differences between the three types of organizational commitment, efforts focused on strengthening affective and normative commitment yield more long-term benefits. Makin, Cooper, and Cox (1996, p. 81) sum it up nicely: "In simple terms . . . people stay with the organization because they want to (affective), because they need to (continuance), or because they feel they ought to (normative)." The better that leaders understand the process of commitment, the more consciously that leadership behavior can be selected that encourages employees to form a commitment. Recognizing commitments made and understanding the dynamics involved in severing or dissolving commitments are also crucial. Otherwise, actions can inadvertently lead to further psychological disengagement of employees from the organization. For example, dissolving a team or closing a service or department may be a wise business decision, but if emotional support is not provided to employees in a way that recognizes the value of their commitment and helps them through this transition, their attachment to the organization as a whole may suffer irreparably.

Continuance commitment is often most emphasized by leadership in organizations during times of workforce shortages, exemplified by strategies such as recruitment incentives, salary increases, and benefit improvements. Yet this form of commitment is weak, and it can actually be harmful. Positive organizational outcomes are more likely attained by focusing on and strengthening affective and normative commitment. These two types of commitment are closely related and more likely to lead to personal and organizational commitment.

Approaches for Building Affective Commitment

How can employees' affective commitment to the organization be strengthened? Affective commitment is based on the employee's emotional and social connections with and within the organization. Studies have shown that a person's experiences during the initial months of employment are perhaps the most crucial in developing affective commitment. Focusing on efforts to ensure that the employee's initial expectations of the organization are met is important. During the early days of employment—a period of tremendous change for the individual—the organization needs to clarify roles and pay close attention to the formation of healthy relationships with new employees.

Still, commitment is influenced by the nature and quality of an employee's work experience throughout his or her tenure in an organization. The work experience is an important socializing force, and it significantly influences the extent to which affective attachments are formed with the organization. Experiences found to influence commitment include the work group's attitudes toward the organization, the organization's dependability and trust, and the individual's perception of his or her importance. In addition, efforts that support the development of healthy working relationships in work groups are crucial in the formation of a strong commitment. Peer relationships are important, but so is the relationship between the individual and the organization's leaders and others with whom interaction is common (such as patients and families, people in other departments, and physicians). (Healthy relationships are discussed in more detail in chapter 6.)

Approaches for Building Normative Commitment

The second form of organizational commitment to emphasize is normative commitment. Building normative commitment involves three essential components, as shown in figure 3-1.

Identifying and working from a foundation of shared values, a common sense of mission, and a shared vision are concrete ways normative commitment can be built within an organization. The degree to which these exist and the degree to which each has meaning for the people involved greatly influence the level of normative commitment in the work group or organization. Shared values, mission, and vision translate into engagement on the part of employees. In a study that examined why nurse managers stay in their role, Mackoff and Triolo (2008b) report that meaningfulness on the job is strongly linked to personal engagement. A key way that managers emphasized their organizations as being cultures of meaning was by "creating mission clarity and perception of the organization's values and fostering alignment between organization and individual values and contributions" (Mackoff and Triolo 2008b, p. 169).

Although the concepts behind values, mission, and vision are relatively simple, actually developing and building an organization-wide commitment

Figure 3-1.   Steps for Building Normative Commitment

Building Normative Commitment

Shared Vision
Our preferred future state
(what we believe we can attain
that is better than our current reality)

Common Mission
Our reason for existence (what we do and for whom)

Shared Values
Deep-seated standards that influence various aspects of our lives

to shared values, a common mission, and a shared vision are rarely easy. Implicit in each of the three concepts is the need for individuals to possess an extraordinary level of insight into what they find personally important in their work so that they can clearly articulate that insight to others. Sharing personal values also requires a high level of trust, and some employees may not feel comfortable enough to participate fully. Once personal values have been shared, the group or organization must then decide which of the values can be deemed important enough that the entire group can commit wholeheartedly to adopting them as the basis for all of their activities. Similarly, a group process is used to develop a statement of the group's essential reason for existing, its mission, and a vision for its future that is meaningful to all. Once the group or organization commits to its shared values, common mission, and shared vision for the future, results can be attained through the joint efforts of the people involved.

Deeply held values, a clear sense of mission, and the ability to develop a vision for the future are personal and leadership attributes rather than specific skills that can be developed. Guided classroom activities may help to clarify an individual's values and beliefs, but such activities cannot help to develop a belief system when it is absent. Usually forged through life experience and influenced deeply by individual personality and spirituality, personal values evolve over time. Most effective people express their values in both their personal and work lives through their day-to-day behavior.

Shared Values

Employee engagement has been linked to the alignment and fit between organizational and individual values (Morgan 2005). Alignment of values shared among leaders and followers and between the individual and the organization is essential to the development of organizational commitment. Values are pervasive, deep-seated standards that affect every aspect of a person's life. Values represent beliefs and determine what a person deems to be worthwhile, such as kindness and honesty.

Most people base their behavior on at least two sets of values: the values they hold as individuals and the values held by the groups to which they belong. These different value systems operate simultaneously.

Group values include the values espoused by the families, societies, religions, and organizations to which one belongs. Societal values are beliefs generally held by most members of a society. Societal values in the United States include the belief in equality, personal freedom, and democracy. Organizational values are beliefs considered to be important by the members of an established entity, such as a medical center, and can include those such as service to others, excellence in provision of services, individual competence, and quality. Family values are beliefs related to what is important within a family unit, such as mutual support, respect, and commitment. Work groups and specialized professions may also share a set of work-related values. For example, physicians and surgeons share a basic value that dictates that they will "first, do no harm."

Alignment of Values

For an individual who experiences a high level of congruence among the different aspects of his or her life, values overlap and are in sync with one another. High levels of energy and enthusiasm for life are the result. Each arena of life supports and reinforces the others. Personal power and effectiveness are at a peak.

Contradiction among values in these different areas creates dissonance, a disturbing experience for an individual. Three choices exist at this point: The individual can take steps to reduce the dissonance, perhaps by redefining the value to make it fit the situation. Another option is to suppress the uncomfortable and possibly painful feelings that arise and deny any discomfort. This happens when the person turns his or her head and pretends not to see a situation that violates a deeply held value. Finally, a person can take steps to change that aspect of life in which unacceptable contradictions in values exist. Such changes can be accomplished by addressing or reporting one's concerns about the situation or even removing oneself from the dissonant situation permanently.

Gilbert, in his book *Strengthening Ethical Wisdom: Tools for Transforming Your Health Care Organization* (2007), shares the dynamic of ethical erosion and cautions about its danger. "Research shows that it is in the small steps and small decisions that lead even well-meaning individuals and their organizations into ethical conflicts—a slippery slope that can ultimately undermine the organization's viability" (2007, p. xiii). Pretending not to see a conflict in values is a dangerous way in which to deal with the situation.

Prioritization of Values

Life is about choices. Many people are continually aware of the values that serve as a foundation for their lives and recognize that a choice must be made. The choices available, however, are not always seen or experienced with great clarity.

In every society, organization, family, or work situation, the values stated sometimes do not correspond to the values truly held. It is easy to let rhetoric drown out the truth. A society may say and believe that it values personal independence but then institute a welfare system that encourages dependence. A health care organization may state that it values service and community when in truth the primary focus of the organization is on its profits and reputation. Recall the hospital with the slogan "Patients first" and how that stated value became a source of great dissonance and dissatisfaction for employees. It takes courage to examine the feelings of discomfort, especially if it is only one's intuition that is saying something is wrong. An individual who has a great deal invested in the current system may find it difficult to admit that his or her values are not in alignment with the organization's values.

A person of integrity acts in accordance with his or her beliefs. If the values of the organization or group do not match those of the individual, he or she first assesses the situation to determine whether it can be changed. Action follows, based on a belief and hope that the situation can be influenced. Perhaps leaders in the organization have not recognized the incongruent messages their decisions are sending. Honest feedback and open dialogue about a perceived mismatch between a stated value and an observed behavior need to occur. When nothing changes, the individual's choice becomes clear: stay or leave. "In the work setting, a lack of congruency between personal and organizational values decreases job satisfaction and work productivity and ultimately may lead to job burnout and turnover" (McNeese-Smith and Crook 2003, p. 260).

In some instances, an individual's assessment of the situation results in a decision to stay so that other highly held personal values may be met. It is not uncommon for individuals who value financial security or stability for their families to decide to remain in a job or at an organization even though their other values are not congruent. Too many times, individuals remain in a dissonant situation and suppress their feelings of rebellion against the incongruent values. Over the long term, however, they may lose sight of their values and tell themselves that those values are not worth leaving their jobs for.

Courage to choose a different path can also be difficult to find when the conflict is between beneficial values. Which is most important? Which choice will be most true to the beliefs held dear by the individual?

Take the example of Jane, a leader in a health care agency. Jane discovered the difficulty inherent in choosing between two seemingly good values. She strongly valued security and stability and had spent most of her professional career in positions that were relatively safe. Fortunately, the positions also provided her with opportunities to meet two other values she held dear: challenge and achievement. In fact, these differing values were very compatible for most of her years in health care. Every challenge she met and every achievement she reached brought higher rewards, greater financial security, and enhanced sense of stability. As a vice president at the corporate level in a home health agency, she most enjoyed the new projects and the service development aspect of her work.

After a new chief executive officer was appointed, Jane gradually became aware that the philosophy of the company had changed significantly since his appointment. Jane's position became responsible for monitoring and ensuring regulatory compliance and advocating with state legislators. Although Jane was highly skilled in these areas, the challenge and sense of achievement she previously enjoyed no longer existed for her in this role. She tried to negotiate a role change so she would be challenged and excited about work again but was unsuccessful. Instead, to make matters more difficult, Jane's salary was increased significantly by the new chief executive officer, and her sense of financial security became stronger than ever. Her choice was difficult: Would she stay and continue to fulfill her need for security and stability, or would she seek another position full of challenge and the opportunity to grow? After much soul-searching, she resigned and became an entrepreneur. Her new business over the years became far more successful than she had initially dreamed possible. Ultimately, challenge and achievement were more important to Jane than security and stability.

Jane's story illustrates the importance of maintaining one's personal values. Values guide daily decision making and provide a sense of direction in day-to-day life. Holding the values of security and achievement simultaneously can lead to a crisis point in a career when situations force an individual to make a choice between remaining in a seemingly secure, well-paying job and seeking a new job with greater challenge. When actions are in accordance with held values, events flow more smoothly.

Results of Shared Values

When values are shared among people, the result is a tremendous feeling of connection and synergy. Achieving such synergy, however, requires that leaders and followers be able to clearly define their values. They must recognize which beliefs are most important in their lives. However, when values are never discussed, a false assumption may be made: either that the values are in agreement or that they differ. Open dialogue about personal beliefs benefits both leaders and employees. When values are shared, people feel united.

The ramifications for a leader who is trying to build commitment to a certain idea are clear. The leader must be absolutely clear about his or her values and how this decision supports those values. When incongruity exists, the leader experiences feelings of dissonance that are telegraphed to employees in subtle ways. When the path chosen is consistent with the organization's and the leader's values and these values are shared by followers, commitment blossoms. The ability to articulate and communicate clearly is critical for this process to succeed. Not only are the technical skills of communication important but also the leader needs the courage to speak from the heart and share his or her deeply held beliefs regardless of the feelings of vulnerability this approach may create.

> The challenge we all face is to find ways to use the workplace as a forum in which to express and embody our deepest values. We can derive a sense of purpose, for example, from mentoring others, or being part of a cohesive team, or simply from a commitment to treating others with respect and care and from communicating positive energy. The real measure of our lives may ultimately be in the small choices we make in each and every moment. (Loehr and Schwartz 2003, p. 140)

Common Mission

"The first responsibility of the leader is to define reality" (DePree 1989, p. 11). In an organizational context, leaders have the task and responsibility of determining both the purpose and the future of their organizations. Beckhard and Pritchard (1992) note that the turbulence of rapid change forces most leaders to re-examine the very essence of the organization along with its basic purpose; its identity; and its relationships with customers (internal and external), competitors, and other key stakeholders. Mycek (1998, p. 26) asks, "What is the true business of healthcare? Is it the 'high-tech, high-touch' blend of dedicated caregivers and state-of-the-art technology that was prophesied in the late 1980s? Or is healthcare purely a commodity—products and services that are bought and sold at the lowest price, on the spot market?" The questions today are becoming more and more difficult. In addition to defining the organization's mission, leaders and employees also need a clear sense of their own personal mission or purpose.

Strong leaders and committed employees have a clear sense of mission; they know why they are here, and they are clear about their purpose. Mission is a reason for existence—of individuals, projects, teams, and organizations. A clear mission defines purpose and gives direction and focus. It enables an individual to decline opportunities that detract from this true purpose. "It's easy to say 'no' when there is a deeper 'yes' burning inside" (Covey, Merrill, and Merrill 1994, p. 103). Ensuring clarity of a mutually held vision is the second approach to building normative commitment.

Over time, each individual's mission in life gradually becomes apparent. People grow into their work roles, including leadership roles, by fully experiencing life and learning its many lessons through reading, talking with and listening to others, traveling, learning new skills, and observing the life around them. Fully engaged workers are continual learners who always look for the lesson in a situation, even when it is difficult or painful.

The link between the person's sense of purpose and his or her daily activities must be apparent. Mackoff and Triolo (2008c, p. 21) report on a study of nurse manager engagement. They found that a manager's "ability to maintain [this] clear line of sight emerged as the crucible in longevity, vitality, and excellence." The notion of line of sight is described as the ability of individuals to understand how their daily activities contribute to the organization's purpose and goals. For health care managers this means creating "a meaningful, ongoing link between their daily management activities and the goals of patient care" (Mackoff and Triolo 2008c, p. 21).

The practice of reflection is growing in popularity today (Taylor 2004). Reflection is a powerful tool that individuals can use to better understand the motivation behind their own actions and reactions, to learn how outcomes are attained, and to recognize what is really important.

Leadership Mission Statement

Every leader needs a personal mission statement. An individual's personal mission statement may or may not include a leadership mission statement. For some people, these are two different but compatible statements. A leader needs to distinguish between his or her purpose as an individual and his or her purpose as a leader. Mission statements cannot be completed in a one- or two-hour period of time. Writing a meaningful mission statement takes "deep introspection, careful analysis, thoughtful expression, and often many rewrites to produce it in final form" (Covey 1989, p. 129). It means sorting through a great deal of extraneous material to reach the core reason for one's existence and how that purpose is to be achieved. The leadership mission statement usually includes the leader's values and often the means by which the mission is to be achieved.

A strong sense of connection between leaders and followers results when leaders openly share their personal or leadership mission statements. Leaders may feel vulnerable or embarrassed at first, because such statements, to be meaningful, must be very personal. However, when leaders sincerely and humbly express themselves, sharing mission statements is a powerful way of making connections with their followers. Even when supporters do not totally agree with or fully value a leader's personal mission statement, mutual understanding can be increased and strengthened from this sharing.

An individual without a sense of purpose is like a rudderless ship buffeted by every strong wind that happens along. People without clear purpose do not make good leaders. Individuals who have no inner sense of direction or understanding of purpose usually find it difficult, if not impossible, to be effective leaders. During periods of rapid change such as the present, it is not enough to simply adopt someone else's purpose because it is politically correct or expeditious to do so. Leaders need a strong inner sense of knowing and a connection to their identified purpose, or the personal mission statement will not serve them during stressful times. A point to remember here is that all employees have the potential of moving in and out of leadership roles, regardless of what their formal positions are in the organization. The concepts related to a leader's mission statement apply equally to an individual employee's purpose statement.

Alignment of Missions

Clarity of personal purpose enables an individual to determine whether his or her values and goals match those of the organization. When the purpose or mission of the organization is diametrically opposed to the individual's purpose, it may not be possible to effectively carry out the organization's mission. For example, assume that one leader believes that encouraging and nurturing employees to function independently and interdependently are important and part of his or her personal mission. However, the leader works in a bureaucratic, heavily hierarchical organization within which no support is provided for empowering employees. This leader will have difficulty feeling successful or satisfied. Or a leader may see his or her primary purpose as developing others, but recent expansions in the scope and span of responsibility have made it difficult, if not impossible, for the leader to serve as a coach for others in the workplace. This leader's primary purpose may no longer be met in this role.

Exemplary health care leaders today demonstrate an abiding sense of personal purpose. Many see themselves as stewards for health care in their communities. Chawla and Renesch (1995) describe this sentiment as a willingness among leaders and managers within health care organizations to become accountable for the well-being of the larger community by operating in service to colleagues, patients, families, and other stakeholders. This enduring sense of operating for the benefit of others and for something bigger than any individual helps create committed partnerships with followers.

As described by Robert Greenleaf in the collection of his private writings, *On Becoming a Servant-Leader*:

> The servant-leader is servant first. . . . It begins with the natural feeling that one wants to serve, to serve first. Then conscious choice brings one to aspire to lead. . . . The difference manifests itself in the care taken by the servant—first to make sure that other people's highest-priority needs are being served. The best test, and the most difficult to administer, is: Do those served grow as persons? Do they, while being served, become healthier, wiser, freer, more autonomous, more likely themselves to become servants? And, what is the effect on the least privileged in society; will they benefit or, at least, not be further deprived? (Frick and Spears 1996, p. 2)

Alignment of purpose between individuals and organizations creates a powerful collaboration. The vision, mission, values, and strategies must represent the best aspirations of the organization and those who work within it.

> The calling to care for and enrich the quality of life for patients, to support their families in times of stress, and to lift the wellness of communities served by the organization, is implicitly or explicitly stated in the vision, mission, and value statements. This calling is the heart of what draws many to healthcare. (Gilbert 2008, p. 3)

Simply ensuring that health care professionals can reach and deliver on their noble purpose is a powerful retention strategy (Ott and Abrams 2008). Both the organization and the individual must have the intention and unwavering commitment to do the right thing, to act with integrity and ethical behavior.

Shared Vision

The third approach to building normative commitment among followers in an organization involves the development of a shared vision. In recent years, vision has become a popular concept in management and leadership circles. Everywhere, managers and leaders are exhorted to have a vision. Example after example of governments, organizations, and people for whom vision made a difference is shared. And all are impressive, but Joel Barker, in the video *The Power of Vision* (1990), raises the question, Does the vision come first, or does the success of an individual, organization, or government lead to a vision? In each instance he examined, the vision came first, and this finding has led him to conclude that "vision has the power to change our lives."

Vision is a crucial attribute of successful leaders. All effective leaders understand vision because of its presence in their lives. It may not be an easily explainable concept, but leaders relate to this idea because they have experienced it. They see the future differently than other people do; leaders see what is possible and dream, while others merely predict. Basically, vision is hope for the future. It is the ability to rise out of the current daily turmoil and see something different for the future.

Developing visions for the workplace is one of the most important functions of leadership. Although the leader's vision of the future may not always be accurate, it is almost always desirable and positive.

The development of a vision for the future is a three-step process. The first step involves describing the vision, the second involves talking about the vision with the others who must help create the new future, and the final step involves putting a structure in place to ensure the realization of the vision.

Step 1: Define and Describe the Vision

A future vision is an idea that the leader has of an upcoming period of time. The power of vision is in its expectancy; it is an idea of a preferred future rather than a forecast of a predicted future. A vision is an illuminated look into tomorrow based on what the leader believes is possible. Vision takes imagination and optimism. "It is the ability to see beyond our present reality, to create, to invent what does not yet exist, to become what we are not yet. It gives us [the] capacity to live out of our imagination instead of our memory" (Covey, Merrill, and Merrill 1994, p. 103).

Some leaders seek or rise to a leadership position because they have a vision of what the future could be, and this vision drives and inspires them to lead. Armed with the vision, they find that it becomes a simple matter to put structures in place to achieve the desired future. Sometimes the position comes first, whether it is a formal leadership position in an organization, an appointment to chair a committee or task force, or an election to an office. The individual discovers that he or she has the responsibility and obligation to take the lead in a situation. Sometimes the sense of mission is clear but the vision of the outcomes is vague.

The first step of developing the vision may be more difficult than it sounds. As in a creative process, following a deliberate, intuitive approach is valuable. The intuitive process starts with preparation by coming to understand as much as possible through reading anything and everything related to the situation, talking with people, and drawing on past experiences. The second step is to let all information and ideas incubate until a spark jumps forward. This revelatory moment brings the leader to illumination, which is the third step. As the vision becomes clear, it is important to create as much detail as possible. Concrete, specific descriptions of a preferred future help others see the vision more clearly. For example, President John F. Kennedy, when he spoke of America's space program in a State of the Union address, did not say that the United States would be the world leader in space exploration in the future. Instead, he said that before the end of the 1960s, America would put a man on the moon and return that man safely to Earth. In other words, Kennedy expressed his vision in explicit and definite terms.

To be inspiring, the preferred future must be a stretch, a far reach from the present. Martin Luther King Jr. (1963) said, "I have a dream that one day this nation will rise up and live out the true meaning of this creed—we hold these truths to be self-evident: that all men are created equal." At the time, in segregated America, this was a tremendous stretch from the reality. Peter Senge (1990) says that once a vision is identified, the greater its distance from the current reality, the more creative tension that exists. Creative tension is the pull between the vision and the present. This tension acts like a giant rubber band, pulling people toward a new future. As Senge warns, when a vision seems too difficult, it is better to extend the time frame for achieving the vision than to scale back the vision to fit the time frame available. In other words, settling for less is the first step toward mediocrity.

Step 2: Engage in Dialogue about the Vision

A leader alone cannot achieve a vision. New realities are created when everyone affected by the vision works together. In a successful organization, multiple visions are encouraged in the same way that multiple leaders exist in different areas and on different levels of the organization. The various visions produce more impact when they are consistent and form a cascade of visions in the organization, as illustrated in figure 3-2. Everyone has his or her own vision of the future, and a shared vision is created when people engage in dialogue about the vision. The different visions are discussed, explored, and modified on the basis of information learned from others. A shared vision occurs when two or more people have a similar picture for the future and are each committed to achieving the vision.

In other words, an organization may develop a vision for itself while a specific department within the organization develops a vision that concretely describes the department's future as it relates to the organization's vision. For example, a health care organization may see itself as the premier health care facility in the region, while the cardiovascular department's vision relates to how it feeds or supports the organization's vision. To be powerfully influential, the visions must be in alignment with each other.

According to Senge (1990, p. 206), "Today, 'vision' is a familiar concept in corporate leadership. But when you look carefully you find that most 'visions' are one person's (or group's) vision imposed on an organization. Such visions, at best, command compliance—not commitment. A shared vision is a vision that many people are truly committed to, because it reflects their own personal vision." When the shared vision reflects personal visions, a deep sense of caring about the future can evolve. Senge (1990, p. 206) describes such shared visions:

> A shared vision is not an idea. It is not even an important idea such as freedom. It is, rather, a force in people's hearts, a force of impressive power.

Figure 3-2.   A Cascade of Visions

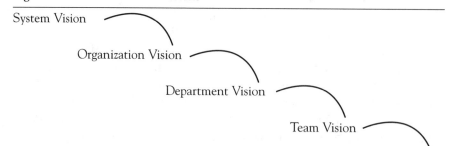

It may be inspired by an idea, but once it goes further—if it is compelling enough to acquire the support of more than one person—then it is no longer an abstraction. It is palpable. People begin to see it as if it exists. Few, if any, forces in human affairs are as powerful as shared vision.

Shared visions do not happen unless plenty of dialogue takes place about the future. Open give-and-take discussions, honest questioning, and stimulating conversations need to happen. Abraham Lincoln is a wonderful example of a leader who understood and applied this concept. "Throughout the [Civil War] Lincoln continued to visit his generals and troops. . . . He always had a kind word for them, frequently telling them his vision of America and how important they were in achieving victory in the cause for which they were fighting" (Phillips 1992, p. 19).

Step 3: Create a Structure for the Vision

Although Martin Luther King Jr. said, "I have a dream" and not, "I have a plan," having a dream without a structure in place will not ensure that a new reality can be achieved. To quote the Noah principle, "No more prizes for predicting rain; prizes only for building arks." The ark in this case is the structure that enables attainment of the desired vision. Some people are great dreamers but are unskilled when it comes to implementing those dreams. Leaders need both skills. "Leaders not only have a vision, they work unusually hard to execute it well. Leaders are implementers, not just strategists; doers, not just dreamers" (Berry 1992, pp. 2–3). Structure includes the steps to be taken to create the future. A person can dream of winning the lottery, but if he or she never purchases a ticket, the dream cannot come true.

Bennis describes vision as "the management of attention," and with this simple statement, he captures the power of vision. With a clearly articulated vision and people who believe in it, the vision itself focuses the attention of the visioning community. Attention keeps people focused on the future, hopeful and expectant about its possibilities. Leaders envision "the destination their followers want, they have the superior skill to guide the journey, and they have the belief to drive the group forward in the face of adversity" (Fagiano 1994, p. 4).

Shared values, a common purpose or mission, and a shared vision together produce the ability to influence others. The personal and deeply held values of leaders and followers influence the direction or mission chosen. And where a strong sense of mission is in place, the possibility exists of visions powerful enough to forge a new future.

Common Pitfalls

Leadership interventions for strengthening employee organizational commitment seem relatively straightforward. However, as with any issue dealing with human behavior and interpersonal interactions, hidden pitfalls and challenges need to be considered. Several of the most common pitfalls are discussed in this section.

Mistaking Compliance for Commitment

Effective leaders grasp the difference between commitment and compliance and do not mistake one for the other. Leadership is more than influencing others to follow a specific direction; it is creating a desire within the employees to do so. Earlier in this chapter, compliance was discussed briefly. Leaders who also have the legitimate authority of a position may be tempted to rely on giving others direction about the needed actions and behaviors and expecting compliance.

At first glance, it may seem easier to seek compliance than to invest in the preparation time it takes to build commitment, as illustrated in figure 3-3. The arrows in the figure represent projects, decisions, or actions that must be implemented. As the figure shows, less preparatory work is needed when the leader simply tells people what to do and people conform. In contrast, a long, intense preparatory period (symbolized by the longer line before implementation) is needed to gain commitment. Preparation includes lengthy conversations, exploration of shared values, refinement of purpose, open sharing of information, collaborative development of the vision and plan, and finally, an internal shift within each person that indicates a deep level of commitment to the outcome.

The paradox, of course, is that when thorough preparation is provided and employees are treated as partners on the journey, the attainment of the desired outcome is actually much faster. In many instances, when mere compliance is sought, leaders find that they have created an open-ended process with no closure because there are always some people who do not understand or agree and who will not comply.

The arrow at the end of the compliance line in figure 3-3 represents the open-ended nature of the situation. Often, leaders must follow up and continually monitor the situation to ensure compliance because people simply have not bought into the concept and do not support it. Unfortunately, it does not take many of these people within the group to create sabotage and undermining behaviors. And, in too many cases, the resistant behavior may be covert and not readily apparent. In either case, full compliance and, thus, closure are never attained.

Figure 3-3.   Comparing Compliance and Commitment in Terms of Time Investment

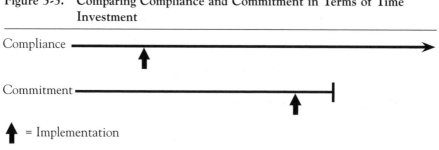

A strong leader understands the difference between compliance and commitment and consciously decides when commitment is needed and when compliance is enough. For leaders without formal authority in the organization, understanding the concept of commitment is essential. Without legitimate authority to force people to comply, these leaders often work to build commitment by following the steps outlined in the preceding section. Commitment is usually needed when following the course of action is going to take a lot of effort or will be difficult in some way.

Failing to Offer Choice in the Work Environment

When leaders understand commitment, the importance of choice is clear. Recall that, according to Brickman, Wortman, and Sorrentino (1987), commitment includes a positive element, a negative element, and a bond between the two. This idea implies that multiple alternatives are to be considered and evaluated. When there is no choice, there can be no commitment because there are not two elements between which a bond can be formed. Choice, then, is essential to the concept of commitment (Waterman 1992). The opportunity to exercise choice is an important construct in American culture. "For Americans . . . making a choice provides an opportunity to display one's preferences and, consequently, to express one's internal attributes, to assert one's autonomy, and to fulfill the goal of being unique" (Iyengar and Lepper 1999, p. 350). As discussed in chapter 2, choice is also one of the intrinsic motivators for work.

Commitment cannot be forced. Therefore, leaders must face the possibility that people may choose not to follow them. "If the most competent and trusted people won't commit, the leader should take another look at the cause itself. It may be ill-conceived or stated in a misleading way" (Waterman 1992, p. 299). Research has also demonstrated that people are less open to receiving new information once they have made their choice (Brickman, Wortman, and Sorrentino 1987). Because forcing a choice prematurely is risky, leaders must be comfortable enough to allow employees to come to their decisions about making commitments in their own time. More information is needed to change a decision than to make one. Demanding compliance on a course of action that requires the full engagement and support of employees is hazardous because it may preclude the possibility of ever achieving true commitment.

Probably the most important ramification of providing choice has to do with understanding why emphasizing continuance commitment is so damaging. When salary and benefits levels are high, employees perceive fewer alternatives to continued employment; that is, it would cost them too much to leave the organization. An employee who feels trapped, even by positive circumstances, is less likely to be positively engaged. Although competitive compensation packages are desirable, other rewards such as job variety, promotion opportunities, increased autonomy, and co-worker support are probably more effective (Iverson and Buttigieg 1999).

Communicating Insufficient Information

Recognizing that making a commitment involves a rational decision-making process underscores the critical importance of communication. Information is crucial in any decision-making process because it forms the basis upon which the decision is made. Recall the earlier recommendation supporting an open flow of information about the leaders' and employees' individual values and missions as well as the organization's values and mission. Involving employees in the development of a shared vision of the organization's future helps create enthusiasm and commitment. Honest and sincere dialogue between a leader and followers helps further shape and enhance the vision. As Senge (1990) points out, only when the vision is shared is true commitment and engagement possible.

How does a person move from thought to action? The choices available may seem overwhelming. Rational decision making requires accurate information. What are the alternatives? What are the consequences of choosing different alternatives? "The essential conflict between rational thought and functional behavior can be put very simply. Rational thought requires consideration of all available alternatives. Effective action requires the pursuit of one alternative, not necessarily the best one, and the ignoring or suppressing of the others" (Brickman, Wortman, and Sorrentino 1987, p. 51). Decisions must be made and action taken even when compelling arguments exist on both sides of the issue. Being rational requires individuals to choose the better alternative. Thus, a key issue in rationality is whether the individual is aware of the alternatives and his or her reasons for choosing one over the other.

The influence of commitment needs to be respected. "To whatever extent people are rational, they are less so following commitment" (Brickman, Wortman, and Sorrentino 1987, p. 35). When circumstances result in the dissolution of commitments, especially those that people have been asked to make, rapid resolution of the emotions involved cannot be expected. A recent example illustrates this. In a small Georgia community, two hospitals with a long history of fierce competition were set on a course toward merger. The chief executive officers in both facilities worked diligently to gain the commitment of employees, physicians, and the community. Their strongest argument was that this course of action was the only hope for the survival of both facilities. People were persuaded that the argument was true, and they became quite committed to the merger. Imagine the difficulties and resulting emotions when the merger fell through.

Missing the Opportunity to Escalate Commitment

Another key aspect to understand is the concept of escalation. Escalation is related to the need for self-justification. The concept has been studied widely in social psychology. "Escalation is self-perpetuating. Once a small commitment is made, it sets the stage for ever-increasing commitments. The behavior needs to be justified, so attitudes are changed; this change in attitudes influences future decisions and behaviors" (Aronson 1995, p. 192). Many savvy telemarketers use the concept of escalation by beginning their sales pitches with questions to which a person can only respond positively. This sets the person up for subsequent positive responses. Thus, when a leader is able to gain even a modest commitment, that commitment sets the stage for more significant commitments later.

Summary

Employee compliance with the directions issued by leaders and managers is not enough during these difficult and demanding times for health care organizations. Whether they hold formal or informal authority, exemplary leaders know how to build a commitment to action among employees. They also understand the different forms of organizational commitment and how to capitalize on these to create a positive work environment.

In successful organizations, effective leaders focus their efforts predominantly on building affective and normative organizational commitment. Developing shared values, a mission common and relevant to all, and a shared vision for the organization are specific ways in which a leader can build normative commitment among followers. Affective organizational commitment occurs when healthy relationships and a strong sense of connection exist among people in the workplace. When these two forms of commitment are present, employees do not just comply with the direction set by leaders; they want to follow the recommended path. Together these efforts inspire passion and provide the energy and courage to create a new reality.

Gilbert (2008, 1) identifies having a noble purpose as one of the disciplines of everyday practice that strengthens organizational integrity and ethical health care:

> Noble purpose is the calling of healthcare expressed in the vision, mission, and values of an organization and those who work in it. It is a powerful, unifying force. A focus on it brings together different parts of the healthcare community who might otherwise find themselves in conflict. It diminishes their differences and mobilizes powerful collaborations for change.

This concept holds true beyond health care as well. Kanter (2008, p. 44), in her analysis of some of the world's largest companies, found that clarity of mission and values serves as a guidance system for these global giants: "Employees once acted mainly according to rules and decisions handed down to them, but they now draw heavily on their shared understanding of mission . . . they more readily think about the meaning of what they do in terms of the wider world." Kanter (2008, p. 45) also found that values in these global companies are truly a primary consideration: "Values turn out to be the key ingredient in the most vibrant and successful of today's multinationals." Holding common values and standards and having clarity of mission allow people at the front lines to make consistent decisions, even under pressure.

Conversation Points

Organizational Perspective

1. Which form of organizational commitment (continuance, affective, or normative) do you think is the strongest in your organization?
2. Are there times when the organization has not lived up to its stated values, purpose, or vision? How are people treated when they question incongruities? Do employees feel safe raising issues related to organizational values?
3. How does the organization ensure that all new employees are introduced to the organization's values, mission, and vision?
4. Were all levels of employees involved in creating the vision? Or was the vision developed by a small, select group and then presented to the others?
5. What are the consequences when people do not live up to the organization's stated values? What happens? What is an example of this?
6. Are meaningful conversations occurring on a regular basis about the organization's values, mission, and vision? When was the last time this occurred in a significant way in the organization?

Leader Perspective

1. What are your most important work-related values? What do you stand for? How do you treat your co-workers and colleagues? What do you mean by *ethical behavior*? How do you want to be known by others?
2. Once you have a list of your important values, identify the specific day-to-day behaviors you engage in that demonstrate how you live by these values. Are there gaps between what you say you value and how you live your life? What values do you say you hold but express infrequently? What values are neglected during periods of high stress?
3. Think of an example when you had to decide which of your values was more important to you. What was the situation, and how did you resolve it? In retrospect, did you make the right decision? Would you change that decision today if you could?
4. What could you do to ensure that you are living by your values on a day-to-day basis?
5. Describe your personal and leadership missions. Why are you here? What do you do, and for whom do you do it? Take some time to reflect, and then write a personal mission statement.
6. What is your future vision? Where do you see yourself in five years? What will you be doing? How will you get there?
7. When was the last time you had a substantial, meaningful conversation with an employee or a colleague about organizational or departmental values?
8. Are your values, mission, and vision consistent with those of the organization?
9. Which forms of commitment do you see in your department? Continuance, affective, or normative?

Employee Perspective

1. Think of something to which you are committed. How did your commitment begin?
2. What has kept that commitment strong over time? What are the elements of your commitment? Which are the positive elements, and which are the negative?
3. Consider your organization's values, mission, and vision. Are your values, mission, and vision consistent with those of your department, service, or organization?
4. Find people for whom vision has made a difference. Ask them to share their story.
5. What is your vision for your future? Where do you want to be and what do you want to be doing in five years?
6. When was the last time you were involved in a meaningful conversation with someone in the workplace about the values, mission, or vision of the organization?
7. Have you asked your manager or another organization leader what values they hold dear? Are they congruent with yours? Are they substantially different from yours?
8. What do you do when you see the organization or its leaders or employees behaving in a way that is incongruent with the organization's stated values? Do you speak up, or do you ignore it? If you have spoken up and addressed the inconsistency, what was the reaction of others?
9. Do you take time to reflect on whether your and your co-workers' decisions and actions are consistent with the organization's values?

4

Experiencing Happiness and Joy in the Workplace

Jo Manion

When work is a pleasure, life is a joy!
When work is a duty, life is slavery.
—Maxsim Gorky

EMPLOYEES WHO experience joy and happiness through their work and in their workplaces are valuable assets in today's health care organizations. Managers and leaders who understand the concept of positive emotion and are able to apply their knowledge to create a positive work environment are more successful at tapping into intrinsic motivators and building organizational commitment, both among themselves and among their employees and colleagues. This chapter explores recent research from the field of positive psychology and offers concrete, evidence-based suggestions for establishing a workplace in which happiness and joy are key characteristics of the environment.

Positive Psychology

A startling innovation in the field of psychology developed during the late 1990s: the birth of positive psychology. Since the earliest days of modern psychology in the mid-twentieth century, the focus of researchers and practitioners has been on alleviating the misery of people suffering from mental illnesses. Thousands and thousands of research studies have been conducted on depression, anger, fear, hatred, and countless other negative emotions and conditions. Mental illnesses have been examined, defined, and categorized extensively. This research has resulted in tremendous progress in the ability of psychiatrists and clinical psychologists to diagnose and treat clinical depression, schizophrenia, and other serious, debilitating conditions.

However, many behavioral scientists are coming to realize that traditional psychology concentrates on reducing misery but does little to encourage happiness. In other words, even when medications relieve a patient's symptoms of depression, the person may not be happy. Although traditional psychology has made some progress toward understanding the positive emotions in the last half of the twentieth century, that progress seems almost insignificant in the face of its overwhelmingly negative emphasis.

Positive psychology recognizes that people want more out of life than correcting their weaknesses and deficiencies. People want to live lives full of meaning and purpose, and they want to be happy. "Positive psychology studies what is right with people and how people live the good life" (Maymin 2007, p. 1). The explosive growth of positive psychology during the past decade is primarily due to the efforts of several prominent practitioners and academicians. Notable contributors include Martin E. Seligman at The University of Pennsylvania, Mihaly Csikszentmihalyi at the Claremont Graduate University, Ed Diener at the University of Illinois, and Chris Peterson at the University of Michigan. As noted by Seligman (2002, p. xi) in his book *Authentic Happiness: Using the New Positive Psychology to Realize Your Potential for Lasting Fulfillment*, "the time has finally arrived for a science that seeks to understand positive emotion, build strength and virtue, and provide guideposts for finding what Aristotle called the 'good life.'"

Work and happiness? Joy at work? For some people, these terms seem inherently contradictory. Yet the truth is, how a person feels at work and whether he or she is happy at work and in the workplace determines to a great extent what that individual's life is like. Most people spend the majority of their awake and alert hours at work, and if they are not happy there, they often judge their lives to be unhappy. If work is unpleasant, tedious, or meaningless, those involved in it often feel demoralized, demeaned, or unhappy, and these feelings permeate the rest of life. Although many people may try to compartmentalize and segment their lives by telling themselves not to bring personal problems to work or not to take the negativity home, the reality is that the different aspects of one's life are closely interconnected and intertwined. It is virtually impossible to confine unhappiness to one segment or arena of life. Unhappiness will surface, unwanted, in the other parts of life as well.

Csikszentmihalyi, in his book *Good Business: Leadership, Flow, and the Making of Meaning* (2003), explores the relationship between business and happiness in some detail. He points out that "it may seem counterintuitive to argue that happiness and business have anything to do with each other, since for most people work is at best a necessary evil, and at worst, a burden. Yet the two are inextricably linked. Fundamentally, business exists to enhance well-being" (Csikszentmihalyi 2003, p. 21). He goes on to make a historical case supporting this contention. From the earliest of human endeavors, the production and exchange of goods make sense only when those goods improve the quality of the human experience. Good business is not merely related to the generation of monetary profit; it also relates to exchanges that increase and contribute to the happiness and quality of life of humans. Not only does the primary purpose of business seek to improve our lives, but also work is the vehicle through which a measure of happiness may be found. It provides a way for a person to apply his or her strengths and to use his or her positive attributes, and this ability to apply strengths and attributes is often considered the foundation of happiness. In other words, a person is often the happiest when doing what he or she does best.

Positive psychology is not just feel-good, pop psychology or "happiology" characterized by easily repeated platitudes. Nor is it the toys-and-trinkets approach currently popular in many of today's recognition and appreciation initiatives. It is a scientific field of endeavor whose hallmark is research leading to a deeper understanding of the positive emotions. Seligman (2002) sorts the field into three areas: the study of positive emotions, the study of strengths and virtues, and the study of positive institutions.

Study of Positive Emotions

Although the negative emotions have been examined in numerous research studies, prior to the mid-1990s little research was conducted on the positive emotions such as joy, happiness, hope, and satisfaction. Positive emotions include those that are related to the past, the present, and the future.

> The positive emotions about the future include optimism, hope, faith, and trust. Those about the present include joy, ecstasy, calm, zest, ebullience, pleasure, and (most importantly) flow; these emotions are what most people usually mean when they casually—but much too narrowly—talk about "happiness." The positive emotions about the past include satisfaction, contentment, fulfillment, pride, and serenity. (Seligman 2002, p. 62)

Clearly, all three of these temporal aspects of emotion are closely and tightly linked, and although it is desirable to experience positive emotion about all three, it does not necessarily occur this way. For instance, a person might feel proud and satisfied about his or her work and contributions in the past but still feel quite unhappy with what is happening in the present. And this individual might not feel optimistic about the future. Another person may be quite bitter about the past and yet enjoy pleasure in the present. Still another individual may be positive about the future and yet miserable in the present. These seeming contradictions are apparent in ourselves and our co-workers.

Positive Emotions Related to Past Experiences

Positive emotions related to past experiences include contentment, satisfaction, fulfillment, pride, and serenity. When the three temporal aspects of life are sorted out, it is clear that many examples may be found of individuals for whom the three are separate issues. This separation can lead to a feeling of liberation when individuals realize that they are not victims of their past but that they can exert free will and rise above events in the past to experience the present and future by choice.

Positive psychology research has found it difficult to produce evidence of even small effects of childhood events on adult personality, and there is less evidence to suggest that childhood experiences determine adult functioning. According to Seligman (2002, p. 67):

> The major trauma of childhood may have some influence on adult personality, but only a barely detectable one. Bad childhood events, in short, do not mandate adult troubles. There is no justification in these studies

for blaming your adult depression, anxiety, bad marriage, drug use, sexual problems, unemployment, aggression against your children, alcoholism, or anger on what happened to you as a child.

Clearly, Seligman's viewpoint is different from that held by traditional psychiatrists and clinical psychologists. However, Seligman's research should not be interpreted as suggesting that childhood events do not affect the person as an adult; it simply has found that traumatic childhood events are not tightly and causally linked to negative adult experiences.

In the same way, in the work world, negative and even destructive events can happen that are regrettable, but they will affect the future only to the degree allowed by the individual. Instead, what has been found is that people are highly adaptable creatures. When positive or negative events occur, there may be a temporary burst of mood in the expected direction, but within a short time, mood settles back into its set range. Thus, emotions, left to themselves, eventually dissipate, and the person returns to a baseline condition.

It should be noted here that it is very common in health care organizations to attempt to measure employee satisfaction levels under the assumption that high satisfaction is related to employment retention and the creation of a positive workplace. However, at best, these measures can give us only a sense of how people feel about the past. Although such information is important, it is only one of the elements that need to be considered. Just as important and as likely to be related to retention is how the employee is experiencing the workplace during the present and how he or she sees the future.

Fred Lee (2004), in his book *If Disney Ran Your Hospital: 9½ Things You Would Do Differently*, examines the difference between customers who are satisfied and those who are extremely satisfied. From his experience as a Disney cast member and further investigation he concludes that it is the *highly* satisfied individual who becomes a promoter and tells others about his or her experience. Such promotion takes a personal connection and an exceptional event that leads to loyalty and return of the customer. In the workplace this translates as employees who have surprising, positive, and even exceptional experiences. These people are promoters with high levels of loyalty. Simply measuring and accepting general employee satisfaction as the goal will fall short of achieving the level of commitment and loyalty needed in organizations today (Huff 2007). Employees need to have exceptional experiences in the past to translate to loyalty and commitment.

Positive Emotions Related to Present Experiences

Positive emotions in the present include joy, ecstasy, calm, zest, ebullience, pleasure, and flow. (Flow is sometimes defined as a sense of engagement. See chapter 2 for a fuller definition of flow.) Positive emotions experienced in the present constitute what is often referred to as happiness. From the research, Seligman (2002) points out that happiness in the present embraces both pleasures and gratifications. Pleasures are those experiences from which the individual derives clear sensory and emotional pleasure, such as having a good massage, listening to favorite music, or enjoying a special meal. Gratifications, on the other hand, are activities that engage the person fully, often without any clear emotional content, but because they require immersion and absorption they cause a loss of the sense of time and consciousness. Reading a good book, mountain climbing, and having a great conversation with someone are all examples of gratifications. Gratifications last longer than pleasures, they demand thinking and interpretation, and they do not habituate easily.

Although pleasures in life increase our perception of happiness, they are not enough to render us truly happy. People become easily habituated to the pleasures. For example, the second taste of a creamy, smooth, deep-chocolate truffle is not as marvelous as the first. And once the pleasure is over, it is over. The good feelings seldom last. Not only do these pleasures fade quickly but sometimes a negative aftermath is the result, such as a craving or even an addiction to the pleasure. Long-term positive feelings instead often result from gratifications.

This one principle, understanding the difference between pleasures and gratifications, has huge implications for contemporary organizations. Focusing recognition and retention efforts on those things that bring immediate pleasure will yield few long-term gains. Both surprise and disappointment are experienced when people become habituated to such immediate rewards and begin to demand more and more. At this point, it becomes difficult for people to emerge from this state of entitlement. Some of these pleasures (gifts, social events, and so on) can be equated with making people happy, but not substantively.

Understanding the nature of gratification can help organizations design recognition and retention initiatives and focus on creating more enduring positive emotions. For example, using gratification to recognize an employee for positive performance might involve supporting the person's attendance at a professional continuing education event or assisting the person in writing an article for publication. These types of rewards have longer-lasting effects than giving a coupon for a free dessert in the cafeteria or movie tickets for a night out.

Nevertheless, those simple little pleasures are also useful and appreciated by individuals. So, approaching recognition with an either/or approach in regards to pleasure/gratification is not as effective as considering both pleasures and gratifications that the employee might enjoy. Positive emotions in the present come from a balance of gratification and instant pleasure.

Positive Emotions Related to the Future

Positive emotions related to the future clearly affect the person's perception of well-being in the work world. Future positive emotions include faith, trust, confidence, hope, and optimism. Seligman (1998) has studied optimism extensively, and he reports that it can be learned. He defines optimism very differently from the more common but superficial "glass half empty/glass half full" approach. He believes, instead, that each person has a basic explanatory style that includes two dimensions: permanence and pervasiveness.

People who are less optimistic and give up easily often do so because they believe the bad events that happen to them are permanent and will continue to affect their lives. This state of mind is different from the state of mind enjoyed by individuals who believe that the causes of bad events are temporary and will pass.

Pervasiveness is related to whether the person sees the cause of a bad event as universal or specific. People who adopt a universal explanation for why a bad event occurred are more likely to let it permeate other aspects of their lives. For instance, a woman might think, "I lost my job and so I am a bad wife and a bad person." On the other hand, she might assume a specific explanation for the same circumstances: "I wasn't skilled enough to perform this job well, and so I need to improve my skills or learn new ones." In the second example, the job loss would affect the woman's work life but have little impact on her family, personal, or volunteer life.

> People who make permanent and universal explanations for good events, as well as temporary and specific explanations for bad events, bounce back from troubles briskly and get on a roll easily when they succeed once. People who make temporary and specific explanations for success, and permanent and universal explanations for setbacks, tend to collapse under pressure—both for a long time and across situations—and rarely get on a roll. (Seligman 2002, p. 93)

Schwartz (2007) builds on Seligman's work and takes a similar approach. He believes that people can cultivate positive emotions by changing the stories they tell themselves about the events in their lives. He says that a very effective way people can change a story is to view it through any of three different lenses. These are all alternatives to viewing the world from a victim mind-set.

> With the *reverse lens*, for example, people ask themselves, "What would the other person in this conflict say and in what ways might that be true?" With the *long lens* they ask, "How will I most likely view this situation in six months?" With the *wide lens* they ask themselves, "Regardless of the outcome of this issue, how can I grow and learn from it?" Each of these lenses can help people intentionally cultivate more positive emotions. (Schwartz 2007, p. 66)

It can be very insightful for people when they realize they have a choice about how to see a given situation and to recognize that the stories they use to explain things powerfully influence the emotions they feel. When a person learns to tell the most hopeful and positive story, without minimizing or denying the facts, it increases positivity.

It is likely that experiencing the positive emotions of the future has a direct impact on an employee's intention to remain in a job within the organization. When there is little faith or belief that the problems on the job are getting better or that the work situation in the future will improve, the employee is more likely to consider pursuing other opportunities. Work environments characterized by low levels of trust among people are also characterized by less hope for the future. It also seems evident that having less hope or faith in the future has an impact on an employee's commitment to the organization or the work group.

Study of Strengths and Virtues

The second area of positive psychology is the study of the strengths and virtues. Peterson and Seligman (2004) have published a catalog of the virtues, which is based on a thorough study of the primary writings in all of the main religious and philosophical traditions known throughout human history. The virtues identified are those found universally across three thousand years and the entire world. The six virtues are wisdom and knowledge; courage; love and humanity; justice; temperance; and spirituality and transcendence. The list of twenty-four strengths describes the traits of human character through which the virtues can be achieved. For example, the virtue of wisdom and knowledge is related to the following five strengths:

1. Curiosity/interest
2. Love of learning
3. Judgment/critical thinking
4. Originality/ingenuity/creativity
5. Perspective

Thus, a person with the strength of curiosity and interest coupled with a love of learning will more likely develop the virtue of wisdom.

The virtue of transcendence is related to:

- Appreciation of beauty/awe
- Gratitude
- Hope/optimism
- Humor/playfulness
- Spirituality/sense of purpose

Talents should not be mistaken for true strengths. Strengths must be built and developed; by comparison, talents are more like innate gifts. Although talents can be honed and refined, they cannot be learned. For example, a person may learn all about music, but if he or she is tone deaf (i.e., unable to sing on key), no amount of practice is going to make the person a good singer. Each person makes the choice about whether to develop a strength and when to use it.

Every individual has several predominant strengths, called signature strengths. Seligman (2002) believes that happiness comes when a person recognizes his or her signature strengths (those that are strongest for the person) and uses those strengths in both work and personal life. These individual strengths can be discovered by completing the Values in Action instrument on Seligman's Web site (www.authentichappiness. com). This concept is discussed more fully in the section of this chapter titled "Strategies for Increasing Happiness and Joy at Work" in terms of how it can be used in the workplace.

Study of Positive Institutions

The third area of positive psychology involves the study of positive institutions such as the family, democracy, and free inquiry. In his book *Good Business*, Csikszentmihalyi (2003) advances the basic position that business itself is capable of being a positive institution in the world. Whether businesses can rise to the challenge of being models of virtue is questionable, given the dramatic examples of corporate fraud and corruption over the past decade (Easterbrook 2003; Hammonds 2004). Certainly, health care organizations could be considered positive institutions in the community and world.

The formal study of positive institutions is probably the least explored area of positive psychology. However, many books in the popular business press attempt to examine successful organizations and identify their key attributes and characteristics.

Business Case for Happiness

Why be concerned about whether people are happy at work? After all, seemingly more important issues tend to require attention in the workplace, such as increasing productivity, ensuring a high-quality patient/customer experience, and establishing effective working relationships, to mention only a few. The truth is that all of these challenges can be better met by people who are happy and who enjoy their work. After extensive study, Amabile and Kramer (2007, p. 77) "believe strongly that performance is linked to inner work life and that the link is a positive one. People perform better when their workday experiences include more positive emotions, stronger intrinsic motivation (passion for their work), and more favorable perceptions of their work, their teams, their leaders, and their organization." Recent research in neuroscience demonstrates clearly that emotion and cognition are tightly intertwined. Areas of the brain associated with rational thinking and decision making have direct connections to those areas associated with emotions. The business case for happiness is dramatically simple and clearcut, and it is based on solid empirical evidence.

The benefits of a workplace characterized by people who are happy seem almost self-evident. However, many managers and executives assume that having a happy workplace is a luxury and not a necessity to expend excessive time developing. After all, employees are paid, and isn't that enough? Yet clearly, advantages to having happy employees include higher productivity, better outcomes, increased employee retention, healthier employees, and a more positive environment for patients and families.

Higher Productivity

One study measured the amount of positive emotion among 272 employees and followed their job performance over eighteen months. Happier people went on to get better evaluations and higher pay. In a large-scale study of Australian youths across fifteen years, happiness made gainful employment and higher income more likely (Seligman 2002). Myers (1992, p. 131), in his book *The Pursuit of Happiness*, notes that "compared to depressed employees, those with higher well-being have lower medical costs, higher work efficiency and less absenteeism." Csikszentmihalyi (2003, p. 25) points out that "a business organization whose employees are happy is more productive, has a higher morale, and has a lower turnover."

In trying to determine which comes first, happiness or productivity, researchers induced happiness experimentally in the laboratory and then examined later performance. It turns out that when both adults and children are put into a good mood first, they select higher goals, perform better, and persist longer on a variety of laboratory tests, such as solving anagrams. Research conducted by Fredrickson (2003) has also found that people in a more positive mood actually think more broadly and can solve problems more readily. Both of these abilities affect productivity.

Better Outcomes

Positive mood has been directly linked to a range of different performance-related behaviors, including greater helping behavior, enhanced creativity, integrative thinking, inductive reasoning, more efficient decision making, greater cooperation, and the use of more successful negotiation strategies (Marsh 2005; George 2000; Totterdell et al. 1998). A negative mood shifts a person into an entirely different way of thinking than a positive mood. When feeling negative, people seem to become critics of each other; negativity engenders a competitive mode of thinking, a win-lose approach to problems. People concentrate on what is wrong and attempt to correct it. Conversely, a positive mood shifts people into a way of thinking that is creative, tolerant, constructive, generous, open, and lateral. The focus is not on what is wrong but on what is right (Seligman 2002). Patient care outcomes even suffer when employees are unhappy. "Results from a Press Ganey study found that hospitals with the lowest employee satisfaction had the lowest patient satisfaction, and hospitals with the highest employee satisfaction had the highest patient satisfaction" (Strachota et al. 2003, p. 111).

Studies of business teams reveal fascinating data on this subject. Losada (1999) studied sixty business teams that were meeting to determine their annual strategic plans. Fifteen teams were considered high performers, twenty-six teams were medium performers, and the remaining nineteen teams were low performers. The performance categories were based on three criteria: profitability, customer service rankings, and the number of positive performance appraisal evaluations received within the team. The planning sessions were videotaped, and all speech acts were coded for three different attributes: whether the act was positive or negative, whether it involved inquiry or advocacy, and whether it was self- or other related. The results were astounding. The high-performing teams had the broadest range and widest repertoire of behaviors. They had a significantly higher number of positive acts. The low-performing teams had a higher level of negativity, and they lost their ability to question and became stuck in self-absorbed advocacy. They lost their behavioral flexibility all together. The clear conclusion is that the more positive the team, the more effective it is.

Positivity and positive emotions are also related to flourishing, or finding the "good life," as well as to developing a broad repertoire of skills. Barbara Fredrickson has studied positive emotions extensively and has proposed a causal theory of positive emotion (Fredrickson 1998, 2001, 2003). In its study of emotions, traditional psychology has come to conclude that emotions engender thought–action tendencies. For example, anger is a cue that signals the person's boundaries have been invaded and prepares the person to defend himself or herself. Fear induces a reaction that causes a person to remove himself or herself from dangerous situations. Sadness prepares the person for loss. However, the positive emotions have only begun to be understood. Fredrickson's extensive research leads her to suggest that the purpose of positive emotions is to help a person develop resiliency and broaden his or her repertoire of skills. The positive emotions build and deepen physical, emotional, social, and intellectual resources. Positive emotions, therefore, clearly produce benefits in the workplace and lead to better outcomes.

Just one example can illustrate this point. When an individual feels a positive emotion, he or she is more approachable to others and builds good relationships with other people, thus broadening social resources. The impact in the workplace is clear: Improved social resources lead to higher levels of teamwork, cooperation, and supportive behavior. All of these outcomes are desperately needed in today's demanding working environments.

Increased Employee Retention

It is almost impossible to sort out whether higher job satisfaction makes a person happier or a happy disposition leads to more satisfaction with a job. Clearly, however, these two factors are closely interrelated. Happier people are more satisfied with their jobs, and job satisfaction is clearly linked to employee retention. It has been shown that engagement and commitment among employees are both related to the employees' attitude toward their work and have an influence on retention rates (Buckingham and Coffman 1999; Kaye and Jordan-Evans 1999, 2002).

In addition, happier people form more positive connections with others. They are friendlier and others gravitate toward them. A happier workforce clearly leads to a higher level of affective organizational commitment and to an emotional bond between co-workers. This affective commitment and affection for co-workers is one of the reasons that people stay in their jobs. Employees who are happier not only are looking for settings with a good work environment but they are also helping to create that environment wherever they go.

Improved Employee Health

A great deal of research in positive psychology has focused on the relationship between positive emotions and health status. Although health status does not seem to be directly linked to a person's perception of happiness, there is no question that overall happy people are healthier than unhappy people. "Optimism and hope cause better resistance to depression when bad events strike, better performance at work, particularly in challenging jobs, and better physical health" (Seligman 2002, p. 83). Research studies have also shown that happiness and other positive emotions can actually undo some of the adverse physiological effects of negative emotions, such as the effect of adrenalin released in response to fear or threat. Experiments on nonhuman primates have shown that recurrent emotion-related cardiovascular activity injures the inner walls of the arteries and can initiate atherosclerosis. In empirical studies, it has been found that positive emotions reduce the amount of time during which the negative emotion affected the cardiovascular reactivity that occurs after negative emotion (Fredrickson 2003).

Positive emotions also seem to fuel resiliency. A study was conducted on students who had been tested for resiliency and optimism shortly before the terrorist attacks on the United States in 2001. The students were interviewed again within days after the September 11 attacks, and more than 70 percent of the participants reported feeling depressed. Yet those participants who had been identified as resilient during the earlier interviews also expressed strong positive emotions immediately after the attacks and were half as likely to be depressed as those participants who had been identified earlier as being nonresilient. The statistical analysis of the study's results showed that the tendency to feel more positive emotion buffered the resilient people against depression. Resilient participants expressed gratitude about the good things they had learned from the crisis and felt optimistic about the future (Fredrickson 2003).

Study after study has shown that chronic negative emotions, especially anger and depression, correlate with a broad range of disorders and diseases ranging from back pain and headaches to heart disease and cancer. For example, one remarkable long-term study typifies this correlation. The broader study was on aging and Alzheimer's disease. A population of Roman Catholic nuns was included in the study. During early stages of the study it was discovered that decades before, in the 1930s, almost two hundred of these nuns were asked to write a personal essay when they entered the novitiate at the age of twenty. Many wrote about their lives and the reason they chose to become a nun. Their essays were archived and eventually came to light during the 1990s as part of this larger study on aging and Alzheimer's disease. Researchers read the essays and scored them for positive emotional content, recording specific instances of happiness, interest, love, and hope. The findings were quite remarkable: "The nuns who expressed the most positive emotions lived up to 10 years longer than those who expressed the fewest. This gain in life expectancy is considerably larger than the gain achieved by those who quit smoking" (Fredrickson 2003, p. 330). Employing healthier staff translates into a number of advantages in the workplace, including lower levels of absenteeism, less illness and therefore lower medical benefit costs, and potentially longer tenure on the job because of overall wellness.

Improved Patient Care Environment

It may seem obvious that employees who are happier contribute to a more positive patient care environment. Patients quickly and easily pick up on the moods of the people who care for them. Certainly, the quality of interactions among employees in the various departments is also a critical factor in the patient care environment. The research on emotional intelligence clearly documents that emotions are highly contagious from person to person, especially from manager to employee (Cherniss and Goleman 2001; Goleman 1995; Goleman, Boyatzis, and McKee 2002).

Furthermore, some research suggests that happy people are more altruistic than their unhappy counterparts. Happy people are likely to be more giving, not just of money but of time and emotion as well. In laboratory studies, both adults and children who are happy display more empathy and are more willing to donate money to those in need. Although it might seem that people who have experienced adversity in their lives would identify with the suffering of others and behave more generously, this assumption is not necessarily true. When people are happy, they are less self-focused, like others more, and are more willing to share of themselves and their good fortune. It turns out that looking out for number one is more characteristic of sadness than of well-being (Seligman 2002).

The strong business case for happiness at work is clear. In spite of the corporate scandals in today's world and the apparent increasing negativity in the workplace, many organizations work hard to create an environment that is a challenging and enjoyable place to work. "Contrary to common perception, there are many successful executives who understand that 'good business' involves more than making money, and who take the responsibility for making their firms an engine for enhancing the quality of life" (Csikszentmihalyi 2003, p. 34).

Happiness Defined

Happiness in the workplace is important for a variety of reasons, but just what is happiness? The capacity for happiness refers to the ability to enjoy the good things in life if and when they come along. Being happy means experiencing pleasure, enthusiasm, and satisfaction (Seligman 2002). As pointed out earlier, happiness can refer to and encompass positive emotions about the past, the future, or the present. "The experience of happiness in action is enjoyment—the exhilarating sensation of being fully alive" (Csikszentmihalyi 2003, p. 37). Happiness is far more than temporary pleasure. Pleasure is only one component of the complex concept of happiness. As explained shortly, authentic happiness is a desirable goal that requires a full understanding of positive experiences that go well beyond mere pleasure.

Ed Diener is considered "Dr. Happy" by many as he has led and conducted extensive research on happiness for decades. He believes there is no easy way to define happiness and instead talks about subjective well-being. Happiness is not the entire answer to what leads a person to feel psychologically wealthy. Instead, he suggests that many aspects together lead to this feeling of psychological wealth, including positive relationships, spirituality and meaning, a positive attitude, money, involvement in engaging activities, and happiness and life satisfaction (Diener 2008).

Happiness Set Range

Can a person determine or influence the level of happiness experienced? To some degree, the answer is yes. However, extensive research on identical twins has led to the conclusion that every individual has a happiness set point, or more accurately, a set range. Lyubomirsky (2006, p. 54) says that "about 50% of the differences among people's happiness levels are explained by their immutable genetically-determined set points." In other words, similar to the genes for intelligence or cholesterol, the set point that a person inherits has a substantial influence on how happy he or she will be. The studies of identical twins separated at birth have been very revealing. They reveal that the psychological makeup of identical twins is much more similar than that of fraternal twins and that the psychology of adopted children is much more like the psychology of their birth parents than like the psychology of their adoptive parents (Lykken 1999). Simply stated, about half of a person's predisposition toward happiness is genetically influenced.

The happiness set point predisposed by genetics appears to function much like a thermostat. After a happy or negative event occurs, one returns to the previous level of happiness within a short period of time. For example, when a matched sample of twenty-two winners of large amounts of lottery money was studied, it was found that each individual reverted to his or her baseline level of happiness over time. The lottery winners ended up no happier than the twenty-two matched controls who were not winners (Seligman 2002). On the positive side, after a negative event occurs, the mood thermostat will pull the person up out of misery. Conversely, for those with a lower set point for happiness, even very positive events cannot improve their level of happiness over the long term.

> Even individuals who become paraplegic as a result of spinal cord accidents quickly begin to adapt to their greatly limited capacities, and within eight weeks they report more net positive emotion than negative emotion. Within a few years, they wind up only slightly less happy on average than individuals who are not paralyzed. Of people with extreme quadriplegia, 84 percent consider their life to be average or above average. (Seligman 2002, p. 48)

Although 50 percent of happiness is influenced by genetic makeup, individual levels of happiness can be changed by life events and the person's own attitudes. The psychological literature reveals that about 10 percent of the differences in a person's happiness levels can be explained by the person's circumstances—such as the person's level of wealth, health, marital status, and so on. However, 40 percent of happiness is determined by the person's own interpretation of life events. This finding indicates that opportunity exists to increase or decrease one's happiness levels (Kurtz and Lyubomirsky 2008; Lyubomirsky 2006).

Sources of Happiness

Before examining what brings happiness, a review of research findings is presented that may shatter some commonly held misconceptions about happiness. For example, it is widely believed in modern societies that money brings happiness, and yet the extensive data on how wealth and poverty affect happiness clearly indicate that beyond a basic safety net, having more money does not contribute much to subjective well-being.

> Work is undergoing a sea change in the wealthiest nations. Money, amazingly, is losing its power. The stark findings about life satisfaction—that beyond the safety net, more money adds little or nothing to subjective well-being—are starting to sink in. While real income in America has risen 16 percent in the last 30 years, the percentage of people who describe themselves as "very happy" has fallen from 36 to 29 percent. (Seligman 2002, p. 165)

Even among people who live in poverty, levels of satisfaction are high in many life domains (community life, work life, personal life, and so on). It seems that the importance of money to a person, more than the money itself, is what influences the level of happiness for that individual. "Materialism seems to be counterproductive: at all levels of real income, people who value money more than other goals are less satisfied with their income and with their lives as a whole, although precisely why is a mystery" (Seligman 2002, p. 54). In the most basic of terms, rich people are only slightly happier than poor people.

Diener (2008) explains this idea of the counterproductivity of materialism further. The toxicity of materialism is the root of the problem. It is true that everyone needs money to meet their material needs of food, shelter, and other things in life that lead to comfort and a sense of security or well-being. However, when money is dominant and the individual sacrifices other elements of psychological well-being for the pursuit or attainment of "more money," the situation can reduce happiness levels. Consider, for example, an individual who stays with a job because it provides a high level of financial compensation even though he or she does not believe the work to be meaningful and finds the activities it requires mundane and boring. This individual is sacrificing psychological well-being in exchange for a hefty paycheck. Consider as well the harried executive or manager who spends so much time at work that personal relationships suffer and the result is a loss of family and other personal or societal connections. These are examples of the toxicity of materialism. The desire for more money and things often leads to less happiness.

Diener (2008) notes that increased income brings with it a declining marginal utility. The more money an individual receives, the less the additional money matters. Thus, real income matters more at the lower end of the income scale than at the higher end. Increasing a housekeeper's pay scale by $2 per hour brings a stronger response than giving an executive making $400,000 a year an extra $10,000 bonus for workplace achievement.

Poor health, too, is only slightly related to levels of happiness. This finding is probably a tribute to the ability of humans to adapt to adversity. Most people rate their health positively even when they are quite sick. "Remarkably, even severely ill cancer patients differ only slightly on global life satisfaction from objectively healthy people" (Seligman 2002, p. 58). One exception is found with individuals dealing with a disabling disease that is severe and long lasting. It does produce a decline in life satisfaction and happiness for most people. Families that include a member who has Alzheimer's disease also were an exception, and their levels of happiness declined over time.

Although the results of positive psychology research may seem counterintuitive to many people, factors such as educational level, climate, race, and gender seem to have little or no effect on happiness. Similarly, physical attractiveness apparently does not have much effect on happiness (Diener 2000; Diener and Diener 1996; Diener, Sandvik, and Pavot 1991; Seligman 2002).

On the basis of extensive research findings, Seligman (2002) has identified three factors that lead individuals to decide whether they are happy or unhappy. The first is the degree to which the person experiences pleasure in life, the second is the degree that the person feels engaged and consumed by the activities in which he or she participates, and the third is the degree that the person's life is imbued with meaning. Ideally, each of these three elements is present in all areas of life: personal, family, and work. (These levels of happiness can be determined by completing the Approaches to Happiness instrument on Seligman's Web site at www.authentichappiness.com.)

The Pleasant Life

The first of these three aspects, the pleasant life, involves enjoying as much pleasure as possible. Pleasant experiences include short-term, intense sensory experiences such as tasting fresh, ripe raspberries; having a hot bath; or receiving a long massage. Because the memory and effects of such pleasures fade quickly, higher scores in this aspect of happiness do not necessarily lead to greater life satisfaction.

The effects of pleasurable experiences, however, can be intensified or prolonged by mindfully engaging in thoughts or behaviors that amplify or prolong the positive feelings, referred to as savoring. Bryant (2004) of Loyola University in Chicago has identified multiple ways of savoring a pleasant situation. Through his extensive research he reports four main forms. Two are related to the internal self and include feeling pride and luxuriating in the pleasure. In the first of these, the person derives pride and ego gratification from either oneself or others following a personal accomplishment, achievement, or award one has received. Luxuriating involves the process of splurging, indulging, or pampering oneself.

The two other forms of savoring focus on the external world and include thanksgiving, or gratitude, and marveling, or awe. Giving thanks involves the process of acknowledging and expressing gratitude for gifts, achievements, or the good things that come into one's life, and it occurs after an outcome. Marveling, on the other hand, is the involuntary process of being struck with awe by an outside stimulus and of losing oneself in the wonder of the moment while it is unfolding.

Too often, the moments of pleasure and happiness just slip by if the person does not consciously savor them. Being mindful and consciously enjoying the pleasures in life increase a person's perception of happiness.

The Engaged Life

Full engagement in activities and pursuits is more likely to lead to a perception of happiness. In fact, Seligman (2002, p. xiii) is very clear on this point: "Authentic happiness comes from identifying and cultivating your most fundamental strengths and using them every day in work, love, play, and parenting." By engagement, Seligman is referring to the idea of flow. *Flow* is defined as the unselfconscious state entered when a person is totally absorbed in the activity at hand. Time passes without notice because the person is totally engrossed in the task.

Mihaly Csikszentmihalyi (1990, 1997, 2003) was the first researcher to extensively study the concept of flow. Csikszentmihalyi and his colleagues use experience sampling methodology to measure the frequency of flow as well as the activities that lead to flow. In this approach, participants are given beepers that are programmed to beep randomly throughout the day. Each participant records his or her activity and describes what is happening each time the beeper sounds.

Based on thousands and thousands of data points, the analysis has revealed that the experience of flow depends on several key factors, specifically:

- The activity must require skill.
- The activity must require concentration.
- The activity must include clear goals.
- The activity must generate immediate feedback.
- The individual must experience deep, effortless involvement in the activity.
- The individual must experience a sense of control.
- The individual's sense of self must vanish during the activity.
- The individual's sense of time passing must stop during the activity.

Research shows that flow happens only when a person is engaged in a challenging activity that matches the person's skill level. Unfortunately, flow does not occur sitting in front of a television set and watching *The Simpsons* or reruns of *Friends*.

Flow is related to gratification rather than simple pleasure. In fact, in most flow experiences, people report experiencing little or no emotion. If any emotion is mentioned in connection with the experience, it is usually described in retrospect. Another key point to note is that being in flow is a way to build psychological capital for the future. In other words, it results in growth and further development of self.

In one study, Csikszentmihalyi tracked the experiences of 250 high-flow and 250 low-flow teenagers. The results were described in *Authentic Happiness*:

> The low-flow teenagers are "mall" kids; they hang out at malls and they watch television a lot. The high-flow kids have hobbies, they engage in sports, and they spend a lot of time on homework. On every measure of psychological well-being (including self-esteem and engagement) save one, the high-flow teenagers did better. The exception is important: the high-flow kids think their low-flow peers are having more fun, and say they would rather be at the mall doing all those "fun" things or watching television. But while all the engagement they have is not perceived as enjoyable, it pays off later in life. The high-flow kids are the ones who make it to college, who have deeper social ties, and whose later lives are more successful. (Seligman 2002, p. 117)

The results of this study support Csikszentmihalyi's contention that flow is a state that builds psychological capital that can be drawn upon in the future when it is needed.

Dick Richards (1995a, 1995b) explored the concept of artistry and experiencing joy through work. Finding meaning in one's work is directly related to a person's experience of joy, according to Richards. His examples are closely related to the concept of flow as presented by Csikszentmihalyi:

> You know the experience. . . . Sometimes it happens at work. Your report is due tomorrow. You have thought about it, made many notes, and written a first draft. You have only the afternoon to write the final document. Sitting before your word processor, looking at the blinking cursor, it comes to you. Words and ideas flow. The next idea is there when you are ready for it. The perfect word presents itself when you need it. You get stuck, stand, walk down the corridor for a break and another cup of coffee, and the idea you need is there, as if it were waiting in the corridor for you to fetch it. You skip your break; you forget the coffee. At the end of the day the report seems perfect, and you marvel at what has happened. (Richards 1995b, para. 5–7)

Richards is describing the experience of joy, "the kind of joy that ascends during a period of activity that engages the entire self" (Richards 1995b, para. 10). He believes that seeking such experiences is part of the artistry of work and that such experiences occur when a person's whole self is absorbed in the activity. It occurs when "we are THERE: body, mind, emotion, spirit" (Richards 1995b, para. 12).

As a result of beginning his career as a graphic artist, Richards brings a different perspective to the concept of work. He points out that artists live for the experience of joy in their work. Unfortunately, this experience is very different from how most people approach their work. When there is emotional distance from the work rather than full engagement in it, the net result is a lack of joy. And "the net result for organizations is a dangerous lack of the very inventiveness, flexibility, and courage [workers] so sorely need" (Richards 1995b, para. 19).

The Meaningful Life

The third aspect of happiness is the belief that a person's life is meaningful. In the context of happiness, the individual's life is meaningful when he or she is using his or her signature strengths with positive focus in the service of something outside or beyond the self, or a larger cause. Most people understand the importance of a clear sense of purpose, both in individual and organizational life.

In *From Good to Great* (2001), Jim Collins found that values-driven organizations with a clear purpose perform better in the long run than those without a clear purpose. At the personal level, clarity about purpose has been an abiding theme in the self-improvement literature for decades (Covey 1989, 1992; Covey, Merrill, and Merrill 1994; Loehr and Schwartz 2003; Thomas 2000). "The search for meaning and purpose is among the most powerful and enduring themes in every culture since the origin of recorded history" (Loehr and Schwartz 2003, p. 131). Purpose is a powerful, enduring source of energy.

In summary, happiness is a concept of splendid richness. Pleasure is one aspect but not the only factor that brings happiness. Happiness is clearly related to pleasure, engagement, and meaningfulness. And happiness is a major component of a person's subjective sense of psychological well-being.

Case Study: Joy at Work*

The field of positive psychology is increasing the understanding of the positive emotions and suggests concrete, specific interventions that can help raise the amount of happiness in personal lives. But the research also suggests several approaches to applying positive psychology to the workplace.

The rest of the chapter pulls all of the research findings together with applications for health care organizations. But first, the implications of applying positive psychology in the workplace are examined by reviewing a research project that studied health care workers who experience joy through their work. This study by Manion (2002a), one of the initial to specifically focus on positive emotions in the workplace, was conducted in 2000–2001 to answer the question, How do health care workers experience and express joy in their work?

The decade of the 1990s was tumultuous for the health care sector as many organizations experienced significant financial challenges, declining employee commitment, and escalating demands from patients and their families. Every day seemed to bring a new crisis. Seeking ways to create a positive workplace, especially during tumultuous and challenging times, this study included twenty-four employed health care workers who experienced

---

*This section is adapted from Jo Manion, Joy at Work: Creating a Positive Workplace, *Journal of Nursing Administration* 33(12): 652–59. Copyright © 2003 and used by permission of Lippincott Williams & Wilkins.

joy in their work. Findings from these interviews provided insight into why some people are joyful even during difficult times and how joy can be brought into the workplace.

Process

The study used a narrative approach and included face-to-face interviews conducted to solicit accounts of joyful work experiences. The sample was made up of individual health care providers who either volunteered to participate or were recommended by their co-workers. All of the participants were credentialed and/or licensed health care providers. They came from a variety of health care facilities, and only individuals who had worked in at least three different employment settings were included in the sample.

Twelve women and twelve men in two different age groups (Baby Boomers and Generation Xers, or GenXers) participated. Coincidentally, half of the participants were first-line caregivers and half were managers (supervisors and executives, including a hospital chief executive officer).

Participants came from California (one), the Midwest (eleven), the Northeast (three), and Florida (nine). Eighteen worked in hospitals at the time of the interviews; others were employed by a staffing agency, an association, a leadership institute, a hospice, a home health care agency, a community clinic, and a state licensure board.

Questions related to the experience of joy were posed to all participants. (The interview format is reproduced in figure 4-1.) The interviews were audiotaped and transcribed later. The data were reviewed using a category content analysis approach, which entails identifying categories and themes

Figure 4-1.   Interview Format

1. Would you tell me a little about what you do and where you work?
2. Now, let's talk about joy. What does joy mean to you?
3. When you are joyful, what does it look like to other people?
4. How often would you say that you experience joy through your work?
5. Can you tell me about a time that you felt joy through your work?
   a. Was there anything specifically happening when you felt this joy or that led to the joy?
   b. Is there anything you did that led to feeling this joy?
6. How did you express this joy?
   a. Do you remember how others around you responded to your expression of this joy?
   b. How did you respond to them?
7. Do you think that you do anything, either deliberately or subconsciously, that leads to an environment of joy in your workplace?
8. Is there anything your organization does that helps you find joy in your work?
   a. Are there times when it is hard to find joy in your work?
   b. Can you tell me what is going on during these times?
   c. Have you ever worked anywhere where it was hard to be joyful?
9. How important is it to you that you find joy in your work?

as they become apparent through review of the data. The themes and categories were derived inductively from the actual words and phrases of the participants. The assignment of themes and categories was validated by two additional reviewers, who compared the analyses of specific interviews.

Findings

Analyzing the stories and examples to determine common themes was the first level of interpretation. A second, deeper level of analysis revealed that each individual had his or her own unique theme related to the experience of joy. These themes are identified and presented in a later section titled "Pathways to Finding Joy at Work."

Nature of Joy

Participants were not given a specific description of joy. Instead, they were asked to define the term in their own words. Those interviewed described joy from their own perspective and in a variety of ways. Some talked about the experiential component of joy (for example, "having a light and happy heart" and "you're excited about getting up every morning and can't wait to get to work"). Others mentioned the physiological aspects of joy (for example, "you feel warm and fuzzy and glad," "it's kind of a spurt," and "inside I get a warmth, a feeling of excitement"). Others described joy in terms of what brings it about for them ("it's a sense of accomplishment," "when someone says thank you," and "knowing you make a difference").

For most of the participants, joy was expressed outwardly (through specific behaviors such as laughing, smiling, humming, singing, or having "sparkly eyes") and was noticed by other people. The almost universal response of others was positive. Over half of the participants described joy as contagious, noting that their joy led to joy in others. Not all descriptions of joy were of an exuberant nature. Many examples of joy were provided that illustrated a restrained, quiet, or contented feeling.

On the basis of the participants' descriptions as well as on an extensive review of the literature, the study concluded that joy can be defined as an intensely positive, vivid, and expansive emotion that arises from an internal state or results from an external event or situation. It may include physiological reactions and emotional expressions as well as conscious volition. It is a transcendent state of heightened energy and excitement.

Each story of joy described by the participants was analyzed and coded for factors that were related to the experience of joy. Table 4-1 summarizes these findings. Factors related to joy at work were numerous and were experienced differently by each individual. Four general themes were identified: the work itself, people and relationships, the self, and the work environment. Participants mentioned factors related to the work itself most frequently. These work-related factors were categorized into items characteristic of the work or an outcome of the work. The single most frequently identified factor was connection with others, found in the general theme of people and relationships.

Table 4-1.   Factors Associated with Joy

Factors	Number of Times Mentioned	Number of People Who Identified Item at Least Once (N = 24)
The work itself	Total 413	Total 24
Outcome of work	116	24
Represented progress	32	14
Accomplishment	21	13
Achievement	89	21
Characteristics of work	74	21
Appeal of work	37	14
Made a difference	31	16
Helped someone else	13	8
Autonomy		
Was an opportunity		
People and relationships	Total 341	Total 24
Connection with others	178	24
Recognition	89	19
Appreciation	74	21
The self	Total 253	Total 24
Competence	129	24
Self-esteem	89	15
Attitudes, values, and beliefs	45	20
The work environment	Total 99	Total 24
Social aspects	52	18
The organizational culture	47	16

Of all of the various factors, only three were found in every person's stories: (1) The work represented progress, (2) it involved connections with other people, and (3) the work reflected competence on the part of the individual. These factors link directly to three of the five intrinsic motivators identified in chapter 2.

Barriers to Experiencing Joy

People were asked about barriers to their experience of joy in their work. The factors most often identified were co-workers (for example, co-workers who displayed negative, unsupportive, unpleasant, or uncooperative behavior), poor leadership, insufficient resources (such as inadequate staffing or lack of necessary equipment), and unappealing (repetitive, boring, or meaningless) work.

Organization's Role in Creating Joy

When asked whether the organizations for which they worked did anything that increased their experience of joy, most of the participants indicated that they believed that the organizations did not have an active role in influencing their experience of joy. In other words, the presence of joy is an individual issue. Nonetheless, in the participants' examples, factors were identified that described the organization's role:

- Creation of a positive work environment
- Recruitment and retention of good people (both employees and leaders)
- Provision of adequate benefits and compensation
- Dedication to mission
- Provision of adequate resources

Pathways to Finding Joy at Work

The next step in analysis moved from breaking down participants' stories into factors to examining each interview in its entirety. Analyzing the stories on a macro level revealed four distinct individual pathways to joy: connections, love of the work, achievement, and recognition. Each pathway reflects a major theme of the participants' stories and their primary source of joy through their work.

Connections

The connections pathway to joy is based on the bonds made and relationships formed with people in the workplace. Caring for, talking with, relating to, and helping others are frequent aspects identified in this pathway. The primary source of joy is other people and relationships. Eight of the participants exemplified this pathway to joy.

Carl demonstrated this pathway when he said, "I definitely like people and caring for them and working with them." Karen initially described joy as "a feeling of well-being . . . surrounded by people you love or care about." Sally (a physical therapist) and Marie (a director of nursing) both said that one-on-one contact with others and the opportunity for socialization at work were important to them. Dick (a director of nursing) and Jake (a young emergency department nurse) both said that what brought them joy was "working with their peers."

Carl, a young director of nursing, offered several illuminating examples as he talked about his work with patients who had undergone major cardiovascular surgery. In his words:

> I did the heart transplants for quite a while and the by-passes where you work with them for eight hours, trying to recover them, and by the time you got back the next day, they're already shipped out. That's when I started going, "Well, hey, I'm not interacting with them anymore." You dealt with them while you recovered the patient. You got them well through their heart recovery phase, and by the time you got back there on the next shift, they

were already gone. For me, I lost my connection. That didn't give me joy anymore, if that makes any sense. You start becoming more of a, like a front line factory worker, is what you're doing. You're not interacting with anybody.

Most of Carl's conversation about his work in the cardiac recovery unit revolved around the people with whom he worked. He described several of his colleagues in great detail and talked about what a great group they were. He recalled his dismay when the group started to break up and noted that "they're all gone, except for one nurse." He said all of a sudden he realized, "Oh, shoot! I'm the lead guy now! Now I'm in charge! But, hey, I didn't have any really true connections anymore."

Karen, a young nurse, worked "temporary" at another hospital in its float pool. She tried this work on two separate occasions because the money was so appealing, but she simply could not stay with it. Karen indicated that she did not stay with this job because she had "no relationship with the people . . . [she was] working with." Most of the stories of joy Karen shared throughout her interview were clearly related to a sense of connection with other people. She summed up the joy she felt through her work as an emergency department charge nurse by saying, "A lot of it is working with other people. The relationships we form and the fun you get to have with other people, and you really get to know people on a very intimate level when you're working with life-and-death situations."

Love of the Work

A second pathway to joy is through the love of the work itself. Although many other factors were associated positively with their experience of joy, eight of the participants felt a strong connection and identification with the work itself. When they talked about the work they did, they reported that most aspects of it excited them.

These participants often expressed a deep sense of personal mission. Lana, who works on a regulatory board, expressed it well: "I feel fortunate that I get to do what I feel a passion for." In several places in Jane's interview she remarked, "I get such joy out of just being a nurse, I love the essence of nursing, this is why I went into nursing, and finally, I realized I really loved being a nurse." All of Jane's comments projected her love and enthusiasm for the work of nursing. Bob, a respiratory therapist (RT), spent the first fifteen minutes of his interview describing his work as an RT in minute detail.

Those who found their pathway to joy through the love of their work often talked about being excited when they woke up just because they were going to work. Alan, a young manager of outpatient surgery, described joy as occurring when you "enjoy what you're doing. Means I can't wait to get to work and I'm excited about getting up every morning and going to work." Pam, a postanesthesia care unit (PACU) nurse, echoed this feeling: "I wake up in the morning, and I'm happy to get up at five o'clock in the morning, even though I'm tired. And I'm happy to go to work. I'm happy to do my day and I'm happy that I've been given this responsibility."

Participants whose experience fell along this pathway shared rich detail about their jobs and expressed enthusiasm about the actual work. Their accounts were vivid in comparison with the accounts of people such as Jake, the emergency department nurse, who openly declared that nothing about the work itself brought him joy. What brought him joy was working with his peers. Pam, the PACU nurse, on the other hand, was a good example of enthusiasm and love for her work:

> It's funny, because I think everything's joyful. I love watching the cardiac monitors. I like doing the phone calls. I love starting the IVs. I like talking to the patients. I like getting them ready. I like receiving them from surgery. I like giving them their warm blankets, putting them around them, 'cause I can just see them melt, you know? And I like to make them comfortable. Everything, I must say, it really gives me joy to do all parts of my job. I [even] love . . . the paperwork.

Achievement

The third pathway to joy is through achievement. For five participants the emphasis in their stories related to accomplishment or to the attainment of a particular goal. Ellen, a director of education, defined joy as "a job well-done. That I feel good about the work I've completed, that I'm happy to know that I did a nice job for myself or someone else, or completed a project relevant to my work and that made a difference."

John, a lab supervisor, said that joy for him came when he realized that "the results of something that you've done, that has truly made someone else happy, then it makes you happy."

Don, a senior-level manager, defined joy as meeting management challenges ("that's what makes life worthwhile to me"). He provided numerous examples of the improvements and changes he had made over his tenure. His sense of pride and accomplishment was evident.

The stories of these five participants were full of accounts of achievements, accomplishments, and positive work outcomes. Melinda, a nurse manager, described each of her promotions, and Ellen, the director of education, described successful projects that contributed significantly to her organization.

Interestingly, all of the achievement pathway participants worked in management or supervisory positions. Perhaps people who experience joy through achievement are more likely to find their way into management and executive positions, where they have more autonomy, authority, and the specific responsibility for making change happen in their organizations.

It is important to note that for these five people, the world's opinion seemed less important than their internal assessment of their outcomes. Pleasure and pride in the process were not as important as the actual outcome. External trappings of success such as wealth, position, adulation, and awards probably would have made little or no difference to them if they had not achieved positive and meaningful outcomes.

This point was clearly evident during Joyce's interview. Joyce was a chief executive officer (CEO) of a major health care organization. She began her interview by explaining that she did not feel much joy in her current position. A highly competent and successful woman, she had been promoted to chief executive officer four years earlier. She was considered influential, principle focused, and people oriented and was highly respected by all who knew her. An extremely committed and hard-working professional, she looked back over the past four years of her career and could not see any significant forward progress in her organization as the result of her efforts. She admitted that "spinning her wheels" and the lack of forward progress just "drove her crazy." All of her stories reflected a need for completion and applicability of the results in a useful way. Although the outside world would judge her to be an extremely successful person, inside she felt joyless.

Recognition

Recognition is the fourth pathway to joy, and three of the participants illustrated this beautifully. Recognition has to do with the acknowledgment of others, and in many instances it occurs as a result of expressions of appreciation.

There can be little doubt that warm, genuine expressions of gratitude or recognition of a person's efforts bring joy to most people. And, in fact, twenty-three of the twenty-four participants identified these two factors at least once. For example, Betty, a staff nurse at an ambulatory care center, said that compliments from co-workers let her know that they appreciated or valued something about her or what she did. The first story of joy that came to her mind was one about how she had influenced a "grumpy" patient's attitude. In the end, she was recognized for her intervention with a public award.

Although recognition brings most people joy, for these three people it is a primary source of joy. In Dan's interview, the number of times he talked about appreciation expressed by others was striking. He said, "The most obvious reflections of joy occur when physicians or other staff members are complimentary or they recognize a job well done." When asked to share a specific example of a time he felt joy through his work, he shared a beautiful story that drove this point home. He was called into his twelve-hour night shift early, at 3 PM, to care for a patient who was hemorrhaging severely after an aortic valve replacement. Dan, a transplant critical care nurse, shared in vivid detail the intense work of trying to stabilize this patient throughout a sixteen-hour shift. Around 3 AM, the patient's condition improved, and it appeared that he would survive at least for the near term. Dan went on to say:

> But an incredible thing happened like, at six o'clock in the morning. Three of this man's daughters (pause) three of his daughters and his wife, had somehow, at six o'clock in the morning, they found a thank-you card somewhere, and they got this thank-you card and they said, "Thank you for an extremely good job and we realize just how close, you know, everything was."

It was obvious that receiving a simple thank-you card from his patient's family had the power to move Dan (a tough Vietnam veteran) to tears and a sense of joy. Almost every example of joy that Dan shared was somehow related to expressed recognition or appreciation.

The common theme of this pathway involves being recognized by others in the workplace. Recognition includes receiving compliments, expressions of appreciation, or awards; being given more responsibility; being asked to take on a special project; or being accorded the respect of others in the workplace.

Model of Joy in the Workplace

A model of joy at work was developed on the basis of the interview data, as well as a review of the literature. (See figure 4-2.) Factors in the three thematic areas—the work itself, people and relationships, and the work environment—all provide the stimulus for joy to occur when the necessary internal factors (represented in the theme the self) exist within the individual. The internal factors include self-esteem; attitudes, beliefs, and values; and competence. The person places a value on the particular situation or makes a judgment that the situation is positive and concludes (either consciously or subconsciously) that he or she feels joy. The joy may or may not be expressed externally. When expressed externally (by smiling, laughing, singing, or having "sparkly eyes"), others in the immediate environment react positively with a similar or reciprocal experience. Their expression of joy further reinforces the individual's perception of his or her own joy.

Implications for Managers

The model of joy has several important implications for managers who are seeking to create a more positive work environment. A person's attitude is both necessary and sufficient for joy to be experienced. Numerous examples described health care providers who clearly found joy despite a negative or

Figure 4-2. A Model of Joy

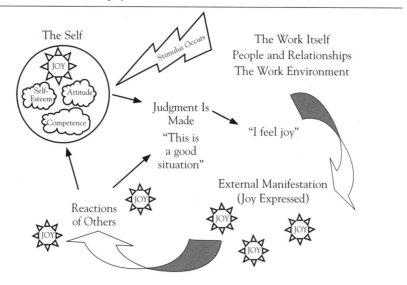

an unpleasant situation. This finding suggests that a predisposition toward joy is sufficient for joy to occur. For example, Karen, the young emergency department charge nurse, described several tragic and painful situations in her department during which she felt joyful because she knew she and her colleagues had made a difference for a patient or a family. She chose to feel joyful when others in the same situation might have been negatively affected.

Furthermore, joy often transcends a particular situation; people who experience joy often retain a positive attitude despite current circumstances. A predisposition toward joy is a positive trait that can be sought in job applicants. Positive emotions are important for anyone aspiring to be a leader. Probing behavioral interview questions that focus on what brings the candidate joy at work could shed light on whether the applicant is likely to experience joy in a specific work setting.

Figure 4-3 illustrates the dynamics evident in an interaction between internal factors that affect individuals and external factors in the work environment. The factors that lead to or impede the experience of joy are diagrammed as a force field. Factors such as attitude (identified by eighteen participants), competency (identified by all twenty-four participants), and accessibility to a favorable primary pathway are more heavily weighted (as represented by the larger arrows). The absence of such necessary factors can actually preclude the experience of joy.

Individual factors (as represented by small arrows) such as progress achieved, appealing work, or the appreciation of others may also lead to joy. These individual factors, however, are not as likely to create the same intensity or sustainability of joyful feeling.

In the same way, inhibiting forces can be significant. For example, incompetence or a negative attitude can lead an individual to feel little or

Figure 4-3.   Factors Supporting or Inhibiting the Experience of Joy at Work

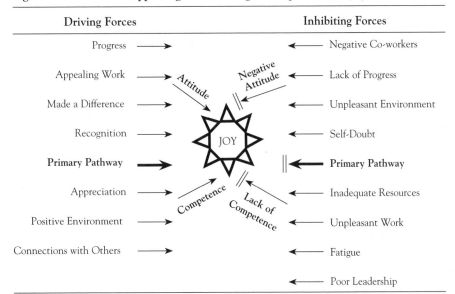

Driving Forces	Inhibiting Forces
Progress ⟶	⟵ Negative Co-workers
Appealing Work ⟶	⟵ Lack of Progress
Made a Difference ⟶	⟵ Unpleasant Environment
Recognition ⟶	⟵ Self-Doubt
Primary Pathway ⟶	⟵ **Primary Pathway**
Appreciation ⟶	⟵ Inadequate Resources
Positive Environment ⟶	⟵ Unpleasant Work
Connections with Others ⟶	⟵ Fatigue
	⟵ Poor Leadership

JOY — Attitude — Negative Attitude — Competence — Lack of Competence no joy. Lack of accessibility to a pathway may result in a lack of joy as suggested in many of the stories. However, the presence of one or two negative factors does not necessarily rob a person of joy. For example, the person who is predominantly joyful, who has a positive attitude, and who has a job and workplace that support his or her primary pathway, is less likely to feel joyless to a significant level in the presence of one or several impeding factors. No workplace is perfect; likely it is the cumulative effect of impeding factors that drives joy out of the workplace.

The reciprocal relationship between some of these factors is more difficult to map, and yet it is relatively easy to understand. For instance, the factor of competence is related to various triggers of joy. For example, if a person is very competent at what he does, he is more likely to receive recognition for it, know that he made a difference, or see desirable progress as a result of his efforts. These factors, in turn, positively reinforce his sense of competence. Conversely, if a person believes she is unable to function in a competent manner because of a lack of training or inadequate resources, she will have trouble experiencing joy. As seen in chapter 2, competence is intrinsically rewarding to people. Understanding this concept can explain employee reactions to changes in policies and practices when the changes have an impact on a person's competence or perception of competence. It can also explain why working in a situation where persistent staff shortages truly impede a person's ability to do a good job feels so negative to people.

From the stories shared by participants in this study, the primary pathway through which an individual experiences joy must be accessed for the person to experience a significant and sustained level of joy. Many participants described work situations in which they had found it difficult to find joy as a result of their inability to access their own individual pathway to joy. For example, Carl, the director of nursing, "lost his connections" and left the job. Dan, the transplant critical care nurse, was miserable in one position because he was treated with suspicion and dislike rather than appreciation and recognition. Joyce, the CEO, was joyless because she was unable to establish forward progress in her organization. People may experience brief periods of joy in their day-to-day work from individual efforts (such as a sincere thank you, completion of a challenging task, or the knowledge that they have helped someone else), but these experiences will not be enough to sustain them in the long run.

Implications for Organizational Leaders

Participants in this study experienced joy through their work despite turmoil and challenges in the work environment. Experiencing joy in their work was important enough that they would seek another position if they were unable to find joy in their present jobs. This finding suggests a direct link to an individual's intent to stay in a job (organizational commitment), which has implications for retention strategies.

The model of joy (figure 4-2) and joy's driving and restraining forces suggest ways leaders can create a more positive work environment. Joy is contagious and transcendent. Study participants provided numerous examples of how joy rubs off on others and creates a reciprocal and reinforcing relationship with those in close proximity. Thus, one person's joy is often shared with others, leading to that second person's experience of joy and, in turn, increasing the original person's feeling of joy.

This finding has major implications for leaders attempting to create a positive environment in the workplace. Evidence from the literature indicates that the moods or emotions of individuals in a particular work team or group are linked to the moods or emotions of others in the same group (Barsade and Gibson 1998; Bartel and Saavedra 2000). Totterdell and colleagues have conducted numerous studies that demonstrate that the moods of individual are often affected by the moods of the people around them (Totterdell 2000; Totterdell et al. 1998).

Organizations can use a knowledge of factors that increase the experience of joy as well as a knowledge of the pathways to joy as underlying concepts for making internal decisions. This knowledge can also be very useful in addressing workforce shortages. For instance, if a person is unable to attain his or her primary pathway to joy, the judgment that "this is a good situation" is not made and joy is not experienced on a significant level. Understanding this concept will help leaders appreciate the full impact of organizational change. For example, skill mix or staffing changes that disrupt relationships may more adversely affect people for whom a connections pathway is important. Changes in work flow that significantly reduce the amount of time spent with individual patients or with co-workers in casual camaraderie can have a negative effect of the development of interpersonal relationships.

For example, one organization implemented a new policy that dictated that employees could no longer use the intranet to transmit information of a personal nature, such as information about baby showers or where friends were meeting over the weekend or who was bringing what to a potluck dinner. The policy change had a much greater impact than anticipated because it directly affected those employees for whom connections were an important pathway to joy at work.

In the same way, during restructuring or work redesign efforts, changes that alter the nature of the work can affect those who love the work they are doing. Many managers today are finding that they have less and less time to be involved in coaching and developing employees. If this is an aspect of their work that they loved, its absence can be dissatisfying. People in the achievement pathway are more likely to be frustrated by meetings that go nowhere, problems that are never solved, an inability to effect substantial change, and meaningless process refinements that have little impact on end results. Those who find joy in recognition want that recognition to be sincere, personal, and frequent. Recognition includes acknowledgment and being treated as a valued contributor. For such employees, the annual employee recognition dinner is probably not enough.

Knowledge of all of the four pathways is helpful for the leader to consider when changes are made. When the potential negative impact on people is appreciated, actions can be taken to recognize and mitigate the potentially damaging effects of the change before the change is made.

Leaders are also instrumental in modeling joyfulness. The participants reported that they purposely monitored their own attitudes and looked for elements in the workplace that created a sense of joy. In the words of the regulatory board member, Lana, "I find things to get joy from." Casey, an emergency department charge nurse, said that she encouraged employees to see the positive side of situations. When complaints were heard about the length of time a patient was held in the department, Casey insisted that they were now that many hours closer to getting the patient transferred.

Strategies for Increasing Happiness and Joy at Work

Joy is a powerful emotion, and when it occurs as a result of the person's work, life is much more satisfying and pleasant. Most people spend more of their awake and alert time at work than they do with their loved ones. To experience the potentially positive impact of joy in one's work requires a tremendous amount of engagement and commitment, but that effort promises to bring fulfillment. In fact, the emotions people feel while they work are likely to reflect most directly the true quality of work life (Goleman, Boyatzis, and McKee 2002).

Each individual is responsible for choosing joy, and the case study above sheds some light on what can be done to find it. The participants in the joy at work study clearly believed that other people can do little to influence the experience of joy and that choosing to look for and feel joy is an individual rather than an organizational issue. Csikszentmihalyi (2003, p. 37) agrees: "Contrary to what most of us believe, happiness does not simply happen to us. It's something we make happen, and it results from our doing our best." Obviously, no one can make another happy if he or she is unwilling to be so; however, strategies can be used by leaders and other individuals to not only increase personal levels of happiness but also influence the level of happiness experienced by colleagues and co-workers.

Several of these proven techniques are explained in the rest of this chapter. Identifying and using a person's strengths is the first strategy. Other techniques are organized by time orientation, that is, by whether they affect positive emotions of the past, present, or future. (Figure 4-4 below summarizes the approaches based on time orientation.)

Figure 4-4.   Approaches to Increasing Happiness Based on Time Orientation

Past	Present	Future
Appreciation	Pleasure	Mentoring relationships
Gratitude	Engagement	Personal legacies
Forgiveness	Meaning	Optimism

Signature Strengths

As mentioned earlier in this chapter, each person has special strengths, and using them in every aspect of life leads to greater happiness and psychological well-being. When one's work calls upon the person's major strengths, positivity in the workplace increases. A person's sense of value and contribution is higher. However, many people are unhappy at work. They may feel underappreciated and overworked. If their work does not call upon their key strengths, they can experience feelings of boredom and apathy. "In worldwide studies of more than 10 million employees, Gallup has found that only about a third can strongly agree with the following statement: 'At work, I have the opportunity to do what I do best every day'" (Rath 2007, p. ii). The beneficial relationship of this question to employee retention, increased productivity, and improved customer service has been clearly demonstrated. Improving the alignment between a person's strengths and the job he or she holds is of crucial importance for organizational effectiveness.

Because using signature strengths leads to so many important organizational outcomes, here are several strategies:

1. **Identify the employee's key strengths.** Multiple approaches may be taken to accomplish this step. Completing the Values in Action character strength instrument on the Authentic Happiness Web site (www.authentichappiness.com) or the StrengthsFinder talent themes test in Buckingham and Clifton's book *Now, Discover Your Strengths* (2001) are two possibilities.

2. **Use the person's strengths in the work setting.** "One thing that seems to differentiate *good* from *great* managers is their ability to recognize the *unique attributes* of each individual and find ways to . . . capitalize on them to ensure individual success" (Vestal 2007, p. 7). This ability represents a huge untapped resource in many organizations.

3. **Coach employees to recognize and use their strengths.** Britton (2007) found that once strengths or talent themes are identified, awareness of them in everyday work and life increases. Finding ways to use and develop strengths is the next step. When a person uses a strength, he or she feels invigorated, whereas when using a weakness, he or she feels drained. The greater clarity and specificity about one's strengths, the more likely work can be geared to these strengths. For example, an educator may love presenting to receptive audiences on topics that are important to her, but she may not like to argue and debate. Having this person facilitate contentious department meetings will be more difficult for her. One way to recognize strengths is to pay attention to what seems to come easily and what tasks in work are more difficult.

4. **Encourage the work group to understand and use each other's strengths.** Clarity about strengths can help the work group tap into and appreciate differences. In some cases, others may perform poorly

not from a lack of responsibility but from a lack of talent or strength. Colleagues in the work group can also help co-workers recognize the important aspects of their various strengths and the way these contribute to overall success of the group.

Results of the strength finder–type instruments can be shared, or employees can simply be asked to think about their strengths and then share the information. Differences in strengths can be used to make decisions on work allocation. Conversation about how to best use each person's strengths can lead to insights that in turn lead to a more effective work group.

Taking the time to identify and capitalize on an individual's strengths is a crucial way in which leaders influence others. The case study at the end of this chapter exemplifies the results that can occur when the focus is on the employee's strengths. Schwartz (2007) says that if organizations want to access the energy of the human spirit, employees must be doing what they do best and enjoy most in the workplace. He goes on to point out that these two are not necessarily mutually inclusive. A person can get lots of positive feedback about something he or she does well but may not enjoy much. Conversely, he or she can love doing something but have no gift for it. As a result, achieving success can require much more energy than is reasonable to invest.

Influencing Positive Emotions Related to the Past

The positive emotions related to the past include satisfaction, contentment, serenity, pride, and fulfillment. Positive emotion about past events can be lost or diminished when the good things that have happened are underappreciated or the negative things are overemphasized through grudges, bitterness, and feelings of injustice. When the value of appreciation and forgiveness is understood, it becomes a relatively simple matter to find ways to begin to mitigate the negative effects of disturbing past experiences.

Appreciation and Gratitude

Some people have the signature strength of gratitude, and they are very aware of the good things that happen to them and rarely take them for granted. Another hallmark of this strength is taking time to express appreciation. Research has found that expressing gratitude and appreciation increases a person's level of happiness. How can this concept be used in the workplace?

Individual employees can apply this principle in a variety of ways. Letting colleagues, physicians, and leaders know when they have done something that is appreciated is important. Few people hear "thank you" too many times, and a sincere thank you can be said in a variety of ways. Often managers and physicians hear fewer expressions of appreciation than other clinical and support staff. Never underestimate the power of simple appreciation. An occasional thank you can really boost the spirits of both the recipient and the giver.

Similarly, the absence of a well-deserved, sincere thank you can also have a significant effect. Consider, for example, this story related by a family practice physician. (This event occurred in the 1950s.) A young family was involved in a serious car-train accident. The husband was taken by ambulance to one hospital, and the wife was brought to the small rural hospital's emergency department where the physician worked. The young woman's condition deteriorated quickly, and it was determined that she was in shock owing to internal bleeding. At that time, the hospital had a walking blood bank that had been organized by the director of the laboratory. During the time this woman was cared for in the small hospital, she received a total of twenty-seven units of blood over a period of thirty-six hours (representing an almost superhuman effort in those days). Neither physician nor hospital staff left her side. Eventually, she was stable enough to be transferred to a large medical center for treatment. She survived and went on to live a full life. More than fifty years later, this physician still remembers that neither he nor any of the hospital staff ever heard a thank you from the patient or the family for their extraordinary efforts.

A great deal of emphasis has been placed of late on managers writing notes to employees to send thanks. Little is said about reciprocity. One participant in a program was complaining about never hearing "thank you" from his boss. He was asked, "When was the last time you thanked her sincerely for something she did?" He got the point.

Many effective management and leadership techniques are based on the principle of appreciation. Most leaders are probably already using one or more of these techniques without realizing it. Appreciative inquiry is an approach to dealing with problems that begins with recognizing and appreciating what is already going right. Another approach based in gratitude is the use of a forward-focused approach in meetings when the discussion is spiraling downward. It brings the group back to focus on what is going right and what it is doing well. The act of simply guiding conversations in the direction of recognition and appreciation of what is good and right is also a way of using gratitude.

Gratitude works because it amplifies the good memories of the past. In some cases, gratitude flows when one simply pays attention. Too often, however, attention is focused on immediate problems: the heavy traffic on the way to work, concern about the Internet sites one's teenage daughter may be looking at, or the heavy workload because John just called in sick. Concentrating on immediate problems and difficulties makes it easy to develop a tendency to forget about all of the things that are going well. For instance, you might forget that you got an early start this morning because the weather was clear and the traffic moved quickly, you might forget that your daughter's grades have improved since she started using the Internet to help with her homework, or you might forget that John's crew works exceptionally well together and will be able to handle the extra work.

A variety of appreciation activities and exercises can be used within a work group. Several have been the object of study to determine their impact on happiness levels. These include the balancing exercise, the gratitude let-ter, and the Three Good Things activity.

The Balancing Exercise
One simple exercise that is based on the value of expressing appreciation is the balancing exercise. It can be used by individuals or groups that are faced with changes in the workplace. The balancing exercise is simple: First, the individual or the leader of the group draws two columns on a flip chart page, white board, or piece of paper. Then the individual or group develops a list of the positive things about the change (what they will gain) in one column and the negative things (what they will lose) in the other. If this exercise is done as an individual exercise and the person finds it difficult to look at the change objectively, it can be done with a trusted friend or colleague. This more objec-tive person sits down and shares his or her perspective and thoughts regarding the change. Chances are, the objective person will think of things not previ-ously considered by the individual facing the change. This exercise is power-ful because it provides a clear reminder that no situation is wholly negative. There are many things to be grateful for, but they tend to be overlooked when one is faced with a difficult change, loss, or challenge.

Simply noticing those things that inspire gratitude is an activity that raises the level of appreciation. Furthermore, two specific exercises from the field of positive psychology—gratitude letters and the Three Good Things exercise, described below—increase the level of happiness in the people who do them.

The Gratitude Letter and Visit
Although the gratitude letter and visit are most often used in the context of the participants' personal lives, they can be modified and used in the work-place. The general idea is to select someone who has been especially kind or helpful in some way but whom the person has never adequately thanked. The person writes a gratitude letter to the individual describing in concrete terms why he or she is grateful. Citing specifics and the effect the helpful person had increases the impact of the letter. The letter is then personally delivered and read aloud to the recipient. In some work groups, this exercise could be effective in a group setting when the members of the group are able to discuss their reactions to the letters after they have been read.

In a study undertaken to determine whether people can become last-ingly happier with simple interventions, participants were sought through the Internet. Visitors to the Authentic Happiness Web site were solicited and 411 participated in the complete study (Seligman et al. 2005). The gratitude visit was one intervention tested. "Participants were given one week to write and then deliver a letter of gratitude to someone who had been especially kind to them but had never been properly thanked. . . . The gratitude visit caused large positive changes for one month" (Seligman et al. 2005, p. 416).

This exercise is not easy for many people, because in Western cultures people tend to shy away from public or open expressions of gratitude. "We do not have a vehicle in our culture for telling the people who mean the most to us how thankful we are that they are on the planet—and even when we are moved to do so, we shrink in embarrassment" (Seligman 2002, p. 74). Yet it can make a profound difference in happiness levels.

In the workplace this exercise can easily be adapted. A common variation is the practice of having employees put the name of each co-worker on top of a blank index card. Then each co-worker writes one thing they really appreciate about working with the individual. The cards are collected and given to each employee. The manager has the option of removing any that are negative. Another variation might involve the department writing a letter of gratitude to another department. Including the signatures of everyone in the work group makes an impact.

Three Good Things

The Three Good Things activity is another simple exercise to increase the amount of gratitude experienced by the individual. Most people spend much of their time focusing on how to correct problems, and they remember failures more readily than successes. Often, people tend to ruminate over bad events more thoroughly than good events, and this predisposition reduces satisfaction levels, elevates anxiety, and deepens depression. Noticing what is going right promotes optimism about the future.

The exercise involves having each individual write down three things just before he or she goes to bed, large or small, that went really well that day. Next to each positive event, the individual then writes an answer to this question: Why did this good thing happen? Even over a short time such as a week, this activity has been found to significantly increase participants' perception of their happiness and reduce depressive symptoms for as long as six months (Seligman et al. 2005).

Variations of the Three Good Things exercise can be used by managers and employees alike. At the beginning of a shift or workday, participants can quickly share something that went well and why since the last time they met. One executive uses this variation of the approach: In a quick team huddle on Mondays she asks everyone present to begin by sharing something good that happened the week before. This exercise, she says, starts the entire week off on a positive note even when things promise to be difficult and challenging.

Many managers use another form of this exercise when they end meetings with a key question such as, What is one good thing you appreciate about the time we have just spent together? This is a positive way to end a meeting and is especially useful when the meeting has been difficult or negative. The exercise can be done quickly, with each individual sharing one thing he or she found positive about the meeting. People leave feeling good about their time together.

Forgiveness

The first way positive emotions about past events are diminished or lost has been discussed: underappreciating the good things that have happened. The second way is by overemphasizing the negative by holding onto grudges, bitterness, or feelings of injustice. To address these negative circumstances, letting go and forgiving are approaches that can increase happiness.

At the individual level, understanding the negative impact of holding onto grudges and grievances is important. Frequent and intense negative thoughts about the past are the raw material that blocks the ability to experience satisfaction and contentment. They make a feeling of peace elusive and serenity impossible. The human brain is wired in a way that gives emphasis to negative emotions, probably because they are often associated with survival instincts. The positive emotions are much more fragile. The only way out of a negative and hurtful past is by changing negative thoughts and rewriting the past, and this can be done through forgiveness and forgetting.

This principle has special ramifications for today's health care leaders. The principle of forgiveness is often called for following times of tumultuous change in organizations. Supporting employees through their grieving during major transitions helps them to let go of the past and the way things were. Addressing transgressions and betrayals and working hard to re-establish trust among employees and between employees and leaders are other examples of this principle at work. Dealing with betrayals in the workplace is important because they can lead to a lack of trust when they are not resolved in a positive way. Organizations depend on trust in order to function effectively. Betrayal destroys the very relationships the organization needs in order to function (Ciancutti and Steding 2000; Reina and Reina 1999). Building a trust-based culture is crucial in today's health care organizations.

Whether at the individual or the managerial level, some important aspects of forgiveness must be considered. Forgiveness involves several pro-social changes that occur within a person who has been offended or damaged by another. To forgive does not mean to pardon, nor does it mean to condone the act being forgiven. Nor is it excusing, forgetting, or denying that a wrong was perpetrated. When a person forgives another for a wrong committed, it usually benefits the person who does the forgiving. It releases much of the negativity that has the power to continue to influence the person's life.

Offering Forgiveness
Robert Enright (2001) suggests a process for forgiving others. The first step is to admit any feelings of anger, betrayal, hurt, or resentment. This can be very painful work. The second step is deciding to begin the forgiveness process. This step often comes with a realization that what has been tried has not been working. The third step is to work toward understanding and compassion for the offender. The last step involves discovery of the intense feelings involved and the suffering that has been incurred. As this step resolves, it leads to a release from the constraints of the negative emotions.

Letting Go of Grudges
Having a specific technique to let go of grudges can sometimes be helpful. The following forgiveness exercise from the field of positive psychology

can be used either by individuals or by managers. This letting go of grudges activity was developed by Karen Reivich, co-author with Shatte of *The Resilience Factor* (2002). Here is the simple process:

1. Choose a person in your life you know fairly well and have a grudge against. On a piece of blank paper, draw a circle in the center of the page and record a few words that capture the essence of the grudge.
2. Fill the rest of the paper with blank circles, at least fifteen of them. The object is to fill each of these circles with a word or phrase that describes something about the person for which you are grateful. Examples include something he or she said to you or did for you or something important about your relationship. Include small or big items, current or past events.
3. Hold the paper at arm's distance and notice how the grudge gets lost in a sea of gratitude.
4. Reflect on how your emotions and thoughts change as you focus on the person now. Are you able to see the person more fully? Do your feelings for the other person change in any way? Did you notice any changes in your mood and how you feel about yourself?

This exercise can be used in coaching individual employees who are holding a grudge. It can also be used with a work group when complaints have been raised about another department or team. Ample opportunities exist in any workplace for a leader to have an active role in coaching others in letting go of grudges and navigating the forgiveness process.

Influencing Positive Emotions Related to the Present

The positive emotions related to the present include joy, ecstasy, ebullience, calm, zest, pleasure, and flow. These emotions can occur as the result of pleasures or gratifications as discussed earlier in the chapter. Three different aspects to consider are pleasure, engagement, and meaningfulness. Understanding these three aspects allows specific interventions in each arena.

Pleasure

Pleasure at work may seem oxymoronic to some people. However, many of us derive pleasure from being at work when the work environment is positive, supportive of efforts expended, and conducive to the fulfillment of natural drives and intrinsic motivators. An important question to ask is, Is this a good place to work? In other words, do people experience pleasure here? Are people excited about coming to work? Do fun and interesting things happen here? What is the environment like?

Anyone can take steps to create the kind of environment in which they want to work. The work environment does not belong to the manager, and building a positive work environment is not just one person's responsibility. It is the responsibility of every employee in the work group. Each individual decides if he or she wants the department or service to be a good place to work, and this decision may start the ball rolling. It has been documented that positive emotion is contagious. Each person has more to do with the climate in the work environment than often is realized.

Take the example of LuEllen, a radiology technician in a community clinic. During an interview she was asked, "What makes your place such a great place to work?" The researcher was genuinely interested in her answer and was shocked at LuEllen's reply. She said in surprise, "What makes you think it's a great place to work?" The interviewer pointed out that she seemed to tell such great stories of the fun they were having at work. LuEllen responded, "Oh, it isn't a great place to work. In fact, it's horrible. We work long hours and we're underpaid. We have a horrible supervisor that everyone dislikes but no one else would take the job. She comes in late and leaves early. The patients and families all complain about her and her attitude. But you know what? We don't let her rob us of having fun at work. We make it a great place to work. Every day we decide that we are going to have fun and enjoy each other and our time together. It's great!" In other words, she meant that she and her co-workers decided to make it the kind of environment they wanted.

For leaders and managers, one of the first steps in conducting an assessment of any work environment is asking the fundamental question, Is this a good place to work? and then following up with, What can we do to improve it?

Many work groups, departments, and organizations have adopted the FISH philosophy for having fun at work. (The FISH philosophy is based on the customer service concepts followed by the employees at the Pike Place Fish Market in Seattle.) In most instances, employees and managers work closely together to ensure that at least a bit of fun is had in each day's work. Humor and laughter at work can greatly lighten the load of the many challenges faced in today's work environment. The manager can certainly set the tone for the department in terms of lightheartedness and humor.

Another important factor to consider in an assessment of the work environment is the physical surroundings. Is the work area pleasant? Is it clean and well organized? Or is it cluttered and messy? Is there space for employees to have a break away from interruptions and the typical demands of the department? What is the noise level? Is the lighting adequate, and are there windows that look out on natural settings? Even in an old facility, measures can be taken to make the physical environment more pleasant. Furthermore, keeping it pleasant is the shared responsibility of everyone in the work group.

Engagement

The second aspect of positive emotion in the present is related to the level of engagement experienced. Work is a wonderful vehicle for the experience of flow, and yet many people find it difficult to experience flow in their workplace. According to data collected by the Gallup organization in early 2001, "less than 30 percent of American workers are 'fully engaged' at work, and some 55 percent are 'not engaged.' Another 19 percent are 'actively disengaged,' meaning that they not just are unhappy at work but they regularly share those feelings with colleagues" (Loehr and Schwartz 2003, pp. 5–6). In some instances the work is tedious or repetitive with little challenge.

Individual employees as well as managers need to consider several issues related to the idea of engagement. One of the first questions to explore is whether the work environment is conducive to a deep level of engagement. In many jobs in today's health care organizations, the physical environment itself is destructive to flow. Many employees carry cell phones so they can be reached (and interrupted) at any moment, and most managers and many employees are expected to be readily available and responsive to interruptions regardless of what they are doing. The noise level alone in many departments is enough to interrupt flow (Sánchez et al. 2008; Brown, Davis-Thomas, and Yessis 2007; Scalise 2004).

Are people being interrupted unnecessarily? If so, what could be done to minimize the interruptions? One of the time management issues for every work group is that its members tend to interrupt each other needlessly. An important activity is for team members to talk openly and honestly about the things they inadvertently do to interrupt fellow team members. Becoming more conscious of these actions allows the interruptions to be minimized. Some interruptions are necessary, and people need to feel they can get help from each other when they need it. Most co-workers would be happy to do what they could to make a colleague's day go better. Batching requests and telephone calls, using message boards, and having short but frequent team huddles for communicating information are all examples of simple ways of reducing interruptions. Avoiding interruptions is just another way for employees and managers to express their mutual respect for each other.

One study of nurses observed that during *one hour* of a typical workday, one nurse worked in eight different locations, changed locations twenty-two times, talked to fifteen different people on twenty-two separate subjects, and spent only one-third of her time delivering patient care (Thompson, Wolf, and Spear 2003). In another, unpublished study, nurses were observed during their normal eight-hour work shifts. During this time, nurses averaged 160 separate tasks, with the average task time totaling 2 minutes and 48 seconds (Wiggins 2001). How can these nurses experience any sense of flow in such work environments? Although the two studies looked at nurses, other clinical professions probably work under similar conditions.

In a study by Tucker and Spear (2006, p. 643), it was found that on an average eight-hour shift, the average task time for nurses was only 3.1 minutes, "and, in spite of this, nurses were interrupted mid-task an average of eight times per shift." If the average task time is so short, surely co-workers and others could wait until the task is completed before interrupting the person's flow of process. Furthermore, the participants in the study linked these interruptions to errors. They found that returning to interrupted tasks "increases cognitive loads because it requires 'recovery time,' during which details about the previously paused task must be summoned for active consideration. This takes time and introduces the risk of one task being confused with another" (Tucker and Spear 2006, p. 654).

Another way to increase the level of engagement is to choose to minimize the amount of multitasking a person attempts. Multitasking is a very popular concept right now, and many people think they can work effectively on several different tasks at the same time. However, the truth is that the human being is not capable of doing multiple tasks as simultaneously as the term implies. Instead, the person is rapidly shifting attention from one task to another and, as a result, fails to give his or her full attention to any one of them. When a person is so inundated with tasks that the primary mode of working must be multitasking, something is going to suffer. Inevitably, mistakes get made and people feel as though they are listened to with only one ear. In health care settings, multitasking may actually be quite dangerous for both providers and patients.

Obviously, most people's work requires some amount of multitasking to quickly shift the focus from one area to another. However, each person must consciously make the decision about when multitasking is an effective way to work and when the task and interactions involved are too important to be given short shrift. Anyone who has developed any kind of listening skills knows the power of simply sitting quietly and listening fully to what the other person is trying to share. When the listener continues to answer the telephone, accept interruptions, or check e-mail during a conversation, the message is quite clear to the speaker: This is not important enough to give complete attention.

Mind-numbing meetings that seem to go on forever can be another source of disengagement. According to Myers (1992, p. 136), one way to increase the flow in work life is by "living more intentionally—saying yes to the things that we do best and find most meaningful, and no to the time-wasting demands." Yet, how many employees feel that they have the option of saying no to meeting requests and other demands on their time?

Flow was discussed in detail earlier in this chapter. A couple of reminders, however, may be in order. "Studies confirm that a key ingredient of satisfying work is whether or not it's challenging. The most satisfied workers find their skills tested, their work varied, [and] their tasks significant" (Myers 1992, p. 133). When hiring decisions are made, there should be an effort to match the candidates and their areas of strength with the work they are going to do. In some cases, a need to redesign jobs may arise to increase the sense of engagement for employees who have been doing the same job for a long time. Sometimes adding new responsibilities to jobs can help employees recapture their sense of flow. "To experience flow we need to find challenge and meaning in our work, and to seek experiences that fully engage our talents. Flow comes when we structure work in ways that summon self-forgetful involvement. It . . . takes both individual and managerial effort to accomplish" (Myers 1992, p. 134).

One of the ways managers and leaders can help themselves and their employees increase their experience of flow is through coaching. Understanding what brings engagement and how to increase it is an important part of coaching. Adversity or boredom can be converted into enjoyment by incorporating some of the ideas developed by the positive psychologists into regular coaching opportunities. The following process, based on the work of Seligman and Csikszentmihalyi, will help leaders develop a work environment in which flow can be experienced:

1. Identify the signature strengths of every employee and manager.
2. Help employees evaluate how they are using their strengths in their work.
3. Encourage employees to set short-term and long-term goals so that they can monitor their own progress.
4. Look for new ways to let employees use their strengths in their work, and offer them opportunities to do so.
5. Encourage them to pay attention to what is happening. Share conversations about their process and success in using their strengths.
6. Share their enjoyment of immediate experiences.

This approach can be effective for workers in any kind of job. Seligman gives an example of a bagger at a grocery store who was bored and felt her work was mundane and meaningless. She completed her signature strength assessment and discovered that social intelligence was one of her strengths. She decided that a way she could use this strength in her work was to make certain that her encounters with customers were the positive highlight of their day. Imagine the difference this made in her approach to her work and her customers. In another example, Seligman was struck by the attitude of an orderly when he visited a severely ill, comatose friend in a hospital. The orderly was changing out the wall hangings in the friend's room and seemed to be enjoying himself immensely. When questioned about what he was doing, his response was, "My job? I'm an orderly on this floor. But I bring in new prints and photos every week. You see, I'm responsible for the health of all of these patients. Take Mr. Miller here. He hasn't woken up since they brought him in, but when he does, I want to make sure he sees beautiful things right away" (Seligman 2002, p. 168).

Csikszentmihalyi's (1990, 1997, 2007) work is also relevant to building engagement. He found there is a direct connection between the level of challenge the task represents and the level of skill of the person. When, for instance, skills are low or poorly developed and the level of challenge is great, as in learning to operate a new piece of equipment or some other technical job requirement, the result may be anxiety. However, when both the person's skills and the level of challenge are low, apathy is the result. It is only when the person has a high level of skill and is meeting a significant challenge that one can reach flow. Typical kinds of activities research participants were involved in during times when they experienced flow included a favorite hobby, work, new tasks, or a learning activity.

Workflow in most health care organizations is characterized by constant interruptions, the need to return to previously unfinished tasks, high levels of environmental noise, and the need to respond to pressing or critical situations (Clancy and Anteau 2008). These factors increase the level of leadership complexity in intervening to increase engagement in today's workplace. It is a worthy goal that demands highly skilled leaders and has become a focus in the corporate world. "People with high flow never miss a day. They never get sick. They never wreck their cars. Their lives just work better" (Marsh 2005, p. 77). Increasingly, organizations are using Csikszentmihalyi's ideas to learn about how they can get the very best out of their workers or create more compelling connections with their customers or those they serve.

Meaningfulness

Emphasizing the meaningfulness of one's work and that of colleagues is another way to increase happiness in the present. Affirming each other and reinforcing the significance of the work by drawing attention to its importance are crucial. Celebrating events such as National Respiratory Therapy Week, Hospital or Long Term Care Week, or Nurses Week demonstrates to people that their work is important. Supporting employees in participating in poster presentations and publication is another. Encouraging people to share their stories of when they made a difference is a great way to increase their sense of appreciation of themselves and the work they do.

Finally, doing everything possible to protect people from tasks that do not add value to their work communicates respect for both individuals and their work. Correcting long-standing problems that eat up time unnecessarily is important. A clear example of this was seen in a small Vermont hospital several years ago. An automated clinical documentation system had been installed as part of an electronic medical record. Physicians were able to retrieve clinical data and laboratory and imaging exam results from their own office and home computers. A handful of physicians refused to use the automated system and instead continued to call the patient care departments to ask the nurses to print off diagnostic results and fax them. This situation was tolerated for two years even though the nurses felt that it showed tremendous disrespect for them and the value of their time and work.

This is an example of what happens when people feel like the work they do has no meaning. The nurses involved became totally demoralized by this situation. The leaders of the organization would never purposely perpetuate it, but not dealing appropriately with it results in significant negative effects.

Intentional Acts of Kindness

Another strategy that produces lasting changes in happiness levels involves doing acts of kindness for other people. "Mounting evidence suggests that prosocial behavior actually has positive outcomes for both the recipient (the person who is benefiting from a kind act) *and* the benefactor (the person doing the kind act)" (Kurtz and Lyubomirsky 2008, p. 30.) Although frequency of kind acts seemed to have little influence on outcomes, the variety of kind acts did affect well-being. These intentional acts of kindness seem to induce happiness in a variety of ways. First, they can enhance the person's self-perception in a positive way. Second, they may capitalize on the person's strengths, which increases a feeling of authenticity. Finally, seeing the effect of unsolicited generosity of spirit simply feels good.

This effective strategy can be implemented in any work group in the organization. Everyone agrees to an additional assignment that entails performing five unsolicited, intentional acts of kindness each week for co-workers. These acts are most effective if they are varied. Of course, none of these acts can put self or others in danger. Anonymous acts are powerful because they avoid a "payback" feeling or a sense of obligation on the part of the recipient.

Influencing Positive Emotions Related to the Future

So at least three ways are available of increasing the amount of positive emotion in the present. The three discussed here are making sure that pleasures are present in the workplace, encouraging engagement or flow in one's work, and recognizing and celebrating the meaningfulness of the work. Furthermore, techniques can be used to increase the amount of positive emotion as it relates to the future. The positive emotions related to the future include faith, trust, confidence, hope, and optimism. Three approaches from the field of positive psychology can have an impact on the level of positive emotion employees experience in relation to the future: utilizing mentoring relationships, appealing to a sense of personal legacy, and embracing optimism.

Mentoring Relationships

A great deal has been written about mentorship in other resources. Suffice it to say that a multitude of mentoring opportunities are available in any health care organization. The opportunities can include mentoring around career and job development as well as simply around how to function effectively in a particular organization. Mentoring implies a more formal relationship than simply being supportive of another person. Mentors generally meet with mentees at specific times for the purpose of conversation and idea sharing. Mentoring is a way of producing positive emotion about the future because it is positive action taken in the present that is focused on the future. As one manager proudly pointed out, "I have birthed ten managers out of this department."

Personal Legacy

Legacy is an important concept in today's workplace. The term refers to "the capacity to find pleasure and satisfaction in caring for and contributing to the next generation" (Mackoff and Triolo 2008a). It is the human need of generativity, or contribution to the world. Although it has special significance for those workers nearing the final stages of their career, it is by no means limited to these people.

One manager was lamenting the decline of one of her better employees, Mary. As Mary neared retirement, her increasing negativity and bitterness were being reflected back to her by colleagues who had grown tired of the complaining and comments. Mary continually told anyone who would listen, "I can hardly wait, sixteen months and I am done! I'm through with this place." Her angry tone left no one in doubt of her extreme dissatisfaction. Her co-workers, fed up with her, were repeating her words: "We can hardly wait! Sixteen months and she will be gone!" The manager was at her wits end for ideas in how to deal with Mary and her increasing negativity. Finally she decided to appeal to Mary's sense of legacy. The manager sat Mary down and gave her honest and direct feedback about her behavior. She pointed out the tremendous contributions Mary had made over the years and asked her how she wanted to be remembered in the department. Mary's realization that she was slowing changing her legacy from a positive, contributing one to a legacy of negativity and bitterness was a wake-up call. Her daily behavior changed remarkably. There were still bumps and bruises along the way, but calling Mary to her sense of legacy gave her a reason to change.

Developing a personal legacy is relatively simple, and yet it demands significant reflection and soul-searching. It involves the individual sitting down and thinking carefully about what he or she would like to leave for his or her colleagues, department, or organization as a result of his or her involvement there. Unlike writing a will, which often sorts through who receives which material possessions, developing a personal legacy focuses thoughts on the less concrete things to leave behind. For example, perhaps a person has been involved in helping create new practices or making changes in the way decisions are made in the department. Or, like the manager who had a substantial hand in helping ten employees move into managerial positions, a person's legacy may be felt for years. Perhaps the individual's important contribution is that he or she taught colleagues how to have a bit of fun at work and not take themselves so seriously, and the memory of the fun and laughter will become an important part of future department events.

When an individual actually writes his or her desired legacy, it helps the person consciously and mindfully consider what he or she wants to leave behind. This encourages a focus on behaviors that make the legacy a reality.

Optimism

Optimism is a signature strength that influences positive emotion about the future. Earlier in this chapter, optimism was briefly discussed. Optimism is based on how a person views the world and his or her perception of whether events that happen are pervasive and permanent or specific and temporary.

At least one way to influence optimism in the workplace is by an activity called "one door closes, another door opens." This simple activity can be used any time something negative happens. It involves simply asking which door has closed and which has opened; that is, what good things may come from this change? The exercise can also be effective when used in retrospect, because events we see as negative may sometimes have a positive element associated with them.

Summary

This chapter explores the role of happiness and joy in creating a positive work environment. Recent findings from the field of positive psychology are included to provide a sense of the research being done and the ramifications of the findings for the workplace. The goal in organizations ought to be to have happy employees and co-workers, in the broader and truer sense of happiness. Happiness is far more than the immediate enjoyment of pleasure through superficial means, such as materialistic pleasures. Instead, happiness is related to pleasure and a sense of engagement and meaningfulness in one's work. The three together can bring light to the eyes and a smile to the face. Recent research findings on how health care workers experience and express joy through their work are also explored. Specific suggestions for interventions in the workplace to support happiness are identified.

Conversation Points

Organizational Perspective

1. How healthy are employees? Are absenteeism rates climbing, stable, or declining? What are the most common health problems?
2. Is productivity at a satisfactory level? Do you see a relationship between productivity results and employee morale?
3. How satisfied are employees? Are there opportunities for improvement in organizational practices, policies, and benefits? Do you measure satisfaction levels frequently enough? Does the tool you use measure only positive emotions related to the past, or does it make an attempt to measure positive emotions in the context of the present and the future?
4. Do formal retention efforts focus predominantly on incentives that bring pleasure, such as gifts and social events? Is the sense of entitlement growing among employees? How does the organization use gratification in recognizing employees?
5. Are your organization's leaders happy people?
6. What are the signature strengths of key organizational leaders?

Leader Perspective

1. How can you help your followers see the deeper meaning of their work? What kinds of leadership interventions may influence their sense of meaningfulness?
2. Is the work environment a pleasant place? Are there ways you can create more fun within your work group? Are there simple things you could do to increase the sense of pleasure both you and your employees feel?
3. What things in your work environment interrupt people's sense of flow? What can you do about them?
4. Who in your work group is remarkably happy? Unhappy? How do you and others react to them?

5. What can you do to influence the level of positive emotion employees feel about the past? The present? The future?

6. What are your key signature strengths, and how do you use them in your work? Are there any you are not fully using? How can you use your signature strengths in new and different ways? Are there key strengths you need to develop to increase your effectiveness in your leadership role?

Employee Perspective

1. What elements or aspects of your work do you find meaningful? How can you increase your sense of meaningfulness?

2. What brings you pleasure at work? How can you increase the amount of pleasure you feel?

3. How often do you experience a sense of flow at work?

4. What kinds of work or activities are more likely to result in flow for you? How can you increase your experience of flow?

5. Are you happy in your work? What things are affecting your level of happiness?

6. What can you do to find more happiness?

7. What are your signature strengths? How are you using them in your work, and how could you use them in new ways?

A Case Study Using Positive Psychology Leadership Principles to Improve Staff and Patient Satisfaction

Thomas M. Muha, MA, PhD

A NEW NURSE manager at a major academic medical center discovered early on in her tenure that there were serious problems with the staff on her units. She had to contend with a core group of extremely toxic nurses who did everything possible to sabotage her by keeping the relationships around the floor as negatively charged as possible.

In her first few months, the rookie nurse manager discovered that this dysfunctional group of nurses had a history of using lateral violence to make life so miserable for new nurse graduates that every single one of them was leaving within a year of starting work. Even long-term staff members who would have liked to see improvements had become so intimidated that they lapsed into complete and total apathy. With other staff members dispirited, the bullies slept on their shift, took two hour lunch breaks, and foisted their work off onto the weaker members of the staff.

The inactive manager who was in charge of the units before the new nurse manager had allowed the negative staff members to become the most powerful people throughout the units. Morale plummeted as the rules of professional conduct were routinely ignored and blaming others for problems became commonplace. As a result, the vast majority of the 200 employees had developed an extremely pessimistic attitude.

Tasked with restoring order on the units, the first-time nurse manager took a tough stance in order to get the staff to comply with the necessary standards of practice. However, this put her into a power struggle with her staff. Negative emotions and behaviors remained rampant. Apathy and bad attitudes were prevalent, even among the "good" nurses. She desperately wanted to find a strategy that would promote a high level of patient care without feeling like she was going into a battle zone every day.

Tom Muha is a practicing psychologist in Annapolis, MD. He and his colleague Linda Burton offer professional coaching services to health care organizations based on the principles of positive psychology through Great HealthCare Systems. He can be reached through his Web site, www.greathealthcaresystems.com, or by phone at (443) 454-7274.

The situation for the nurse manager was frustrating. She had done everything she had been taught to do, only to be devastated when she received the results of an independently administered survey assessing the culture on her units two years after taking over. Staff satisfaction and job retention rates were at 1 percent, while job engagement was at 3 percent compared with a database of hospitals nationwide. Feedback from focus groups indicated that her attempt to turn around the units was seen as poor leadership and as being out of touch with staff members.

The objective of the intervention that followed was to determine whether positive psychology leadership principles could be taught to the hospital leadership and staff through a coaching process designed to make a measurable difference in their engagement and satisfaction levels.

The positive psychology leadership principles used in this case study had previously been identified to be the essential elements driving the performance of a high-functioning Solucient 100 hospital located in a major metropolitan area. The author of this case study and Linda Burton conducted a year-long appreciative inquiry to explore how this hospital had been able to maintain a vacancy rate in the 2 percent range while keeping its turnover rate around 5 percent for more than a decade.

Six leadership principles were found to be crucial. To make them easy to remember, an acronym was created—PROPEL©, or Passion, Relationships, Optimism, Proactivity, Engagement, and Legacy. The research revealed that leaders in the high-functioning hospital lived by six values: (1) generate a passion for being the best, (2) create collaborative relationships, (3) instill optimism, (4) promote staff who are proactive versus reactive, (5) enhance engagement by generating positive energy, and (6) leave a legacy by making a difference in the lives of others.

This case study was a year-long initiative during which one positive psychology coach worked with the leaders and another with staff to teach them the practical application of these principles in their daily work. An independent survey was conducted to measure the level of staff satisfaction, engagement, and retention immediately before and just after the initiative. Vacancy and turnover rates were also measured pre- and postintervention, as were the statistics from the ongoing surveys of patient satisfaction, patient safety, National Database of Nursing Quality Indicators (NDNQI®), and other measures used by this hospital.

Central to the positive psychology coaching process is a strengths-based assessment identifying the unique set of talents that every person has hard-wired into his or her brain. Strengths are developed by combining natural talents with knowledge and skill, a formula that the research has found enables individuals and organizations to function at a peak level of performance. The nurse manager completed several assessments that have been proven to be valid indicators of people's primary character traits and their most effective interpersonal strengths.

Coaching helped the nurse manager to understand that she was experiencing the same emotions as many of the other nurses on her staff, and that to quit would mean the negative people had prevailed. Her coach helped her to see how it was possible for her to use her strengths to become a great leader, someone capable of turning the staff around by working with them to achieve a high level of success and satisfaction. To reach that goal, however, would require that she become a model for transformation by being proactive in using her strengths rather than continuing to allow her negative reactions to dominate her management style.

The transformation process began with the coach helping the nurse manager to create a vision of what an ideal department would look like. She envisioned that the staff would feel a sense of camaraderie, take care of patients through great teamwork, and perform with the highest level of professionalism. However, she felt it was impossible for her to accomplish those goals due to being derailed by the bitter conflicts that resulted from being in the role of enforcer of the hospital's rules and regulations.

To help her see that her vision could be achieved, the coach provided an overview of how optimally functioning nurse managers were using the six positive psychology leadership principles to create high-performing teams. The coaching taught the nurse manager how to apply the six principles to her daily functions in order to develop collaborative relationships and engage in optimistic problem solving.

At the same time, another coach began the crucial work of teaching the staff how to make positive contributions to the change process. A meta-analysis of the change management studies by Hubble, Duncan, and Miller (1999) in *The Heart and Soul of Change* indicates that 40 percent of the success in transforming an organization involves identifying what the people in the system believe is necessary for improving performance.

Another 30 percent of the variance lies in the quality of the relationships between the people involved in the process. The remaining 30 percent of what contributes to successful change is equally divided between optimistic problem solving and leadership skills. These data make clear how important it was for the nurse manager and her team to learn how to develop relationships in which they listened and resonated with the staff's ideas for improvements.

To begin the process of constructively responding to her staff's dissatisfaction, the nurse manager started developing alliances with those people on her staff who shared her resolve to transform the units. To facilitate that process, the coaches met with the nurse manager and her top performers to forge a common vision based on their values of camaraderie, teamwork, and professionalism.

The coaches helped the transformation team to develop a strategy map that defined specific, measurable tasks for transforming their culture. Once the transformation team was able to use the positive psychology principles within their own ranks, they began to talk with others on the staff about how they could also become key contributors in creating positive outcomes. In the meantime, a coach was working with the staff to teach them how to convert their complaints into proactive suggestions that they could present to leadership as part of the collaborative problem-solving and decision-making process.

Prepared with a true understanding of the positive psychology principles and coached to consistently apply their strengths, the core group of change agents became increasingly hopeful and confident in their roles as leaders. As they saw that the six principles could help them to achieve their vision, the transformation team was able to generate a great deal of passion for becoming the best they could be. For example, when they learned that high-performing teams exceed a ratio of five positive interactions for every negative encounter, they made a concerted effort to get the entire staff above that threshold. While they worked together to solve problems, they also maintained a focus on creating positive experiences with every staff member.

Eventually, the nurse manager, her management team, the top performers, and the two coaches were meeting with the entire staff. This brought the positive psychology leadership principles to all levels on the units, creating a whole systems approach. Everyone on staff eventually experienced being an important part of the solution, and nearly all began to accept their fair share of responsibility. Some of the most negative staff members left of their own accord, but the majority of staff embraced the positive psychology principles.

As the staff saw that they could make a meaningful contribution, their perceptions of the nurse manager as a villain and themselves as victims changed dramatically. The more empowered the staff became, the more respect they felt—for themselves and for their nurse manager. Over time, everyone was able to work together to make the vision of improved camaraderie, teamwork, and professionalism a reality.

A year after commencing the study, these units received recognition as among the best in the hospital. The staff came to love their jobs and their co-workers. It was common to hear staff members talking about how well these principles were working in their home lives as well.

At the conclusion of the study, the independently administered surveys found that overall staff satisfaction soared from 1 percent to 85 percent. Employee engagement also rose substantially, increasing from 3 percent to 84 percent. The nursing staff's retention rate scores improved from 1 percent to 49 percent. The unit's Rand Patient Safety and NDNQI scores also improved dramatically.

Studies of U.S. hospitals have shown that a patient's satisfaction with his or her care is directly linked to the satisfaction level of the people providing that care. The research also revealed that increases in staff and patient satisfaction combine to produce a substantial benefit to a hospital's bottom line. This certainly proved to be true in this case study, with the Press Ganey Patient Satisfaction (HCAHPS) scores for nursing continuing to show significant and sustained improvement—having risen by 43 percent in the year following the initiative.

In addition, the hospital realized substantial savings as a result of nearly eliminating the use of agency and experiencing a 75 percent drop in the use of sick leave. The turnover rate of newly graduated nurses on the units studied had been at 100 percent the year prior to the positive psychology coaching. This turnover had been costly in terms of its negative effect on patient satisfaction and the hospital's bottom line. A 2008 *Journal of Nursing Administration* study estimates that to turn over one nurse costs between $82,000 and $87,000 (Jones 2008). Since the start of the case study, the turnover rate among new graduates improved by 80 percent.

As a direct result of this initiative, the hospital estimates it has been able to contain more than $816,000 in costs per year for the units that participated in this study. Most importantly, all of the improvements cited have been sustained for more than two years.

II

Strategies and Interventions
for Creating a Positive Workplace

Part I provides foundational information on the complex and dynamic subject of organizational behavior. Special emphasis was placed on understanding the importance of employees' engagement with their work and commitment to the organization. Chapters 1 through 4 also make a case for focusing on retention programs in addition to well-established, solid recruitment practices. The reasons people work are reviewed from both historical and contemporary perspectives. In chapter 3, the issue of personal and organizational commitment is thoroughly examined, and recent research from the field of positive psychology is summarized in chapter 4. It is noted that understanding the emotions of happiness and joy as they relate to workplace productivity and well-being helps managers and leaders develop more positive organization or department environments. And, for employees, this information provides insight into why an individual may or may not be happy in the workplace.

Part II focuses specifically on the strategies and interventions individuals and organizations can undertake to increase their effectiveness. As in the first four chapters, the suggestions offered in chapters 5 through 10 are meant to apply to individual employees, managers, and executives, as well as more broadly to organizations. Chapter 5 introduces the various approaches to creating a positive workplace, and subsequent chapters examine specific strategies in more detail.

5

Creating a Culture of Engagement

Jo Manion

We need more than a culture of retention,
we need a culture of engagement and contribution.
It's not enough that you've stayed here for 20 years,
it's "What are you giving? How are you contributing?"

—Jo Manion

DIRE PREDICTIONS for the future seem to dominate every discussion of workforce issues in today's health care organizations. Even if the organization, department, or work group is not currently facing a shortage of key personnel, given the rapidly approaching retirement of the Baby Boom generation, every health care organization needs to actively take on the challenge of maintaining a vibrant workforce in the near future and for some time to come. The importance of the manager's role in creating a culture of retention began to emerge even before the Health Care Advisory Board exhorted managers to see themselves as chief retention officers for their departments (Advisory Board Company 2000). This recommendation was reinforced by the Gallup Organization's conclusion that employees do not leave their organizations, they leave their managers (Buckingham and Coffman 1999). Other research has also linked the retention of employees to the existence of a positive relationship with their managers (McNeese-Smith and Crook 2003). Today, managers are being held accountable for retaining valuable employees. Yet retention programs continue to take a shotgun approach to decreasing turnover rates rather than implementing focused and effective strategies. How do managers and leaders actually create a positive work environment and a culture of retention? This chapter presents the results of a study conducted to answer this question.

The Issue

Identifying the manager as chief retention officer serves to emphasize the importance of focusing on the retention of valued employees. However, assigning titles and responsibilities without an adequate assessment of the capacity of the individual to accept or carry out that responsibility is likely to

Portions of this chapter are adapted from Jo Manion, Nurture a Culture of Retention, *Nursing Management* 35(4): 28–39. Copyright © 2004 and used by permission of Lippincott Williams & Wilkins.

result in a no-win situation. First-line managers need adequate preparation for the role of chief retention officer and need increased capacity through provision of adequate resources. They also need to be delegated appropriate levels of authority for accomplishing meaningful results. Exceptional managers may be successful even without such support, but their success often comes at great personal cost. And for most managers, the situation is likely to lead to a sense of failure and frustration, which can only serve to further escalate the turnover rate for health care managers themselves.

The senior executives to whom the managers report play a major role and have a key responsibility in providing meaningful support for their first-line managers. The truth is that creating a culture of retention and engagement in the organization is a shared responsibility. The manager must work with employees as well as with senior executives and key stakeholders for retention programs to be successful on the organizational level. Engagement of employees is the primary goal, which leads to increased retention. But what specific actions can a manager take?

The Study

A qualitative study was undertaken to determine exactly what successful health care managers do to create a culture of retention (Manion 2004b). Managers who had successfully done so in their areas of responsibility were recommended for inclusion in the study based on a variety of criteria. These managers' department showed some combination of the following criteria: low turnover rates; high patient, employee, and physician satisfaction levels; good patient or customer outcomes; and overall positive working relationships among employees. Many of the managers in the study reported having a waiting list of applicants who were seeking positions in their departments.

Interviews were conducted with thirty-two managers from health care organizations throughout the continental United States. The participants managed a number of inpatient and outpatient services including respiratory therapy, pharmacy, radiology, admissions, physical therapy, oncology, perioperative services, critical care, surgery, emergency care, and medicine. About half of the managers were responsible for two or more departments. The span of control ranged from 42 to 170 employees; half of the participating managers had fewer than seventy-five direct reports, and half had more than seventy-five.

To confirm the accuracy of the managers' self-reported information, interviews were conducted with focus groups made up of the participating managers' employees and direct supervisors. Remarkable consistency was seen in reported behaviors, and the conclusion was drawn that the managers' self-reports were accurate.

The Culture of Retention

To begin, participants were asked to describe a culture of retention in their own words. Typical responses included the following:

- "It's creating an environment where people want to stay."

- "It means people enjoy their work so much and the people they work with that they want to stick around and get involved. Everybody is trying to make it a great place to work."
- "It's an environment that meets peoples' [sic] needs."
- "When people come to work, they enjoy being here, [and] they feel good about being here. They feel safe. They can trust each other [to make sure] that the job will be done and done well."

The results of the study made it clear that the way to create a culture of retention is to first create a culture of engagement and contribution. It is this type of culture that makes a workplace people want to work in. It is not enough that an employee stays in the job for twenty years. The employee must continue to make meaningful contributions throughout those twenty years. Reed (2007) describes this concept as discretionary effort on the part of the employee. He defines *discretionary effort* as the difference between performing adequately and performing in an outstanding manner. Discretionary effort cannot be mandated; it is the employee's choice to give.

Leadership Strategies

The managers' responses to the question, "What do you do to create this culture of retention?" were recorded, transcribed, and analyzed using a categorical content analysis approach. In other words, the categories and themes emerged from the participants' own words and stories. More than twenty factors emerged, and the factors were sorted into five primary themes: (1) Put employees first, (2) forge authentic connections, (3) coach for and expect competence, (4) focus on results, and (5) work in partnership with employees. These simple and yet powerful interventions are discussed more fully here and illustrated with the participants' words and stories. (See figure 5-1.)

Figure 5-1.   Major Themes of Effective Managerial Interventions in Creating a Culture of Engagement

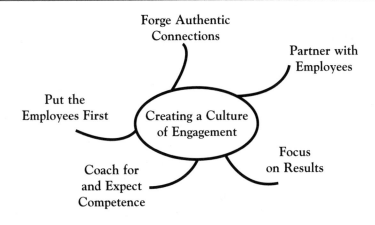

Put Employees First

The successful managers who took part in the study clearly believed that their job was to put the employees first so that their employees could put their patients or customers first. Typical responses included the following:

- "My staff comes first, not the patient first. Because if I make my staff feel valued and respected and good about what they do, then they're going to give the best care in the world."
- "I know that if I am looking out for them, they will look out for the department. They know when they need me I will be there for them."
- "I put my employees first so they will put the patients first."

Putting employees first may sound simplistic, but it can be complex and difficult. The following example illustrates this point. A critically ill patient was brought into the emergency department of a medium-size community hospital during the early afternoon. When it became apparent that the patient's death was likely to occur within several hours, a supervisor was called to facilitate the patient's transfer to an inpatient nursing unit, where the environment would be more conducive to a peaceful passing for both the patient and the patient's family. The supervisor called the nurse manager of the inpatient department and requested assignment of a room. The nurse manager responded that no rooms were available and that she would call back when one became available.

Surprised at the information about room availability, the supervisor waited for about thirty minutes before deciding to go to the department herself to determine whether any beds had become available. She found that there were several suitable rooms to which the patient could be transferred. Somewhat startled, she sought out the nurse manager and questioned her about using one of the empty rooms. The nurse manager surprised her by admitting that she had refused to accept the patient because of concerns for her staff. In her words, "They have had just an awful day. It has been crises and problems one after another all day long, with patients admitted and discharged in a steady stream. They are exhausted. They've had no breaks or meals. This close to the change of shift, I just didn't have the heart to ask them to do one more thing."

In the supervisor's mind, this case was an example of the nurse manager putting her staff first but to the detriment of a patient. What could she have done then? Override the manager's decision and insist that the patient be transferred? A less-often-considered response would have been to ask the question, "What can we do for your staff so that they would be able to accept this patient?" Asking this question could have led to productive problem solving that considered the employees' needs as well as the patient's needs. For instance, it might have been possible to have a nurse from the emergency department stay with the patient and family until the change of shifts had occurred. Alternatively, a float nurse could have been assigned to the patient temporarily. Maybe lunch needed to be brought to the department for the staff so they could have a brief meal break.

Furthermore, very few organizations have mottos that say, "We put our employees first!" Almost all would say that their mission is to put the patient or the customer first. However, putting employees first is a means to the desired end. Spiegelman (2007) says that building brand loyalty begins with cultivating employees first. Patient loyalty is based on people who have developed the passion and commitment that results in the staff putting patients first, and to do this, the managers put the staff first. Davies and Chun (2007) believe that organizations must first be agreeable to their staff; then the positive attitudes will rub off and boost customers' opinions and satisfaction levels.

Other studies have reported similar findings. In recent research by Mackoff and Triolo (2008c), nurse manager engagement was studied. This qualitative study found that specific behaviors were related to long-term, high-performing nurse managers and their organizations. These managers invested in creating a positive work environment that translated into the way their staff interacted with patients. One manager noted, "I see my responsibility as also creating a healing environment for all the staff that work here so that they are taking care of themselves in a way that they are energized and have what they need to take care of patients and families and give their best" (Mackoff and Triolo 2008c, p. 23).

The specific ways the managers in this study put their employees first included:

- Caring about them as people
- Meeting their needs
- Providing support
- Listening and responding to them
- Treating them with respect and high regard
- Expressing appreciation and recognition liberally

Care about Them

One striking finding of this study was the depth of authentic feeling and caring the participant managers expressed for their employees. This did not mean the manager always liked everything individual employees might do or how they might behave, but the love and caring for them as individuals far transcended any negative incidents. Some of their comments include:

- "It's caring about people and not just their work."
- "It's understanding that they have a life outside the department."
- "They know I love them. I have fallen in love with my employees!"

Managers who were told early in their careers that they should avoid getting too close to their employees, keep their distance, or stay uninvolved and unemotional may find these comments surprising. However, the care and positive regard these managers held for their employees was striking, and it was demonstrated through many of the other behaviors the managers reported.

These findings support a new awareness of the presence of and even the need for strong emotion in our workplaces (Henry and Henry 2004). Furthermore, "We are refocusing on the deep longing we have for community, meaning, dignity, purpose, and love in our organizational lives. We are beginning to look at the strong emotions of being human, rather than segmenting ourselves by believing that love doesn't belong at work, or that feelings are irrelevant in the organization" (Wheatley 1999, p. 14). Champy (2003, p. 135) notes that "the caring part of empathy, especially for the people with whom you work, is what inspires people to stay with a leader when the going gets rough. The mere fact that someone cares is more often than not rewarded with loyalty." Caring in health care organizations is often discussed in relation to patients and their families and only rarely in relation to employees and co-workers. Perhaps the need to minimize love in business and work relationships exists because it can lead to uncomfortable feelings of vulnerability (Sherwood 2003).

Meet Their Needs

Another way to put employees first is by meeting their needs. The participating managers reported talking to their employees about how they as managers could do a better job and how they encouraged employees to reveal what was important to them in the workplace. Basically, the successful managers treated employees as though they were their customers.

Scheduling practices were some of the most frequent examples of meeting employee needs. Using a self-scheduling approach was very common, and this concept was also applied to make it easier for employees to attend classes, facilitate child care, or arrange days off.

However, meeting the needs of employees goes well beyond scheduling issues to understanding each employee's individual situation. Many of the managers' comments supported this idea, for example:

- "I try to be responsive to them. If they need to cut down their hours for some reason or another, not letting that be a long process but really making that a very short process for them."
- "I try to remember when people are going through stressful times, especially personal [problems], as to what's going on. Undergoing treatment for breast cancer, or a parent that's dying, or a very sick child."

Again, although such simple managerial interventions were common, they fly in the face of the advice most managers receive at an early point in their careers: that managers should not become involved in their employees' lives and that employees and managers should leave their personal problems at home. The managers in the study gave many examples of intervening and assisting employees with personal issues when those issues had an impact on the workplace. However, the managers indicated that they were always careful not to overstep and violate appropriate professional boundaries.

For example, Susan, one of the managers who participated in the study, told the story of an employee, Mary, who had been an excellent worker before the quality of her work began to slip significantly. Mary was a Russian immigrant who had come to the United States after marrying an American man—she was the modern-day equivalent of a mail-order bride. Susan sat down with Mary to discuss the performance problems only to discover that Mary was being abused by her husband. Mary did not know what to do.

Susan helped Mary by referring her to the employee assistance program and a support group at the hospital. In her own explorations of the problem, Susan discovered a local law firm that specialized in this type of case. Although Susan never became personally involved in Mary's problems, she certainly went further than many managers would have. Katzenbach, in *Why Pride Matters More than Money* (2003), notes in another publication that "getting involved in the everyday problems of your people may violate the HR rule-book, but it's also the single best way to build an emotional bond with your employees" (quoted in Byrne 2003, p. 66).

This strategy has led to some remarkable programs in the workplace. More organizations are seeking to create environments that are healthier for staff. At a New Jersey hospital, critical care nurses are encouraged to take advantage periodically of a former storage area remodeled as "an oasis of peace and quiet—a 'sacred space' where they can replenish their flagging spirits" (Weber 2005). In other organizations, massage therapists make rounds, offering brief massages to employees. Programs such as multidisciplinary retreats are offered to provide staff with the energy to tap into their inner strengths when dealing with stress, pain, and conflict.

Support Them

Support is another way that the managers in the study put their employees first and demonstrated their caring. Support encompasses a variety of behaviors, including:

- Advocating on behalf of the employees
- Ensuring the availability of support staff for the department (for example, clerical staff, department-based educators, clinical specialists, social workers, case managers, and specialty pharmacists)
- Creating a nonpunitive environment that treats mistakes as opportunities to learn
- Helping employees deal with irate or difficult physicians, customers, and patients' families
- Making educational funding available
- Supporting individuals during personal crises and difficult times

Another important way to show support is by recognizing the need to balance work and personal life. In a survey conducted by the Families and Work Institute in 2000, a nationally representative group of 3,400 employees was surveyed to determine what they considered very important in their current jobs. The second most important factor identified was a balance between work and life (Barney 2002). When managers fail to recognize the importance of work-life balance for employees, a tremendous opportunity is lost, not only to demonstrate understanding and compassion but also to provide appreciable help in what has become a significant challenge for most people. "Twenty-seven percent of American workers say their organizations don't understand the tremendous need for work-life balance. . . . People wonder about whether they have enough time to do a good job at work but also do a good job at life" (Anonymous 2002, p. 27).

The past decade has seen a growing appreciation of the various values and needs of employees from different generations. Work-life balance has been identified as a primary concern of Generation Xers (or GenXers), and organizations are being warned that some common practices need to be changed in order to successfully recruit and retain individuals from this age group. GenXers "think they should have a life. The classic shift-weekend-holiday rotation will not cut it with this group. They are looking for a workplace that offers flexible scheduling, liberal vacations, daycare centers, workout rooms, on-site dry cleaning, florists, and the list goes on. They will pick the job that allows them to get the most fun out of life" (Cordeniz 2002, p. 247). In addition, many Baby Boomers are rapidly reaching a time in their lives when they will become more concerned about work-life balance simply because they are tired of working the extra shifts and being on call. After decades of putting up with difficult work schedules, they are ready to call it quits. Like it or not, this issue must be faced. Chapter 11 discusses intergenerational issues more fully.

Listen and Respond to Them

Listening carefully to what employees say and share was identified by most of the managers as essential in how they related to their employees. Although the managers described using effective listening techniques (such as making eye contact, listening reflectively, and paying full attention), what was most striking about their comments was that when asked how people knew their managers were listening, the managers said that the employees knew because "something changes as a result of [the manager's] listening to them." In other words, people knew they had been heard when some follow-up or resolution to their problem occurred as a result of the conversation. It may not have been the answer they wanted, but it was an answer nonetheless. Atchison (2003) reports hearing similar comments in his interviews of health care leaders.

Contrast this sentiment with the admonition delivered to one of the participating managers by an executive: "Just because we haven't done anything doesn't mean we are not listening to you." To the manager, who felt frustrated with the organization's lack of response to her repeated pleas for help, nonresponse meant exactly that: that she was not being heard.

Once again, these examples may seem like very simple interventions, and yet the managers in the study went further than just listening when people asked for their help. They often asked probing questions such as, What took you too long to do today? What are you doing that is just plain silly? What is holding you back from doing your best work? What keeps you up at night? What could we change to make your work easier or more fulfilling? Contrast such authentic questioning with the more typical (and understandable) behavior of a manager who wants to run and hide when a troubled or troublesome employee appears. Other comments made by the participating managers underscore the value of listening:

- "They are the ones with the gems. They will come to you with their problems. You'll know what needs to be fixed, 'cause they'll tell you what's broken."
- "[When] I address issues they have brought up, it surprises them sometimes."
- "I may not have the answer right away because I like to go back and process things, but I always get back to people and they really appreciate that."
- "Listening is probably one of the most important things I do. I repeat what they said and then I get back to them on it."

Listening to people is the first leadership intervention presented in the popular book *Love 'em or Lose 'em* by Kaye and Jordan-Evans (1999). The recommendations in that book focus on what managers need to do to keep good people. Managers and supervisors cannot assume they know what their people want. Kaye and Jordan-Evans advise to look them in the eye and ask, "What can I do to keep you? What do you need? What do you want?" (Kaye and Jordan-Evans 1999). The responses to such questions can be powerful.

Treat Them with Respect

Expressing respect and a high level of unconditional regard for others clearly constituted one of the ways the managers in the study treated their employees. For example, some of the managers' responses were:

- "They have the right to challenge me on any decision."
- "I always respect their opinions, and I don't judge them. I listen to what they are telling me."
- "I am just in awe of what they do. I am just stunned by it."
- "I trust that they are honorable people. If they tell me they need something, I believe it."

One manager told a story about an applicant whom she later hired. The employee told her, "You know, the reason I took this job is because when you toured me in the department, you introduced me to the housekeeper and you not only knew her name, but knew her grandkids by name and told me several things about her. I came here because you clearly respect everyone!"

Show Appreciation and Recognition to Them

Each manager in the study used unique methods for recognizing and appreciating people. Just a few of the methods included:

- Arranging for reports of employees' accomplishments to be printed in a newsletter
- Obtaining funding for employees' attendance at educational events
- Sharing thank-you notes and cards by mounting them on bulletin boards
- Planning department events during national recognition weeks (Respiratory Therapy Week, Hospital Week, Long-Term Care Week, Nurses Week, Nurse Assistant Week, and others)
- Displaying evidence of employee accomplishments (such as mounting employee certification plaques on a wall in the department)
- Creating and using recognition and retention tool kits with giveaway items such as movie tickets, T-shirts, and discount coupons for the gift shop or cafeteria
- Distributing thank-you notes and special-occasion cards
- Taking pictures of employees and posting them in the department
- Acknowledging employees for special accomplishments or service anniversaries at department gatherings

Admittedly, these kinds of activities take time and attention. For instance, if a decision is made to recognize employees by sending birthday cards or employment anniversary cards, managers need to be consistent and send out cards for every employee without exception. What begins as a seemingly simple intervention can become an overwhelming chore over time. Most of the managers in the study undertook such activities in partnership with their employees. Responsibilities were shared so that the burden did not fall too heavily on any one person. For example, some people thoroughly enjoy buying and giving greeting cards, and accepting the responsibility for seeing that everyone in the department gets a birthday card at the right time may be a true pleasure for them. Many of the managers talked about asking a small group of employees to create recognition opportunities for the department.

Forge Authentic Connections

Taking time to connect with employees is important. The managers in the study believed that every employee needs to have a personal, individual connection with the manager. Examples of the managers' comments included the following:

- "Sharing some of myself with them. Letting them know I care about the same things they care about."
- "I take time to connect with my people and listen to them."

A variety of managerial behaviors build the foundation for developing strong connections with employees. Examples include getting to know them, creating a sense of connection and community in the department, hiring the right people, and having fun together.

Get to Know Them

Even managers with a large span of control believe that it is essential to know the people with whom they work, not just the direct departmental employees but also housekeepers, security officers, and anyone who comes into the department on a regular basis. Knowing each individual includes understanding something personal about them and calling them by name. One nurse manager described a situation experienced by a patient care technician (PCT) she had just hired. The PCT had completed an intensive six-month training course at another hospital and then had promptly resigned. When the nurse manager asked her why she had left the first hospital after they had paid for her education, the PCT replied, "After six months they still didn't know my name!" In *Execution*, Bossidy and Charan (2002) explain that an essential leadership characteristic is knowing your people as well as you know your business.

The managers who participated in the study were not necessarily the most social people at the holiday party, nor did they always join employees for pizza and beer after work. But they took the time to know something special and unique about each individual. Here are some examples of the managers' responses:

- "It's understanding what's important to them outside the institution. That they're human, that they have important lives and need to feel valued."
- "I know all of them. I know their names, their families, their dogs, what they like to do."
- "I invest time in them, I make rounds, I ask them—what's going on? What's important to you? The investment in them makes them feel wanted. It creates a bond and a rapport."
- "I try to have lunch with my staff once a week—not more often because I want them to have plenty of time to talk with each other."
- "They need to know who I am. I have pictures of my wife, my kids, my cat on my desk. I let them know who I am."

Several managers described taking note of major events that affected individual employees, such as the loss of a loved one. One manager mentioned that she had lost her sister years ago, and she described how good it made her feel when someone asked her, "How is it going without Marie?" So she keeps track, and on the anniversary date of the loved one's death, she finds the employee and asks, "How are you doing? Are you thinking about your Dad?" And she said, "I don't do it as a strategy. I do it from my heart, and I know it makes a huge impact on them. Because I remembered and they're not alone in their memory." This manager went on to share that she was not the most socially inclined person at the department parties and that she really was more of an introvert. However, it is almost certain that her employees realize that she cares deeply about them.

A pharmacy director who participated in the study reported using a job-shadowing program. He routinely spent a half day shadowing an employee to stay in touch with both the employee and the work issues that were typical during a shift. All of the managers who took part in the study described their own unique approaches to gathering this kind of firsthand information.

Create a Sense of Community

Many of the managers' stories involved examples of an extraordinary sense of community that had been created in their departments. Examples included employees who rallied together to support a colleague experiencing a tragedy or very difficult times. Several described situations in which an employee had been injured in an accident and was unable to work for an extended period of time. One emergency department put a jar out at the central desk to collect donations, and more than $3,000 in cash was collected for the individual. Another common example involved co-workers who donated their own vacation or paid leave time to other employees who were experiencing significant difficulties.

In addition, managers who took part in the study described the camaraderie experienced during special occasions such as weddings, graduations, and other life events. In one work group, the young department secretary was planning to move in with her boyfriend. The couple wanted to marry, but they felt that they could not afford a wedding. The secretary's co-workers pulled together and created a beautiful wedding for the couple. The department social worker offered her home for the wedding and reception, two colleagues sewed the wedding dress, another co-worker sang and played the music, the department manager (who was also an ordained minister) performed the ceremony for free, other co-workers brought food, and a physician donated a night in the honeymoon suite of a local hotel. The manager laughingly told the young woman, "You're having a nicer wedding than I had!" What a delightful way to celebrate and reinforce strong connections at work.

As in other healthy communities, the work environments described by study participants were inclusive rather than exclusive. In other words, no one was deliberately left out, and every attempt was made to include as many people as possible. Anyone in proximity to the department was drawn in, including patients and their families, physicians, and workers from other areas of the organization. An exclusive community is more like a clique, and cliques depend on having narrow membership requirements to maintain their exclusivity. Establishing community is an effective strategy for enhancing retention (Manion and Bartholomew 2004) and is addressed more fully in chapter 7.

Hire the Right People

One way of forming strong connections involves taking care to hire the right people for the department. The importance of careful recruitment practices is a relatively common theme in the business literature (e.g., Buckingham and Coffman 1999). In Jim Collins's words, "you have to get the right people on the bus" (Collins 2001). Interestingly, the managers in the study did not emphasize the importance of finding the right technical skills and cognitive intelligence to fill vacancies. They focused instead on the candidates' attitudes, behaviors, and emotional intelligence. The following comments were typical:

- "I look for optimism. I look for perky. I look for people who are very comfortable with themselves."
- "I look for emotional intelligence. How they deal with interpersonal problems in the workplace, how assertive are they?"
- "We look for people who are passionate about their work."
- "We look for people who really have the energy and the sense of humor that fits with our group."
- "We want someone who is going to contribute, participate on committees, be a part of what's going on."

One manager said that her favorite question to ask during selection interviews was, "How has life treated you?" From this, she claims, she can tell a great deal about a person's perception of his or her life and whether he or she has a victim mentality or is optimistic and does not let negative events and other people get him or her down. This managerial approach is strongly validated by the recent findings in the field of positive psychology. The study and understanding of resiliency, or a person's ability to bounce back after difficult circumstances, reinforce these concepts.

The managers who participated in the study also described the involvement of employees in helping select their new colleagues. A variety of approaches were used for involving co-workers in this process, and the managers found employee involvement in hiring to be very effective. Even employees reported that, although technical expertise was important, it was not the key attribute they looked for in a new colleague. More important was the person's ability to fit in well with the work group.

Have Fun Together

Whether they featured making cookies or popcorn in the middle of a busy shift or giving a prize to the person who most closely guessed the correct number of syringe caps in a jar, the workplaces described by the participating managers were full of humor and fun. Several actually reported setting up employee committees whose only purpose was to plan lighthearted activities for the staff. Some described using the FISH philosophy based on the now-famous Pike Place Fish Market in Seattle, where fun is considered an important component of everyday work life (Whiley 2001).

In one department, three different employee committees were responsible for fun activities. One committee handled the events and activities that were held in the workplace, such as birthday celebrations, fun contests, and activities that stimulated and brought enjoyment to the staffers. Another committee was responsible for off-site activities, which included summer golf tournaments; picnics; and trips to nearby cultural, sports, and theatrical events. No one was bothered when some employees chose not to participate, recognizing that for some people another night away from their family would not be perceived as fun. However, for many of the young people and singles for whom work represented an important part of their social life, such activities were considered a real treat. The third committee was responsible for the bulletin boards in the department; they designed the boards along a new theme every month. Their creative ideas delighted everyone who saw them: employees, physicians, patients, and patients' families and friends.

In some cases, managers talked about having to feed the committees ideas in the beginning, but most of the work was accomplished by employees. This is an important point because the staff members felt more ownership when they played an instrumental part in the process. All of the managers said that it was important to create a positive work environment by making certain that the workplace was fun, but they also said that they made sure that work got done. Comments about the importance of fun included the following examples:

- "We try to keep it lighthearted in the department. I have a good sense of humor. Employees see that, and it sets the tone for the department."
- "I use humor and fun to emphasize the things I think are important. For example, we always celebrate the end of orientation. I take the new employees to breakfast and the preceptors out to dinner."
- "We have so much fun at our parties. We started having these little cookouts every month. One of the employees brings his grill and we'll do hamburgers and hotdogs around 6 p.m. so oncoming and offgoing staff can have some. We invite everyone."

Coach for and Expect Competence

The third way successful managers create a culture of retention is by focusing on the growth and development, both personal and professional, of the people with whom they work. As noted in an earlier chapter, competence is a key intrinsic motivator for work. Thus, it is no wonder that supporting employee development was identified as a major leadership intervention in the study. Highly effective workers are rarely impressed with glitzy perks and increased fringe benefits. "What keeps them around are extensive training and career-development programs that offer valuable benefits to both workers and employers" (Dobbs 1999, p. 51). Organizations that recognize that their best employees are eager to develop their careers realize that development opportunities are some of the best perks around. The factors in this key theme include setting high standards and expectations, coaching and supporting development, modeling behavior, and managing performance.

Set High Standards and Expectations

The managers who participated in the study set high standards, for both themselves and others, and helped people achieve those standards. Performance expectations for clinical and technical performance as well as for interpersonal behaviors were made clear, and people were held accountable for meeting them. For example:

- "My leadership team and I actually look for and create new goals every year so that people are always feeling challenged. So we're always on the cutting edge. You cannot be satisfied with what you did last year."
- "I have very high standards and expectations for participating in performance improvement efforts [and] committee work and for practicing their profession in a high-quality way."
- "I don't expect anything of them that I wouldn't do myself."

Support Development

The managers in the study talked with pride about having helped develop the skills of individual employees who were later promoted to other positions in the organization. They took pride in the accomplishments of their employees. Coaching is a common approach, but successful managers also employ other strategies, including:

- Supporting attendance at national conferences and educational programs
- Encouraging and helping employees present posters at national meetings or co-write articles
- Obtaining reference materials for the department
- Implementing strong orientation and development programs
- Encouraging employees to take advantage of tuition reimbursement programs
- Encouraging membership in professional associations

Managers in the study offered the following comments:

- "I take a personal interest, finding out what they want to do is important. And then not just delegating and dumping, but really giving them growth opportunities."

- "I constantly look for opportunities for them."
- "Each employee has particular strengths and it means recognizing those and asking people what they would like to develop. They may like teaching others, or improving their clinical skills, or being charge or a case coordinator. So what kinds of experiences would be beneficial to help them prepare for that role?"
- "I get them involved in things. First of all I solicit what they are interested in. I ask, 'if you're interested in doing other things, let me know.' Then when opportunities arise, I ask them."

These successful managers talked extensively about the need to be proactive in identifying people's interests. Opportunities that arise are evaluated and shared with others. The Gallup Organization reported years ago that when employees do not have at least one or two conversations about career planning with their manager every year, they conclude that their manager does not care about them (Buckingham and Coffman 1999).

Model Behavior

An important way the managers in the study coached and developed others was by serving as a role model. They modeled the behavior they wanted to see. Acting as a role model includes living up to the expectations they hold of others, staying positive, using a nonpunitive approach to problem solving, remaining calm in the midst of chaos, and persevering in the face of extreme difficulty. Typical examples of the managers' comments included the following:

- "I have faced many situations that would get most people down, but I don't let it. I'm choosing my attitude every day and I want my employees to see that."
- "You have to lead by example. We have to help each other. This job is difficult enough as it is. We need to be supportive of each other. If you see someone is sinking and having a really tough day, help them out."
- "I try to model the behavior that I think most employees want—they want honesty, they want fairness, and they want to see that I treat everyone the same."

A beautiful example of role modeling was shared by a manager during a conversation. A very unpopular decision had been made in the organization, and employees were unhappy and upset about it. Throughout the day a great deal of complaining went on. Early in the afternoon, an assistant manager finally said to her manager, "I simply cannot believe that you are not upset about this." The manager replied, "Oh, don't mistake me. I'm very angry about this decision, but that doesn't mean I have to spew all that negativity out and infect everyone around me! I can control my emotions and not let them infect everyone else." What a wonderful example for others.

Manage Performance

Performance management is a critical element of coaching for competence. Performance management was specifically mentioned by more than 80 percent of the managers in the study. The managers recognized and rewarded positive behavior and dealt with problem behavior immediately. They had learned the hard way that managers cannot ignore problems, and they understood that their own credibility with staff would be jeopardized if they ignored performance problems. Here are some examples of what they said:

- "I hold people accountable for their behaviors. We follow a process. It's time-consuming, but you know what? They either comply or move on."
- "Here's the bar. It's set right here, and if you don't get up to that bar, then there are consequences. Too many people are afraid to discipline, afraid to counsel, because there are workforce shortages. But the reality is you can't keep bad apples. You really dilute the quality of care and morale in the work group."
- "If things have to be addressed, then I address them. It doesn't do any good by waiting for it to go away, 'cause it doesn't."
- "When employees bring these problems, they want to see that they are taken care of. They want to trust that something will happen."

A major issue for most of the managers related to their working relationships with the human resources department in their organizations. Some of the managers reported that the support they received from human resources was exquisite, but other managers indicated that they needed to work around a weak or poorly functioning human resources department that was more a roadblock than a support.

For example, one nurse manager of an orthopedic service was the fifth new manager for the department over a five-year period. When she began in her position, she identified several toxic and dysfunctional employees who acted as highly skilled saboteurs within the department. They not only attempted to block virtually every positive step she initiated but they also used bullying behavior in a way that made life miserable for their co-workers. The manager was on the verge of resigning. She had worked extensively with an organizational development specialist from human resources to initiate team building and begin setting expectations within the department and among employees. The manager had also begun counseling and disciplining the most toxic of these negative employees, because she was determined to deal with their unacceptable behavior. As a result, she found herself in trouble with the human resources staff, who saw themselves as employee advocates. Roadblock after roadblock was thrown in her way until the internal organizational development consultant sat down with her human resources colleagues and said, point blank, "If you don't help her deal with these toxic employees, you are going to be hiring manager number six for this department and nothing will have changed." The human resources staff had been unaware of the extent to which they had become employee advocates rather than organizational advocates in a manner well beyond what was appropriate.

It is not uncommon for toxic employees to find a safe and comfortable home in a department where manager turnover is the norm. The challenge is to recognize poor performance and then deal with it appropriately. Threatened lawsuits, fear of aggression, fragile race relations, and workforce shortages are just a few of the reasons managers may be reluctant to deal with poor performance. Yet when such problems are ignored, the employees who leave are usually the good ones, the ones needed to create a positive culture, and not the employees with substandard performance or bad attitudes. The best workers simply do not need to put up with a dysfunctional environment; they can and will find another place to work. Even when they do not walk with their feet, they walk with their heart. Managers and executives lose a tremendous amount of credibility among the decent, hardworking employees in the organization when poor performance is tolerated. (Chapter 10 addresses this subject in more detail.)

Focus on Results

The fourth group of leadership strategies for creating a culture of engagement involves focusing on results. The managers who took part in the study worked hard to solve problems, and they achieved improvements in their departments, often with the help of the people with whom they worked. Four factors are related to the focus on results: solving problems, empowering and involving employees in decision making, providing adequate resources, and providing a pleasant environment.

Solve Problems

Solving problems is an important way for managers to gain and maintain their credibility among employees and colleagues. The managers in the study reported that they continually asked for input on what needed to be fixed and then they acted on that information. Some of the bigger systematic problems took longer and results often took more time, but the managers always gave feedback to their employees on what was being done to address the problems. As a result, employees felt as though progress was being made. Examples of the managers' comments included the following:

- "I try to deal with whatever they need in a very timely manner. I try and be responsive to them. They don't have to come back to me again and say, 'Whatever happened to . . . ?'"
- "People know they've been heard when the problem is solved."
- "Taking action quickly is crucial. Delay, delay, delay will kill them and the manager's reputation and credibility. If they bring something forward or you see something wrong, take care of it now."

The managers in the study also talked about the importance of establishing trials during implementation of major projects so that the bugs and glitches can be worked out early in the process. Examples of difficult system issues included:

- The speed of patient throughput
- The delays caused by neurology residents who insisted on using emergency department beds to do patient workups
- The conversion of the pharmacy distribution system to a new approach
- The implementation of electronic medical records
- The initiation of work redesign projects

Simpler problems included malfunctioning equipment and insufficient supplies.

Empower and Involve Employees in Decision Making

One of the most influential ways the managers in the study had for getting results involved using employee empowerment and participation in departmental decision making. Many of the managers' stories mentioned exemplary examples of employee involvement and participation and increased levels of autonomy and decision making among staff. Using a department council structure, encouraging and supporting employees' involvement in committees, establishing problem-solving task forces, and delegating responsibility for specific tasks were examples. The following are some responses from individuals in managerial roles:

- "A big role of the leader in this environment of retention is that you start by giving up as much power as possible. I measure my success by how little they need me anymore!"
- "I want to create more leaders in my department, people that can take the ball and run with it instead of always feeling like they have to come to me. My goal is to get them so self-sustaining that they don't need me anymore."
- "Micromanaging kills you. You've got to let go. You think you're going to do it all, but you can't. It will kill you. You've got to have everyone helping you."

The managers also reported instances when employees were empowered to deal with interpersonal issues and conflicts, order equipment and supplies without the manager's signoff, make decisions about where temporary staff was needed most, determine work schedules, and decide what types of employee education were needed. Contrary to common complaints about the unwillingness of employees to participate in department activities, the successful managers who took part in the study seemed to have little or no difficulty finding people to take on extra responsibilities. The advice they offered for other managers was that if increased staff participation in departmental activities is a goal, the participation has to be valued and supported.

If the manager asks someone to participate on a committee, for example, but fails to follow through in terms of helping that individual get the time off to go to the meetings, the result is likely to be increased frustration and decreased commitment on the part of the employee.

Empowerment of employees and managers was a dominant theme for the nurse managers in Mackoff and Triolo's (2008b) research findings. Empowerment was related to the participants' perception that their organization fostered a culture of regard. Employees and managers described being encouraged to implement their ideas and indicated that senior leaders helped this implementation by removing barriers. The managers described having the flexibility and autonomy to make decisions for their departments, knowing they would be supported by their own senior manager.

Provide Adequate Resources

A focus on results is dependent on resources. As one manager said, "It's the little things that tick people off . . . like when you go to get some linen and there's not enough there. Or you go to find a PCA [patient-controlled analgesia] pump and we don't have any." Many of the managers in the study considered it an important part of their job to make sure that employees had everything they needed to provide high-quality service. Nothing is more frustrating to employees during times of short staffing than knowing that they waste incredible amounts of time tracking down equipment (Lanser 2001), calling for supplies, or following up with co-workers and support staff who have not done their work properly. Addressing such problems requires managers to pay attention to the resource issues employees raise and to take appropriate action as quickly as possible.

Provide a Pleasant Physical Environment

Results are also dependent on the physical environment and the working conditions provided by it. In a recent study conducted by the Federation of Nurses and Health Professionals, 56 percent of the respondents cited working conditions as the biggest problem with their job (Menninger 2001). The successful managers in this study discussed improving the physical environment in ways that increased retention. Such improvements can be achieved through structural changes in the department's facilities as well as through process changes in the way services are delivered. The managers noted, for example:

- "One of the things that draws them to this department when they're being interviewed is the physical environment. That it looks clean. It's organized. It's not outdated."
- "I'm a huge gardener, so I bring in flowers and put them on tables and around the department."
- "We created a new cardiovascular inpatient department where our open-heart patients stay in the same bed throughout their stay. . . . It's rewarding for the caregivers."

- "We created a quiet room. It's beautifully decorated, has music, and an easy chair. [Employees] can go in and put their feet up and relax for a few minutes."

Partner with Employees

The last theme in leadership interventions for creating a culture of engagement relates to the way managers work with their employees. Most of the managers who participated in the study described using leadership styles based on partnership and the concept of servant leadership. They stressed the idea of working *for* their employees. Examples of the managers' comments included the following:

- "My job is to facilitate their work. I make a joke about it, but really the truth is that I work for them. They don't work for me. . . . I work for them."
- "It's understanding that it's never about me. . . . It's about we. I'm not retaining people, we are."
- "All of these things create a sense that I'm working for them and an environment where there's mutual respect between us."
- "My job, and I can never forget this, is to provide service to these employees. That's my job. I'm working for them."

These successful managers were clear that they alone could never produce a positive workplace environment, but that they must work interdependently with others. They worked together to create an environment in which people felt liberated and were willing to take risks to accomplish innovation and progress.

The type of environment the managers described is very similar to a workplace culture of coherence as described by Ponte and colleagues (2004, p. 173): "Developing a sense of coherence depends on the existence of mutual trust, a commitment to the process of working together, and a shared responsibility for practice and professional development." A culture of coherence depends on how individuals perceive their individual place in the department and the department's place in the larger organization. Coherence is a pervasive, enduring, and dynamic feeling of confidence that a person's internal and external environments are predictable, that even when the day starts badly, it is highly probable that things will work out well by the end of the day.

The key factors related to the partnership approach to engagement include high levels of visibility and accessibility to employees; clear boundaries between managers and employees; and open, positive, and direct communication.

Be Visible

Visibility was crucial for the managers in the study. In many cases, visibility was not limited to being present and being seen, but included jumping in and helping out when and where they were needed. Making patient rounds was the most common example in the patient care departments, but visibility also meant being present for employees on every shift. For these leaders, spending most of their time out in their departments was a priority—most purposely scheduled time to be visible. For example, one pharmacy director and his assistant made certain that one of them was at work early enough to see people on the night shift and the other was there late in the afternoon to overlap with people on the evening shift.

The way each of these managers pitched in and helped their employees was unique. Some were still clinically or professionally skilled, while others simply answered the telephone, got coffee for family members, brought food for employees during extremely busy times, helped out with uncomplicated work, or picked up a mop when needed.

- "Whenever I can just jump in and help out, that's a good opportunity to be with that employee."
- "I spend time out at the desk. . . . I take as much of my work out there as I can. Just to be around the people."
- "I make it a point of getting out at least once a day, making rounds and seeing everyone."

One very astute manager noted that presence does not always mean physical presence. "It's getting back to people, following through, answering their phone messages, leaving them a note in their mailbox; even if I don't have the answer, it's staying connected in all of these ways." In contrast, a factor that seemed to have a devastating effect on both managers and employees was employees seldom seeing their managers or experiencing any sense of managers' presence in the workplace.

Be Accessible

Accessibility is closely linked to visibility; however, a manager can be accessible without being visible. The managers in the study talked about how important it was for employees to have someone available to talk with about their concerns and issues. Frequently mentioned strategies included having an open-door policy, occupying an office located within the department, being available by pager, responding promptly to voice messages and e-mails, holding frequent and convenient employee meetings or team huddles, and attending to people. *Attending* means actively observing, listening, and making a concentrated effort to be present, open, and available (Clarke 1999). Examples from the interviews with the managers for the study included the following:

- "I'm out there with them. I tell them, 'I'm available. . . . This is what I'm here for. If you need me or need to talk about something, I'm here.'"
- "Things like where your office is are important. What you wear to work. If you come in dressed to work with them or you are in business

attire. Wearing the proper clothing sends the message, 'if you need my help, I'm ready.'"
- "I post my schedule on the door so people will know where I am at all times. If they want to talk to me and don't know where I am or when I am coming in, it creates a lot of frustration. This way, they know."

Maintain Clear Boundaries

Even though the managers in the study were visible and accessible to employees, they also set appropriate boundaries between themselves as leaders and their employees. Several noted that employees want a leader who clearly is a leader and not their friend. Maintaining a connection while keeping an appropriate distance was an area to which these successful managers gave attention. This concept has been validated in subsequent research on why managers stay in a position. "Boundary clarity is defined as the capacity to build strong connections with others—without losing the sense of self" (Mackoff and Triolo 2008a, p. 122). Mackoff and Triolo's research identified three dimensions of boundary clarity. These included cultivating strong internal boundaries, creating a sense of emotional buffering through disengagement, and modeling and displaying appropriate boundary management to others.

A significant issue for these leaders was balancing accessibility and visibility with a level of focus on their own tasks that allowed them to utilize their time where it would make the most difference for the department. One nurse manager described being told by the chief executive officer that she was not delegating enough. He pointed out that whenever she was in the department, people freely came up to her and asked for her input or for a decision on an issue that did not really need her level of authority. Her initial reaction to his comment was anger and defensiveness.

With reflection, however, she came to see that he had a point. To address the problem, she put a note in the department's communication book and asked people to go to the charge nurse with issues first but to feel free to come to her with problems that the charge nurse was unable to handle. The nurse manager made it clear that it was not that she did not want to hear about problems, but, in her words, "you don't ask the general if you want a weekend pass, you go to your commanding officer." She told her employees that her past level of accessibility had made it difficult for her to focus on the bigger problems in the department. The manager was surprised to find that no one on her staff had been insulted by the change or felt that she was distancing herself from them. They understood and were eager to help because they wanted her to continue to act as a strong advocate for them in the wider organization.

Provide Open and Honest Communication

It is no surprise that open and honest communication characterized the relationships between the successful managers and their employees. Participants in the study talked not only about their methods of keeping people informed but also about their philosophy of communication. For example:

- "I don't hide anything from my staff that they need to know. I hold no secrets from them."
- "We post data every month to show where we are."
- "I approach things from a 'no surprise' perspective."

These effective managers talked about the importance of creating a climate in which employees were able to give each other as well as the manager direct feedback about issues, concerns, and even the manager's performance or behavior. The managers believed that when their employees felt liberated, they would hear about problems much sooner than anyone else did. Thus, issues can be dealt with more quickly, which can keep small issues from escalating into large problems.

Open and honest communication is the foundation for all of the leadership strategies for building a culture of engagement. Listening, for example, is one way to put the employee first, and listening is clearly a specific communication skill. In the same way, focusing on results and coaching for competence would be impossible without effective communication skills.

Summary of Strategies

In the end, the effective strategies reported by managers who have successfully created a culture of engagement and retention are not complex; neither are they glitzy or expensive. In fact, they can be deceptively simple practices that, when authentically expressed, can create a workplace in which people want to work. (Figure 5-2 summarizes the interventions discussed in this chapter.)

Jim Collins's (2001) research on organizations that make the leap from being good, solid companies to being great companies has increased understanding of how to achieve excellence on an organizational basis. During an interview, Collins was asked whether he could put his finger on what really differentiated good from excellent companies. His response is telling and applicable to the research on positive workplaces: "The people in the good-to-great companies did things that seemed so incredibly obvious, straightforward, simple . . . the comparison companies may have had very smart people, brilliant, but they saw things as complex, and they had elaborate plans and complicated strategies" (Flower 2002, p. 19). In other words, the people in the organizations that never made the leap to excellence might be brilliant and capable but could not seem to grab onto simple strategies that would actually work.

The findings in this research study substantiate the foundational work presented in the first part of this book. The major themes that emerge from these data are clearly related to many of the intrinsic motivators as well as to the various forms of organizational commitment. Forging strong connections relates to the intrinsic motivator of healthy and positive working relation-

Figure 5-2.   Managerial Interventions for Successfully Creating a Culture of Engagement

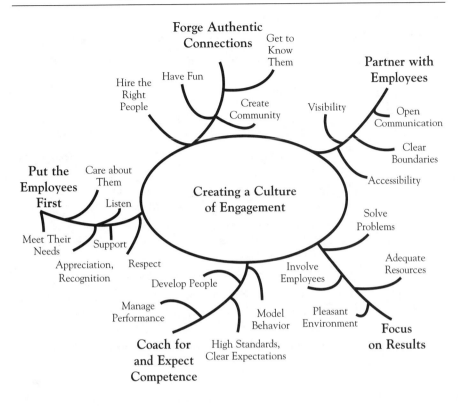

ships and forms the basis for affective commitment. The manager's focus on results produces improvements and changes in the workplace, which are clearly related to the intrinsic need to see progress as a result of efforts.

Furthermore, a key way the managers in the study obtained results was by empowering or delegating responsibility (along with an appropriate level of authority) to employees. Autonomy is an intrinsic motivator for work as well. The theme of coaching for performance and developing people supports the intrinsic motivator of competence. All five major themes as well as the factors within them demand managers and leaders whose behavior reflects the specific values held by the individual. When the managers' values are congruent with the values held by the employees, the possibility of normative commitment emerges.

One way to use the results of this study is through an assessment instrument (see figures 5-3 and 5-4). This questionnaire can be completed by the manager or supervisor of a work group or department and simultaneously by employees. Scores can be compared and where there are discrepancies, there are opportunities for conversation. This conversation can support the partnership between employees and managers in making forward progress on creating a culture of engagement in their workplace.

Figure 5-3.   Creating a Culture of Engagement Manager Survey

Directions: When you complete this questionnaire, think about your department(s). Answer by circling the number that best describes how strongly you believe the following statement describes you or the people with whom you work.

Y = Yes, Strongly Agree   S = Agree Sometimes   N = Strongly Disagree

Y   S   N   1.   I encourage the employees who report to me to challenge me in any decision I have made.

Y   S   N   2.   I trust that the employees who work with me are honorable people, and if they tell me they need something, I believe it.

Y   S   N   3.   I believe, as a leader in this organization, that I need to put the employee first.

Y   S   N   4.   I continually look for ways to show my appreciation through special gestures and events.

Y   S   N   5.   Employees in my department regularly recognize each other and participate enthusiastically in any department recognition events.

Y   S   N   6.   I continually ask employees, "What's important to you?"

Y   S   N   7.   We work hard at keeping scheduling in our department as flexible as possible in order to meet both customers' and employees' needs.

Y   S   N   8.   My employees believe I listen to them when they come with their concerns and issues.

Y   S   N   9.   The employees in this department know they have been heard when they see action taken on their issues and concerns.

Y   S   N   10. Employees feel supported by management.

Y   S   N   11. I believe each employee needs to have some kind of personal, individual connection with his or her manager.

Y   S   N   12. I believe that it is important to share something personal of myself with my employees.

Y   S   N   13. I know the names and something personal about each and every one of my employees.

Y   S   N   14. There is a strong sense of connection, of community, among people in the department.

Y   S   N   15. When an employee is having problems, other people in the department rally around and help in constructive ways.

Y   S   N   16. When interviewing job applicants, I consider the personality and "fit" of the applicant a priority for hiring.

Y   S   N   17. When seeking potential employees, I believe that technical skills are secondary to other characteristics and interpersonal skills.

Y   S   N   18. Department employees are involved actively in the hiring and selection process of new employees.

Copyright © 2009 Jo Manion. All rights reserved.

Figure 5-3. (Continued)

Y	S	N	19.	Employees in this department enjoy coming to work.
Y	S	N	20.	We enjoy spontaneous fun as well as planned fun together on a regular basis.
Y	S	N	21.	The standards for performance are very high in this department.
Y	S	N	22.	The expectations and standards are clearly articulated and communicated to everyone.
Y	S	N	23.	A strong, consistent network of coaching is available to employees in this department.
Y	S	N	24.	Development of employees is a key goal in this department.
Y	S	N	25.	I am continually asking employees, "What are you interested in learning," and "What opportunities are you interested in?"
Y	S	N	26.	I am continually aware that I must model the behavior I expect to see in my employees and colleagues.
Y	S	N	27.	I am always on the lookout for great performance so I can recognize and reward it in a concrete and immediate manner.
Y	S	N	28.	I hold people accountable for their actions, dealing with inconsistent or inadequate performance and problems immediately and consistently.
Y	S	N	29.	I deal with problems immediately and do not let them fester.
Y	S	N	30.	When employees bring me problems of an interpersonal conflict, I use my judgment about whether they should resolve the problem or whether I should intervene.
Y	S	N	31.	Most of the improvements in our department over the past year have come from ideas and concerns shared by employees.
Y	S	N	32.	I continually ask the employees, "What needs to be fixed?"
Y	S	N	33.	If a problem brought by an employee cannot be solved, I at least get back to the employee in a timely manner to let him or her know what I have done.
Y	S	N	34.	We have a specific structure for involving employees in decision making in this department (department council, governance structure, problem-solving teams, etc.).
Y	S	N	35.	Employees are instrumental in helping make decisions that affect the department.
Y	S	N	36.	Our department's committees, councils, and teams are robust and active.
Y	S	N	37.	If I ask employees to participate in a committee or task force, I make certain they have the time scheduled off to attend the meeting and I actively coach them so they are prepared for their participation.

Copyright © 2009 Jo Manion. All rights reserved.

(Continued on next page)

Figure 5-3.   (Continued)

Y	S	N	38.	I consider an important part of my job is making certain that employees have the necessary equipment and supplies to do their job.
Y	S	N	39.	Employees are authorized to obtain adequate supplies and equipment, even in my absence.
Y	S	N	40.	I work to ensure that the physical environment of our department is clean, organized, and pleasing.
Y	S	N	41.	I believe that my most important job as leader is to facilitate the work of the employees.
Y	S	N	42.	I believe that I work for the employee, rather than the employee works for me, regardless of my status or positional authority.
Y	S	N	43.	I regularly see employees on all shifts.
Y	S	N	44.	I jump in and help out employees with their work on a regular basis.
Y	S	N	45.	Employees know when I am available or how to find me when they need something.
Y	S	N	46.	I am readily visible throughout the department throughout the day.
Y	S	N	47.	I don't hide anything from my employees that they need to know. I don't believe in secrets.
Y	S	N	48.	We have multiple methods of communicating important information within the department.
Y	S	N	49.	We have regular department or staff meetings that include active dialogue on current issues and concerns.
Y	S	N	50.	My employees are comfortable giving me direct feedback.

Scoring Directions: Count up the number of Ys, Ss, and Ns. Each Y is two points, each S is one point, and each N is zero. Total the number of points by clusters of ten questions.

Total for Questions   1–10   _____   (Put staff first)

Total for Questions 11–20   _____   (Forge strong connections)

Total for Questions 21–30   _____   (Coach for and expect competence)

Total for Questions 31–40   _____   (Focus on results)

Total for Questions 41–50   _____   (Partner with employees)

        TOTAL   _____

Interpretation: If your total score is 90–100, your workplace is likely to have a culture of retention; if your score is 70–89, you have opportunities for strengthening the environment. If your score is 69 or below . . . get going! Either get going to try and change things, or just get going!

Copyright © 2009 Jo Manion. All rights reserved.

Figure 5-4.   Creating a Culture of Engagement Employee Survey

Directions: When you complete this questionnaire, think about your department(s) and the employees with whom you work. Answer by circling the letter that best describes how strongly you believe the following statement describes your situation.

Y = Yes, Strongly Agree   S = Agree Sometimes   N = Strongly Disagree

Y   S   N   1.   We feel free to challenge any management decision in a respectful way.

Y   S   N   2.   Management believes that I am an honorable person, and if I tell my manager I need something, he or she believes me.

Y   S   N   3.   My manager puts the employee first when making decisions and solving problems.

Y   S   N   4.   My manager continually looks for ways to show his or her appreciation through special gestures and events.

Y   S   N   5.   Employees in my department regularly recognize each other and participate enthusiastically in any department recognition events.

Y   S   N   6.   Employees are frequently asked, "What's important to you?"

Y   S   N   7.   We work hard at keeping scheduling in our department as flexible as possible in order to meet both customers' and employees' needs.

Y   S   N   8.   My manager listens to me when I come with my concerns and issues.

Y   S   N   9.   Employees in this department know they have been heard when they see action taken on their issues and concerns.

Y   S   N   10.   Employees feel supported by management.

Y   S   N   11.   Each employee has some kind of personal, individual connection with the manager.

Y   S   N   12.   I know something personal about my manager.

Y   S   N   13.   My manager knows the names and something personal about each and every one of the employees who works here.

Y   S   N   14.   There is a strong sense of connection, of community, among people in the department.

Y   S   N   15.   When an employee is having problems, other people in the department rally around and help in constructive ways.

Y   S   N   16.   When interviewing job applicants for this department, we consider the personality and "fit" of the applicant a priority for hiring.

Y   S   N   17.   Technical skills are secondary to other characteristics and interpersonal skills when we seek new employees.

Y   S   N   18.   Department employees are involved actively in the hiring and selection process of new employees.

Copyright © 2009 Jo Manion. All rights reserved.

(Continued on next page)

Figure 5-4.   (Continued)

Y	S	N	19.	Employees in this department enjoy coming to work.
Y	S	N	20.	We enjoy spontaneous fun as well as planned fun together on a regular basis.
Y	S	N	21.	The standards for performance are very high in this department.
Y	S	N	22.	The expectations and standards are clearly articulated and communicated to everyone.
Y	S	N	23.	A strong, consistent network of coaching is available to employees in this department.
Y	S	N	24.	Development of employees is a key goal in this department.
Y	S	N	25.	Managers frequently ask employees, "What are you interested in learning," and "What opportunities are you interested in?"
Y	S	N	26.	Our manager models the behavior he or she expects to see in employees and colleagues.
Y	S	N	27.	My manager is always on the lookout for great performance in order to recognize and reward it in a concrete and immediate manner.
Y	S	N	28.	My manager holds people accountable for their actions, dealing with inconsistent or inadequate performance and problems immediately and consistently.
Y	S	N	29.	My manager deals with problems immediately and does not let them fester.
Y	S	N	30.	When employees bring the manager problems of an inter-personal conflict, the manager uses his or her judgment about whether he or she should resolve the problem or coach and encourage the employees to do so.
Y	S	N	31.	Most of the improvements in our department over the past year have come from ideas and concerns shared by employees.
Y	S	N	32.	Employees are frequently asked, "What needs to be fixed?"
Y	S	N	33.	If a problem brought by an employee cannot be solved, the manager at least gets back to the employee in a timely manner to let him or her know what has been done.
Y	S	N	34.	We have a specific structure for involving employees in decision making in this department (department council, governance structure, problem-solving teams, etc.).
Y	S	N	35.	Employees are instrumental in helping make decisions that affect the department.
Y	S	N	36.	Our department's committees, councils, and teams are robust and active.
Y	S	N	37.	If employees are asked to participate in a committee or task force, the manager makes certain they have the time scheduled off to attend the meeting and actively coaches them so they are prepared for their participation.

Copyright © 2009 Jo Manion. All rights reserved.

Figure 5-4. (Continued)

Y	S	N	38.	The manager sees an important part of his or her job as making certain that employees have the necessary equipment and supplies to do their job.
Y	S	N	39.	Employees are authorized to obtain adequate supplies and equipment, even in the manager's absence.
Y	S	N	40.	The manager works to ensure that the physical environment of our department is clean, organized, and pleasing.
Y	S	N	41.	The manager believes that one of his or her most important jobs as leader is to facilitate the work of our employees.
Y	S	N	42.	Our manager believes that he or she works for us employees, rather than the employees work for him or her.
Y	S	N	43.	Our manager regularly sees employees on all shifts.
Y	S	N	44.	Our manager jumps in and helps out employees with their work on a regular basis.
Y	S	N	45.	Employees know when the manager is available or how to find him or her when they need something.
Y	S	N	46.	The manager is readily visible throughout the department throughout the day.
Y	S	N	47.	The manager doesn't hide anything from employees that they need to know. The manager doesn't believe in secrets.
Y	S	N	48.	We have multiple methods of communicating important information within the department.
Y	S	N	49.	We have regular department or staff meetings that include active dialogue on current issues and concerns.
Y	S	N	50.	Employees are comfortable giving the manager direct feedback.

Scoring Directions: Count up the number of Ys, Ss, and Ns. Each Y is two points, each S is one point, and each N is zero. Total the number of points by clusters of ten questions.

Total for Questions 1–10	_____	(Put staff first)
Total for Questions 11–20	_____	(Forge strong connections)
Total for Questions 21–30	_____	(Coach for and expect competence)
Total for Questions 31–40	_____	(Focus on results)
Total for Questions 41–50	_____	(Partner with employees)
TOTAL	_____	

Interpretation: If your total score is 90–100, your workplace is likely to have a culture of retention; if your score is 70–89, you have opportunities for strengthening the environment. If your score is 69 or below . . . get going! Either get going to try and change things, or just get going!

Copyright © 2009 Jo Manion. All rights reserved.

Organizational Ramifications of Positive Leadership Strategies

It is clear from the findings presented in this chapter that simply expecting more and more from today's managers without providing ways to increase their capacity is a no-win situation for everyone. The participants were asked how their organizations supported them. Although at least half of the participating managers felt a strong level of support from within their organizations, too frequently comments like this one were heard: "It's hard to keep doing this for employees when no one does it for me." When organizations are serious about improving their work environment and reducing costly turnover, one approach they can take is simple: Provide the same support to managers that the managers are expected to provide to their employees. Complaining that the organization cannot afford to take these steps is shortsighted and ultimately destructive. An organization cannot afford to ignore investing in practices that help it keep its best people.

When the managers in the study were asked the question, "What would make your job easier?" the responses were not surprising. The managers asked for adequate administrative support, more visibility from senior leadership, more manageable spans of control, and the cooperation of physicians in retention efforts. Put simply, the managers needed everyone to do what they are supposed to do. They said:

- "There is a lack of insight into just how much they've asked us to do. Unrealistic deadlines, meetings, expectations. It's just overwhelming."
- "What would help? Having support for some of the mindless details that have to be taken care of."
- "Even a day or two a week of secretarial support, 10 to 12 hours, just to help with the paperwork."
- "Physicians have to understand that their behavior affects people. Their outbursts, their sarcasm, their flippant remarks. Staff take it to heart."
- "If I had any support. I don't feel like I can trust anyone."
- "If every department would just do what it's supposed to do."

Support from Senior Leadership

Managers need support, and to provide effective support, senior leaders (in this case, any leader to whom managers report directly) must examine the evidence rather than rely on anecdotal experiences or interventions that were effective in the past.

What can senior leaders do to support employee engagement and retention efforts? The research suggests the following recommendations:

1. Understand which leadership behaviors make the difference, and support managers in implementing those behaviors.

2. Help managers deal with polarities in their leadership practice.
3. Negotiate for a strong supportive partnership role from the human resources department.
4. Remove organizational barriers to getting results.
5. Encourage managers to develop a support network.
6. Listen to what the managers tell you.
7. Encourage managers to learn from each other through appreciative inquiry.

Support Effective Behaviors

Although executing many of these simple interventions appears to be within the direct control of front-line managers, too many mixed messages from the organization sometimes make managers reluctant to take action. For example, how can managers ensure their own visibility and accessibility when they are scheduled to spend six to eight hours every day in meetings outside their department? How can managers form authentic connections with their staff when they have a hundred or more direct reports? How can managers put their employees first and focus on results and employee development when they are bogged down with administrative responsibilities such as managing payroll, tracking absenteeism, verifying certifications, filing new policies in binders, and finding information for other departments?

In many health care organizations today, the demands placed on managers border on being unrealistic and overwhelming, and one glaring example of a significant inconsistency is in the availability of administrative support for managers. Most departments in hospitals employ secretaries who work closely with department managers to support administrative functions; however, patient care departments are a clear exception. Most nurse managers have minimal or no dedicated administrative support even though nurse managers, like their counterparts in other departments, are expected to run multimillion-dollar business operations, manage large numbers of people who often work from multiple locations, and basically deal with one of the most complex organizational systems known.

Each patient care department usually employs a full-time support person, called a unit secretary, to serve as the department's receptionist and coordinator of traffic, to support patient care, and to provide clerical assistance for the physicians who flow in and out of the department every day. However, most unit secretaries are too busy to provide consistent, dependable administrative support for nurse managers. This issue simply has not been addressed adequately by most health care organizations.

Numerous examples were given of nurse managers in this study who, when asked by an executive, "What can we do to make your work easier?" responded by saying, "I need consistent, qualified secretarial support." The response to this request in almost all of these instances was some variation of, "Nurse managers in this organization will never have their own secretaries." This response may well reflect the reality in most organizations, but if it does, it suggests that organization executives are not listening to what the managers are saying. In the end, they are likely to continue to see a high level of nurse manager turnover at a time when it is critical that every health care manager is able to function at the highest capacity possible. Keep in mind that turnover is not limited to physical departure. How can a person continue to stay committed to an organization that seems to misunderstand and devalue the work they do?

One participant in the study discussed her extreme frustration with this situation. Karen was a second-career nurse who came to the health care field with extensive business experience. Because of her performance and skills, she rose quickly to a management position. At the time of her initial interview during this study, she was the manager of two inpatient orthopedic departments. During her tenure as a manager, she repeatedly communicated her needs for support and felt increasingly frustrated at the lack of response to her requests. Eventually, she resigned, much to the consternation of the nurse executive and the chief operating officer, both of whom recognized that Karen was probably the most competent manager they had. At their request, she met with the chief executive officer to discuss her concerns before she made the resignation final.

In her meeting she challenged the executive directly in his thinking: "You keep talking about health care as a business and telling us that we have to be good business people. Give me an example of a business where a manager has responsibility for eighty employees, two geographical locations, and a multimillion dollar annual budget but is told that she cannot have a secretary!" The executive was unable to rebut her argument, and he could not think of an example of a business that would organize itself this way. The end result? Karen was given permission to use the unit secretary's services for a specific, dedicated amount of time each week. This was hardly a satisfactory solution. The decision meant a reduction in the amount of support available to the rest of the department. At the end of the year, Karen was given a $10,000 bonus in her paycheck. She was furious and returned the money with the response, "I didn't ask for more money, I asked for help!" Her case became just another example of senior management not hearing what a manager was desperately trying to communicate.

Because effective managers are the key to creating a positive work environment, organizations ought to be looking for anything they can do to increase their managers' capacity. To do so requires conducting a careful review of each manager's activities, implementing up-to-date technological support, and providing consistent administrative support. Senior leaders need to open-mindedly consider the key factors that lead to a manager's success and then honestly ask themselves whether the organization is providing the resources the manager needs to be successful.

Help Managers Deal with Polarities

The manager is a bridge between operational and administrative practices in the organization. A bridge is a sturdy structure that provides a path between two widely separated banks. Organizationally, bridges ensure the open flow of energy, information, knowledge, and other resources between the various parts of the organization. To keep this flow moving requires a lot of support. All five of the interventions identified through this study require judgment in their application. Issues such as visibility and accessibility are not problems to be solved but rather polarities to be managed.

For example, within the nursing profession it took years to transition from the "head nurse in white uniform" image to the nurse manager dressed in business clothes who appears more managerial than clinical. Yet the managers who took part in this study strongly believed that it was better for them to appear for work in clinical uniforms, at least part of the time. For some nurse managers, returning to clinical garb may seem a step backward. However, what the successful managers in the study were saying is that if their primary responsibility is the management of a clinical function, some very real requirements had to be met for presence, comfort, and ability to fit into a clinical environment, even to the point of occasionally performing clinical services. Dressing in clinical garb every day may be inappropriate for occasions that require business attire. And always appearing in business attire can result in distancing from the clinical staff. Whether the manager is a director of nursing, a director of pharmacy, or a director of physical therapy, the same principle holds true.

These other interventions all entail polarities to be managed:

- How to get to know employees and forge strong connections without becoming too personally involved
- How to set high standards and expectations and yet know when standards, policies, and practices can be bent to create a more humane workplace
- How to be accessible to staff without becoming fragmented and distracted
- How to support and become involved with people dealing with personal problems without developing or encouraging codependent relationships

Managing the polarities entailed in a managerial position is easier with the support and guidance of trusted senior mentors and coaches.

Negotiate a Supportive Partnership Role with Human Resources

It is very clear that if first-line managers are to successfully create a culture of engagement, they must be able to manage employee performance effectively. Performance management concentrates on eliminating unacceptable performance. Although some of the managers in the study identified human resources as one of their key supports, many others characterized human resources staff in a much more negative light, with comments ranging from "they are no help at all" to "they are a barrier to effectively managing performance." Many managers also referred to the damaging effects that their inability to deal effectively with employee performance issues had on their credibility and the credibility of the organization as a whole.

In some organizations, it is not reasonable to expect individual managers to negotiate a positive relationship with human resources alone. Senior leaders, often at the executive level, must insist on an effective working partnership between the manager and the organization's human resources department. It has to be an expectation that is supported at the highest levels in the organization.

Remove Organizational Barriers that Hinder Results

For managers to be credible in the eyes of their employees and physician colleagues, they must be perceived as efficacious in getting problems solved, issues dealt with, and improvements made. Today's health care organization is so complex and interdependent that many of the problems in a department are really system issues, or at least have ramifications for the broader system. This situation makes it more difficult for a single manager to effect needed results. The more processes in health care organizations can be simplified to enable managers to solve problems, the better.

Managers not only need the skills and competencies to resolve issues but they also must have the authority they need to act. Providing this authority is a powerful way to support managers. Granting clear authority or giving permission is necessary when expecting managers to deal with issues. In some instances, problems require the intervention of individuals with higher levels of authority. When this assistance is readily available, the manager is more likely to feel supported. For example, a manager may have tried dealing with a fellow department manager about a problem situation, yet nothing has been resolved. When the manager brings this problem forward, those at higher authority levels in the organization need to recognize that this issue is being elevated and may require the involvement of those with more authority to help solve it. Continuing to expect the two department managers to "just work it out" is not supportive, nor always appropriate, behavior.

Standardizing methods of process improvement and preparing all employees with these techniques are other ways of removing typical organizational barriers. When the manager has a cadre of employees who understand and are capable of using process improvement methods, real results can be obtained. Tolerating problems leads to a sense of futility on the part of everyone.

In some instances, removing organizational barriers is as simple as communicating with other people in the organization to let them know who is accepting responsibility for dealing with an issue. Asking others to support this individual is a way of garnering organizational support. For example, the managers of the emergency department and the admitting department are named as co-chairs of a process improvement committee to resolve the issues surrounding patient throughput. When this announcement is made by the executive team, the message is clear: These people have been delegated this responsibility, and it is necessary for everyone to respond to their requests as if they had been made by senior leadership.

Encourage Managers to Develop a Support Network

Research conducted by AbuAlRub (2004) recognizes the importance of social support for coping with stress in the workplace. Managers should be encouraged to develop support networks consisting of their peers. One manager told of getting together with her peers for lunch every Friday afternoon. After debriefing the week and sharing issues, the lunchmates leave for home and an early start to the weekend. In other organizations, the encouragement of senior leaders may be needed before managers feel comfortable taking an afternoon away from their departments—even though most first-line managers already work significantly more than forty hours per week.

In some cases frustration was expressed by study participants who reported that there was simply no time to keep in touch with their peers, much less talk through issues and provide support to each other. Of even more concern was the finding that in some health care organizations, exemplary managers are ostracized by their fellow managers who are afraid that their colleagues' success makes them look bad in the eyes of other people in the organization. One young manager who had taken over a toxic, dysfunctional department worked hard at turning around the negative culture. She was successful, much to the dismay of her colleagues, who told her, "Stop it. You're making us look bad! If you can do [it], we're going to be expected to do it as well."

Listen to Managers

Successful managers in the study reported that one of their most important responsibilities was listening to their employees. In the same way, if the frontline managers are to feel supported, senior leaders must listen when the frontline managers tell them about their difficulties. Individuals will not feel as though they have been heard until something is done with the information they communicated. Senior leaders need to ask probing questions to learn what needs to be fixed and where the managers' frustrations lie. In fact, several managers identified feeling supported by behavior that demonstrated that they had been heard:

- "I have always been able to say what I needed to say."
- "They give me the latitude to be who I am, they want to know who I am."
- "I feel supported by my boss, and it's okay to make mistakes. She says, 'We trust you in that position to do what you do. Tell me what you need me to do.'"

Encourage Managers to Learn from Each Other

Appreciative inquiry is an approach to organizational learning that assumes something is already going right in the organization, for example, that some managers implement effective strategies that lead to employee engagement and retention. Finding those who are successful and then encouraging other managers to learn from their practices is a useful intervention. However, it requires finesse and tact to avoid making the successful manager uncomfortable and creating unnecessary tension among colleagues. Treating success as an opportunity to learn and openly discussing what the manager has done that led to success can increase the level of organizational learning in the group. Remember, however, that all managers need not do things in the same way. Finding a unique approach that works for each department is the key to success; applying cookie-cutter approaches can yield unanticipated negative results.

For example, Joan, a manager who participated in the study, described her anger at the standardized approach used by her organization in response to very poor employee satisfaction ratings. Based on the recommendations of a popular consulting group, Joan received an e-mail telling her that in the future she would be required to "write down who [she] sent thank-you notes to on the staff. It was insulting!" She was furious when she was required to attend a three-hour in-service to learn how to write thank-you notes. Joan's response: "I've been sending people handwritten thank-you notes for years." She added that to make matters worse, within two weeks after the mandatory educational program, she had received handwritten thank-you notes from both her executive and her director. Having never received a thank you from either of them in the past, much less a handwritten note, it was clear to Joan that she was merely an assignment to them, which just added fuel to her fury.

The sad truth is that although leaders have access to the hundreds of success stories in hospitals across the United States, they often fail to capitalize on what successful managers already know. Appreciative inquiry is an opportunity to learn from other managers. (This process is discussed more thoroughly in chapter 8.) If the organization was a true learning organization, systematic ways would be in place to learn from internal successes, and perhaps, less need would arise for expensive external consultants. The trap in relying on external help is the tendency to implement their recommendations without taking into account the unique culture and people in the organization.

Summary

Developing and retaining good managers are critical in today's health care organizations. The credibility of the manager and his or her capacity to establish effective relationships with employees is a central factor in employee commitment and engagement. Understanding which managerial and leadership interventions lead to a positive workplace based on management and leadership evidence is crucial. Once the key strategies available are understood, first-line managers can be encouraged to adopt effective management practices that lead to employee engagement and retention. Specifically, coaching for these skills in frontline leaders can help them attain higher levels of success and make their work more enjoyable. Organizations and senior leaders who are serious about improving the work environment and reducing costly turnover can use the recommendations outlined in this chapter.

Conversation Points

Organizational Perspective

1. If a research team approached your organization and asked for the names of exceptional managers to participate in a study of how they have created a culture of engagement, how many would be recommended? How many first-line managers have successfully created a culture of engagement and retention in their departments?
2. Most organizations claim that people are their most important asset, and yet the organizations' behavior does not reflect this philosophy. What organizational behaviors and practices do you see that demonstrate the idea that employees should come first (so employees will put their patients or customers first)?
3. Do well-received, positive forms of recognition and demonstrations of appreciation occur on a regular basis in your organization? Are some of the activities celebrated in an organization-wide event, such as an employee recognition night or a summer picnic, as well as at the individual level? Do employees perceive these efforts as authentic demonstrations of appreciation? How are these varied from year to year?
4. How are healthy working relationships encouraged in the organization? Do executives and other senior leaders have good working relationships with employees? How much hierarchical thinking and behavior take place?
5. Are managers listened to when they express concerns? Are they encouraged to be honest about their needs?
6. Is there a concrete, specific plan for the retention of managers?

Leader Perspective

1. Have you created a positive workplace in which a culture of engagement exists among employees?
2. What do you do to demonstrate that you put your employees first? What are examples of concrete behavior?
3. What is the quality of your working relationships with your employees? Do you genuinely care for them? Or is this emotion uncomfortable to feel and express in the workplace? Do you know the names and interests of all of the employees in your department?
4. What progress have you been able to achieve in the past four months on problems that make working in the department difficult? Have you seen any substantial improvement in the issues you and your employees are dealing with?

5. How much time during a week do you spend deliberately coaching employees on their development? When was the last time you sat down with each of your employees and had a conversation about their career plans or job aspirations?
6. What level of support do you feel from senior leadership or the organization as a whole? Have you had a conversation with the person to whom you report about your need for more or different support? What was the reaction? What is your next step?
7. What would make your job easier? Have you communicated this information to anyone?

Employee Perspective

1. On a scale of 1 to 10, with 10 being the most positive, how would you rate your work environment? What would it have been three years ago (that is, if you worked there then)?
2. What specific things do you do to help your manager create a positive workplace?
3. Do you put the patient (or customer) first? What are the barriers, if any, to doing so? Do you feel like employees are put first by your manager?
4. What is the quality of relationships within your department? With people in other departments? What could you do to improve those relationships?
5. Do you see any signs of progress in your work area? Are long-term problems being addressed? Do you anticipate changes that will help you do your work more effectively in the future?
6. Do you feel as though you are treated as a partner by your manager? Do you see senior leaders on a fairly regular basis?

6

Building Healthy Relationships in the Workplace

Jo Manion

Few can walk alone.
—Mary Wollstonecraft

PEOPLE EXIST in webs of relationships, the quality of which directly affects the richness of life and the degree to which an individual perceives himself or herself to be happy. In chapter 2, the presence of healthy relationships is identified as a motivator, and chapter 3 examines the role of healthy relationships in forming commitment. Although a few people in health care organizations do work primarily alone, they are still immersed in a complex network of relationships in which others rely on them or they rely on others to carry out their work. Interdependence is the nature of relationships in any health care organization. For this reason, a primary strategy for creating a positive workplace is the formation and cultivation of healthy working relationships among people.

Simply the number and range of relationships to be considered make them a complex issue. The relationships among co-workers in the same work group, among people in the same department on the various shifts, among co-workers in different job categories, and between employees and their manager must be considered. In chapter 5, the importance of a positive relationship between the manager and the employee was discussed and identified as being of primary importance in retention. In addition, the relationships between employees and other key stakeholders such as physicians, vendors, and people from other departments must be considered. Not to be left out, relationships between employees and customers or patients are also critical. Thus, an issue that may seem relatively straightforward can become overwhelming owing to its sheer magnitude.

This chapter explores aspects of healthy relationships between individuals. Chapter 7 explores the importance of group or collective relationships, and the impact of teams and the importance of a sense of community in creating a positive workplace are addressed. The basic principles of relationship formation remain the same and can be transferred from the individual

This chapter is adapted from *From Management to Leadership: Practical Strategies for Health Care Leaders*, second edition, by Jo Manion. Copyright © 2005 Jossey-Bass Publishers. This material is used by permission of John Wiley & Sons, Inc.

level to the collective level; however, several additional aspects should be considered when the relationships involve members of the same team. Clearly, the formation of healthy working relationships among individuals often precipitates the development of community within the work group.

Leadership Relationship

The relationship between manager and employees is the one most closely examined in this chapter. Because managers play a pivotal role in the creation of a positive workplace, they are the focal point of this chapter. Bear in mind, however, that the principles explored apply to all relationships. Also note that although both the terms *manager* and *leader* are used, they are not synonymous. Not all leaders are managers; many of the effective leaders in health care organizations do not hold formal management positions. Simply attaining the position of manager does not make a person an effective leader (Manion 1998, 2005). However, for the manager to be fully effective in creating a positive workplace, the basic nature of his or her relationship with employees is that of leader to follower. Thus *leader* and *manager* are used interchangeably in the context of this chapter even though they may not be used synonymously in the context of a work environment.

Leadership exists only within the context of a relationship. It is an intensely personal experience, a process of relating to another person who becomes a follower. All definitions of leadership include the ability to influence others to do what needs to be done. Leadership is a dynamic interaction between the leader and the follower, and, as a result, both are changed irrevocably. It was noted earlier in this book that emphasis is increasing on the importance of the relationship between the leader and the follower for the formation of a positive workplace environment that leads to a culture of engagement and retention. Yet few managers today have been taught or prepared in how to develop close interpersonal relationships with their employees. In fact, as Wall (2007, p. 66) notes, "Many leaders choose to hold their direct reports at arm's length. Building relationships takes time and the desire to get to know, and become known, at a personal level. Some argue that personal distance makes it easier to hold people accountable." Other experts, such as Gottman (2007, p. 45), disagree with this attitude: "managers need to connect deeply with followers to ensure outstanding performance, and we celebrate leaders who have the emotional intelligence to engage and inspire their people by creating bonds that are authentic and reliable."

Research in the area of emotional intelligence clearly demonstrates that the emotions of the leader directly affect the atmosphere as well as the quality of the leader's relationships with others. The emotionally intelligent leader is described as one who is able "to generate excitement, optimism, and passion for the job ahead, as well as to cultivate an atmosphere of cooperation and trust" (Goleman, Boyatzis, and McKee 2002, p. 29). Leaders need competencies in four different domains: self-awareness, self-management, social awareness, and relationship management. Figure 6-1

Figure 6-1.   Emotional Intelligence Competencies (Cherniss and Goleman 2001)

	Self (personal competence)	**Other (social competence)**
Recognition	**Self-awareness** Emotional self-awareness Accurate self-assessment Self-confidence	**Social awareness** Empathy Service orientation Organizational Awareness
Regulation	**Self-management** Emotional self-control Trustworthiness Conscientiousness Adaptability Achievement drive Initiative	**Relationship management** Developing others Influence Communication Conflict management Visionary leadership Catalyzing change Building bonds Teamwork/collaboration

Reprinted from *The Emotionally Intelligent Workplace*, edited by Cary Cherniss and Daniel Goleman. Copyright © 2001 Jossey-Bass Publishers. This material is used by permission of John Wiley & Sons, Inc.

presents these four domains as well as the competencies that exist within them. Closely intertwined, these competencies form the basis for effectiveness in the workplace.

Emotional intelligence was first described by Mayer, Salovey, and Caruso (2000, p. 396) as "the ability to perceive and express emotion, assimilate emotion in thought, understand and reason with emotion, and regulate emotion in the self and others." The emotionally intelligent individual has a high degree of self-awareness and is able to recognize his or her own emotions. Not only is this self-awareness accurate but, importantly, the individual is able to regulate his or her response to the emotion. The example used in the preceding chapter of a manager who was confronted by several employees in the department about her seemingly neutral response to a recent administrative decision about which the employees were very angry is a good illustration of this point. They confronted their manager, surprised she was not angry about the situation. The leader's response took them by surprise when she replied, "Oh, do not mistake me, I am very angry about this decision, but that doesn't mean I have to spew all that negativity out and infect everyone around me! I can control my emotions and not let them infect everyone else." In her brief words, the employees were given a beautiful role model of an emotionally intelligent leader capable of emotional self-regulation.

But emotional intelligence is not limited to the individual and personal levels. The leader also is competent in relationships with others, both in social awareness and in relationship management. These competencies build on the personal competencies of recognition (emotional self-awareness, accurate self-assessment, and self-confidence) as well as self-regulation (emotional self-control, trustworthiness, conscientiousness, adaptability, achievement drive, and initiative). The social competencies related to social awareness include empathy, service orientation, and organizational aware-ness (Cherniss and Goleman 2001). Having social skills means knowing what to say and when to say it so that interactions with another person are effective and both parties get what they want. Effective leaders have well-developed social skills.

The quality and depth of the relationship between the leader and the follower directly affect the abilities of the leader. Without a strong foundation for a healthy relationship, the aspiring leader cannot attain extraordinary outcomes. Although troubled leaders seldom return to the basic components of a healthy relationship when they are frustrated by followers who do not follow, but the answer to their difficulties often lies within this basic concept.

Developing and maintaining healthy relationships among people seems like it should be a simple proposition, and yet there are many ramifications for those seeking to do so in an organization. First, people who work together must share an understanding of what precisely is meant by a healthy relation-ship. Unfortunately, many people would not recognize a healthy relationship if it was staring them in the face. Misconceptions abound regarding what comprises a vibrant, dynamic relationship. For some people it means not making waves, going along to get along, and being accommodating to the other person. For others it means not being direct and honest about how they feel in a situation because it may hurt the other person's feelings or the other person may not agree with them. The first step is to be clear about what is meant by a healthy relationship in an organizational context. Figure 6-2 presents a sample of behavioral expectations that clearly address the compo-nents of a healthy relationship. This list was developed by an organization in an attempt to define and communicate clearly what it meant by a healthy working relationship.

Second, once clear about the meaning of a healthy relationship, all employees must be told, "You have two responsibilities to the organization. The first is to do the work for which you were hired, at the quality we expect. The second is to create and maintain healthy working relationships with the other people in this workplace." Too many employees and managers believe that healthy working relationships in a work situation are the responsibil-ity of the manager. The manager is expected to deal with interpersonal conflicts, communicate negative or constructive feedback, and generally act as the spokesperson for the department when difficulties arise. In posi-tive workplaces, the creation and maintenance of healthy relationships are accepted as everyone's responsibility, and the level of understanding is con-sistent about what a healthy relationship entails. Once these expectations have been clarified and accepted, then everyone is held accountable for his or her own behavior.

An important organizational ramification for those interested in cre-ating a positive work environment is the recognition of the relationship

Figure 6-2.   Sample Behavioral Expectations

In this organization, we expect the following of all employees:

1. To develop and maintain positive and healthy interpersonal relationships with others in the workplace
   a. Communicates openly, directly, and honestly with other employees
   b. Gives both positive and negative feedback in an affirming, supportive manner
   c. Shares ideas and opinions in a positive and honest manner even if these differ from peers or managers
   d. Maintains a positive attitude toward others (and speaks positively of others in their absence)
   e. Follows through on commitments and promises made
   f. Assumes other people have positive intentions
   g. Shows respect for and values the diverse skills, abilities, and characteristics of other employees
   h. Expresses appreciation of others
   i. Shares work-appropriate information openly with others on a need-to-know basis
   j. Accepts and respects differences (in approach, styles, and personalities) of co-workers
   k. Has a will-do attitude
   l. Seeks mutually beneficial solutions when solving problems or resolving issues
   m. Maintains confidentiality and does not talk about co-workers' sensitive or personal business to others

2. To work interdependently with co-workers and employees from all departments
   a. Looks for ways to help others and makes self available
   b. Works at a steady pace and carries an equitable share of the workload
   c. Supports the goals of the organization and department by behaving and acting in a manner that helps achieve these goals
   d. Participates positively and successfully completes any needed cross-training
   e. Is willing to learn new skills and grows in ability to take on new responsibilities
   f. Keeps co-workers and manager informed so they can work as effectively as possible
   g. Focuses on similarities between co-workers rather than using differences to separate and isolate
   h. Cooperates with others
   i. Shares responsibility and delegates appropriately
   j. Does what needs to be done for good patient care or customer service regardless of whose job it is
   k. Shares knowledge and expertise openly with other people

3. To participate actively and positively in ongoing department and team processes
   a. Attends department and team meetings
   b. Initiates problem-solving activities when issues or problems occur repeatedly
   c. Supports the department's decisions even when they disagree personally
   d. Works with co-workers and manager to achieve the department's goals and outcomes
   e. Works to help the department and organization succeed

between managerial span of control (the number of direct reports, etc.) and the quality of the leader–follower relationship. Establishing meaningful and healthy relationships with all employees is time-consuming and demanding work. Clearly the number of direct reports affects the ability of a manager to accomplish this feat. One large, integrated health system decided to determine if span of control really mattered or if it was just an excuse used by managers for falling short of expectations. The results revealed that managers with small spans of control had higher levels of shared problem solving, helping and cooperation, mutual respect, and shared goals and knowledge with their employees. "Managers with larger spans of control managed at arm's length, enforced standards and rules, and had less positive interactions with direct reports" (Cathcart et al. 2004, p. 396). The organization's researchers used Gallup measures to determine levels of employee engagement and found that engagement scores dropped most noticeably as work group sizes grew larger than fifteen, and then again as work group sizes grew larger than forty.

As a result of this study, the organization modified its management structure, reducing the span of control for managers who had more than eighty employees reporting to them directly. The addition of management positions resulted in an overall 30 percent to 50 percent reduction in the span of control for managers. The study was repeated a year later and revealed that in each area where the span of control was reduced, a positive change was observed in the employee engagement mean score. The organization concluded that span of control does matter.

Definition of a Healthy Relationship

Although these concepts may seem self-evident, Dr. Phil McGraw's psychological self-help television show would not be so popular today if more people understood and embraced the simple elements of good relationships. Those people who have an inherent ability to relate comfortably to others often take this talent for forming relationships for granted. The naturalness and spontaneity in relationships result in mutually beneficial outcomes. When a particular situation is not going well, the relationship-centered individual often reflects first on the quality of the connection with the other person to determine potential problem areas. And, because this person is already skillful in the relationship arena, the assessment process is not likely to produce undue anxiety. If, however, the individual is not naturally talented at forming strong relationships, discomfort may be experienced during this assessment process. The good news is that it is possible to develop relationship-building skills or strengthen them if the innate talent is already present.

Three essential elements are identified here that are needed in a successful working relationship between individuals: trust, mutual respect, and communication. These three elements are described as essential because the absence of any one of the three can damage or reduce the effectiveness of the relationship. (See figure 6-3.) It is readily apparent that the circle in figure 6-3 would not be complete without all three elements. Each of these elements is discussed below in some detail, with a primary focus on the leader–follower relationship, especially the manager–employee relationship. However, the concepts likely apply to all relationships, whether personal or professional.

Trust

According to *Webster's Encyclopedic Unabridged Dictionary*, one who enjoys trust can rely on the "integrity, strength or ability of a person or thing. Confidence implies conscious trust because of good reasons, definite evidence or past experience." The importance of trust in the leader–follower relationship is clear. Without trust or confidence in the person attempting to influence them, people do not follow the leader's direction. In organizations, when the leader also holds legitimate positional authority, the relative health of the relationship can be deceptive. People may do what the manager wants, not because they agree or believe in the direction set or the request made, but because they believe they must comply in order to avoid painful or undesirable personal consequences.

Understanding the concept of trust is important for understanding relationships, but it is imperative for anyone aspiring to lead others. Yet little academic preparation is offered for health care professionals devoted to helping new managers build and sustain trust with their staff (Rogers 2005). Warren Bennis offers a concrete, applicable framework for understanding trust within the context of a leadership role (Flower 1990). He defines three essential

Figure 6-3. Three Essential Elements of a Healthy Relationship

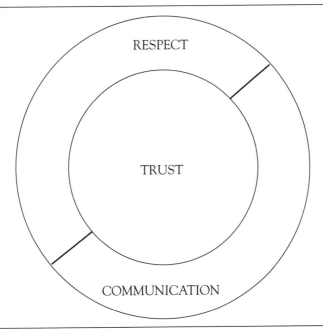

ingredients of trust: competence, congruence, and constancy. (See figure 6-4.) Examination of these three components of trust provides a guide for anyone seeking to more fully understand his or her personal effectiveness.

Competence

Webster's defines *competence* as the possession of required skill, knowledge, qualification, or capacity. The application of this definition in a leadership context is clear. Supporters must believe that the leader has the skill and knowledge to do what is required. "Whenever we step in front of the crowd and say, 'Follow me,' the implication is that we know where we're going and what we want to achieve and that we're committed to giving our very best efforts" (Melrose 1996, p. 20). Confidence in a leader develops from working with that person and from evidence of the leader's past performance demonstrating competence. Both skill and knowledge are included in this definition. Knowledge alone is insufficient. The leader may know that followers need accurate information and clear communication, but an unskilled leader is greatly hampered if unable to articulate information clearly and in a manner that ensures shared understanding.

For this reason, turnover of key leaders in organizations can result in a troublesome situation. It takes time to establish trust and confidence in new leadership and to build solid relationships. Nevertheless, many health care organizations embarking on major changes choose to alter the managerial and executive structure by eliminating or combining positions without solid reasons. Entire departments find themselves in a new reporting relationship. Leaders in these new positions are then expected to lead their followers

Figure 6-4.   Components of Trust in a Healthy Relationship

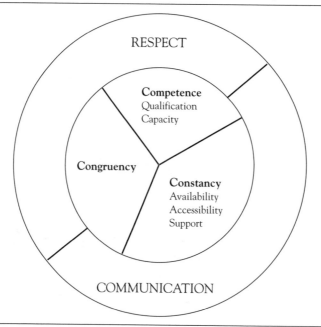

through the changes, and yet they are severely disadvantaged because they must first form a trusting relationship with their followers. Certainly, in some instances, this sequence of events caused by organizational change is appropriate; however, its impact on the time required to change should be carefully considered. In one midwestern hospital, for example, the chief executive officer routinely changes reporting relationships every couple of years because he likes to keep people off balance, in his words, "to shake things up a bit." What he fails to see is the effect on productivity and the cost in terms of relationships of such frequent changes in leadership.

Qualifications are an interesting factor in competence. Health care places a notable emphasis on technical expertise as a necessary qualification for managers. Some people simply do not follow an individual unless the person has a particular qualification believed to be important, such as a particular clinical discipline background or a certain academic degree. Whether the qualification actually prepares or enables the manager to function competently is a moot point. From the perspective of the employees, the absence of such qualifications can become a critical issue with significant repercussions. Organizations that have consolidated departments and replaced two or three managers with one manager often encounter significant obstacles when the new manager no longer shares the background or expertise of the employees in the department. Although this situation is not an insurmountable obstacle, it can take longer for the new manager to establish a trust relationship with employees because of his or her need to prove his or her competence in the face of what appears to be a significant qualification issue.

Capacity issues also influence the level of trust in the leader. When a leader is seen by others as simply having too much to do, too many responsibilities—juggling too many balls—a question of trust may arise. Does this leader have the competence to handle the current situation? Will it be too much? What if it pushes the leader over the edge? When managers appear frazzled and out of control, employees become uneasy. Personal endurance and a phenomenal capacity for work often go hand in hand with effective leadership. The motto "Never let them see you sweat" may be appropriate, but it should not imply that a good leader never lets followers see the reality of a difficult situation.

In one West Coast hospital where significant organizational consolidation of leadership roles was under way, a newly appointed executive had a personality style characterized by spontaneity, impulsiveness, and a high degree of self-disclosure. As the initiative progressed, this vice president was given more and more responsibility because she was very capable. She quickly reached the point of overload and began manifesting counterproductive behaviors such as volatility, extreme distractibility, and pure panic. Her communication patterns became dysfunctional as a result of her intense anxiety. Her erratic behavior with her followers clearly transmitted her anxiety, and she began to lose their trust. In this instance, skill, knowledge, and qualifications were not at issue. Instead, her followers feared she could not handle the heavy workload.

Congruence

The second of three key ingredients of trust within a leadership role is congruence, meaning consistency or agreement between the leader's verbal messages and his or her behavior (Lorimer and Manion 1996). A manager with a high degree of congruence between what he or she says and does is perceived as more honest and trustworthy by employees. If the leader says one thing but does another, the result is an enormous credibility gap; leaders must "walk the talk." The integrity and character of the manager are important. Employees need to believe that their leader's acts are in accordance with what their leader said or is known to believe. This belief in the leader's ability to be congruent in speech and action is more important than agreeing with the leader's beliefs. "Effective leadership . . . is not based on being clever; it is based primarily on being consistent" (Drucker 1992, p. 122).

Lack of congruence can be thought of as a discrepancy. Discrepancies are common in any work setting. For example, one department director in the hospital maintenance department established employee work teams and assured team members that they would have input into any decisions that affected their work. After almost a year of working together as a team, they were joined one day by two new team members whom no one on the team had expected. Their manager had hired the additional members without including the team in the decision. Consequently, the team members felt betrayed by the manager, and the ensuing breach of trust was difficult to repair. They wondered what other decisions the manager had made without their knowledge or input.

One of the most serious problems with congruency is that inconsistent messages are often inadvertent. The leader usually does not purposely engage in behavior contrary to previous messages sent but instead, without realizing it, acts in direct contradiction to the oral and written messages delivered. This example of incongruence occurred in one organization where competence was a stated organizational value, clearly printed on the back of all employee identification badges. When the organization needed to determine which employees would be laid off during an economic downturn, tenure was the key selection criterion, not competence. Tenure and competence are clearly not the same thing, and many employees were offended and angered by what appeared to be a decision-making criterion inconsistent with a stated, and often touted, organizational value. When this decision was questioned, the senior executive leading the initiative became defensive and angry but eventually listened to the feedback and changed the decision-making criteria. Tenure was used as a final determining factor only when the employees in question first met the criterion of competency.

A similar situation in another hospital was handled differently. When confronted with the incongruity between using the stated organizational value of competence versus tenure as a selection criterion, the administration retained tenure as the deciding factor. The senior executives reasoned that this was not the appropriate time to correct problems with employee competency issues that had not been dealt with previously by managers.

Although it may sound reasonable and senior leaders felt better because they had a reason for their decision, their choice created a major credibility issue. They were basically admitting that they had never held true to the organization's stated value of competence by saying that managers had never dealt properly with unacceptable or poor employee performance.

Any leader concerned about influencing others must scrupulously examine his or her behavior to avoid the appearance of incongruence, although it is virtually impossible to avoid all discrepancies. It is especially important for a manager to promote openness and honest feedback from employees. An executive team in one northeastern medical center worked diligently to establish an open environment by making certain that employees knew their leaders wanted feedback when their behaviors appeared incongruent. The leaders knew that their initial reaction to feedback would determine the amount and usefulness of future feedback, and they were very careful to listen fully and react nondefensively when discordant messages were brought to their attention. In some instances, behavior deemed incongruent was changed to fit the leader's message. In other cases, communication was unclear, and through sharing additional information the problem was resolved. This openness did not occur overnight. Many employees were— and some still are—hesitant to provide feedback because of fear of reprisal. This fear is a common obstacle for managers who hold a hierarchical position and have legitimate power over employees.

Giving the leader feedback on incongruent behavior is much more difficult than it may appear. Many employees simply say nothing when they feel a leader is about to make a mistake, and employees who were not well received when they did speak up in the past are unlikely to speak up again in the future. Some of this reluctance to speak freely and honestly is related to early socialization messages. According to Chaleff (1996), young people are taught from an early age to obey authority, to say "Yes, sir" and "Yes, ma'am," and this conditioning runs deep. It takes work to overcome these deep internal messages. "We are afraid that if we question authority we will be viewed as a nuisance, pushed out of the loop, overlooked for promotion, even fired. We fear the consequences of speaking up far more than we are afraid of the more serious consequences of not speaking up" (Chaleff 1996, p. 16).

Another way to view congruence involves congruity between how a leader conducts himself or herself in his or her personal and public lives. People who do not live up to commitments to their family or who cheat their neighbors often hide behind the belief that what happens in their personal life should not affect their leadership roles. Like it or not, if untrustworthy personal behavior is observed by followers, the level of trust in the leaders is adversely affected.

Constancy

Constancy is the third and last ingredient of trust as identified by Bennis (Flower 1990). Constancy implies that the leader is reliable, dependable, and consistent. A good leader keeps commitments and follows through on promises. When it becomes clear that a promise or commitment cannot be met, the leader communicates openly and honestly with people to inform them of the changed circumstances, ideally before they are confronted by it.

To many people, availability and accessibility are part of constancy. For leaders to be most effective, they must be accessible to followers at more than prescheduled, formal times. Some of the best dialogues occur in a completely spontaneous fashion and in informal settings. When the leader is also a manager or an executive, the formal trappings of the role may serve to distance the leader from the followers. Common examples are isolated office locations or the presence of secretaries who see their role as protecting or buffering the leader from others. Although impossible to remain available twenty-four hours a day, neither should the leader be completely inaccessible to followers. A balance must be found, because the perception that the leader is available is a potent one in creating a positive, collegial relationship with others. The importance of this concept was underscored by the results of the research reported in chapter 5.

Visibility of the leader has long been suggested by many authors as a key way that managers create a positive work environment. Peters and Austin (1985) refer to it as "management by walking around" or MBWA. This practice suggests that the closer a leader is physically to followers, the more a sense of connection and understanding is established. The leader who sees a situation with his or her own eyes is certainly better informed than one who hears about it from a third, potentially biased, party. When managers are present, they are more likely to be made aware of issues and problems in getting the work accomplished and, as a result, they can identify when problems require a system-wide solution rather than a more local approach (Tucker and Edmondson 2003). Unfortunately, as time pressures increase, managerial visibility and availability are often sacrificed. Whatever constraints may exist, they are never as serious as the threat to a leader's effectiveness from employees who do not feel a sense of connection and, as a result, do not follow.

These ideas may seem like common sense or intuitive knowledge. However, availability and accessibility are difficult to achieve in these demanding times. The rapidity and breadth of change occurring in health care today creates an environment filled with uncertainty, and people have many questions. Employees may not perceive every change as positive and may be very unhappy, even deeply angry, about the current direction of the organization. Every manager today knows how daunting it is to face a crowd of antagonistic employees, and it is a natural tendency to avoid these situations and withdraw from contact with people during these times. This area demonstrates one major difference between the excellent leader and the not-so-effective leader: The excellent leader stays more visible and involved, more accessible and available to followers during bad times. In a sporting event, when a team has fallen behind, it finds inspiration from the coach and the fans look for it from the cheerleaders. The excellent leader, like both a coach and a cheerleader, knows the importance of being present when there is significant unrest. Such leaders understand that their mere presence is a message of support to uncertain and unhappy people.

Being able to count on the presence of the leader is important, although some leaders feel uncomfortable when they do not have answers to the complex or difficult questions that may be raised. Many managers have been socialized to believe that the manager's job is to have answers. A good leader, however, understands and accepts that it is impossible to have all of the answers all of the time. It takes remarkable courage for leaders to stay present with others when they are being looked to for answers they do not have. Yet people respect leaders who are not afraid to admit that they do not have the answers. People are encouraged when a leader communicates belief that the answers will be found by working together. This presence during trying times is a tremendous gift the leader gives to others.

When the three elements of trust are present (competence, congruency, and constancy), credibility in the leader and his or her actions is possible. Kouzes and Posner have studied credibility extensively. They believe credibility relates to how a leader earns the trust and confidence of his or her constituency. In their studies they have found that "people want leaders who hold to an ethic of service and are genuinely respectful of the intelligence and contributions of their constituents. They want leaders who will put principles ahead of politics and other people before self-interests" (Kouzes and Posner 1993, p. xvii). Credibility is a way of maintaining or regaining people's faith in their institutions and the individuals who lead them. In *Strengthening Ethical Wisdom*, Gilbert (2007) proposes a blueprint for success for organizations and individuals who are committed to achieving exceptional performance while aspiring to the highest levels of organizational and personal integrity. He demonstrates throughout his work that "high levels of integrity are critical to reaching and sustaining higher levels of organizational performance in safety, care, patient and employee satisfaction, retention, and financial health" (Gilbert 2007, p. xiii).

Constancy of support offered by the leader is a vital issue affecting the quality of the leader–follower relationship. (This idea was identified in the research presented in chapter 5.) To provide support means to nurture or to give sustenance. Support is a two-way street within this context, going from followers to leaders and from leaders to followers. Consistency of support is critical; without it, trust wavers. If support is offered only when everything is going smoothly and then withdrawn during vulnerable times, it is of virtually no value because the person cannot count on it. The net result in the relationship is one of uneasiness, of being uncertain whether the support will be there this time. It is ironic that support is most needed during the times when it is most frequently withdrawn, that is, when mistakes occur and when poor decisions or errors in judgment are made. In a healthy relationship, support is consistent, offered freely, and visible to the receiver.

A manager's response to mistakes or errors is often the clue employees have to the consistency of the support extended by the leader. When punitive consequences are the norm, people do not feel supported. Punitive consequences for mistakes can occur in the form of shaming, blaming, humiliation, or reduction of future opportunities. Simply stepping in and taking over, relieving the individual of responsibility for correcting the consequences that resulted, can also be perceived as a lack of support. Interestingly, when the manager is observed behaving in a negative, punitive way with any employee, it is enough to damage trust even among those who were not directly involved. Of course, this is not to imply that appropriate actions should not be taken for a person making the same mistakes repeatedly.

Constancy may also refer to the stability of personal characteristics. The manager who experiences extreme fluctuations in mood, who is quick to anger, or who responds with knee-jerk reactions is very likely to have trust problems with employees. Take, for example, the individual who is excessively positive about ideas, unrealistically optimistic about the chances for success on a project, and effusive with praise one day, but the next day is exactly the opposite. Employees are left with an uncomfortable feeling of uncertainty, and trust is impaired. One person said, in referring to the two personalities of a union leader: "We wonder which one will show up today!" It is next to impossible for a leader to be completely balanced and thoroughly predictable. However, leaders who avoid such surprising changes in behavior can enhance the level of trust in their relationships.

Strategy for Repairing Broken Trust

Each ingredient of trust—competence, congruency, and constancy—offers challenges for healthy relationships in the workplace. When mistrust becomes evident, examining these three areas can help the leader to sort out probable causes. When mistrust is apparent in relationships, one possible approach to the solution is to ask followers, "What has happened to damage trust?" Leaders with the courage to ask this question are often rewarded with insight. Unless the question is asked sincerely, however, people may be reluctant to discuss situations in which they believe they were let down by a leader. Bennis (1989) points out that good leaders encourage respectful dissent so that they can know the truth about a situation even when it is not what they want to hear. In fact, good leaders need people around who have contrary views and can serve as devil's advocates.

Rogers (1994) identifies three steps for repairing broken trust: acknowledging the problem, apologizing for the problem, and making amends.

Step 1: Acknowledge the Problem
The first step, acknowledging broken trust, is tough for many managers. Few leaders purposely set out to destroy trust, and it is difficult to admit that something has happened to damage the relationship. In fact, some people prefer to call it something else, anything else, rather than accept it as a lack of trust. Some managers and executives believe acknowledging a lack of trust implies a personal fault of some kind, and this belief makes it especially onerous for them to honestly examine these situations.

For example, Susan was a senior vice president in a community hospital in Texas. In her organization the hierarchy was very rigid, and the rules and policies were plentiful. One expectation was that employees, including managers and executives, submitted time cards. For years employees were required to have their time cards signed by the individual to whom they reported, but this practice did not include managers and executives. Problems developed when one executive began submitting questionable entries and inaccurate records of sick and absent time. As a result, Susan began to require that all managers and executives get their time cards signed. The reaction was predictable. People felt they were no longer trusted. Susan was adamant that her requirement for the double check on the time cards was "just corporate compliance policy," but her assurances did nothing to assuage their feelings. When pushed, she finally admitted that it was because of problems with one individual. Even when confronted directly, she continued to deny any trust issues. It was clearly a lack of trust (albeit well deserved) in the one individual who had been found altering and falsifying time cards. Because of her unwillingness to deal directly with the individual who had the problem, the situation resulted in damage to her credibility as a leader and her relationships with those who reported to her.

Step 2: Apologize for the Problem

Apologizing for a breach of trust is difficult for many people. It does not mean accepting fault for something that is not the manager's responsibility. If it is clearly the manager's behaviors or actions that are responsible, the apology may sound like this: "I made a mistake and I am sorry" or "I am sorry that my decision has caused these difficulties for you." If the manager is not culpable, the apology may sound different: "I am sorry to hear that you feel this way; the decision was right for this situation," or "I am sorry that is what you heard. Let me try explaining this again." Another possibility is simply to say, "I am sorry that happened."

Apologies are very difficult for some people because they believe it diminishes their stature or damages the respect held by the other person. Many managers and executives have been socialized in a hierarchical system in which formal leaders just do not admit mistakes to employees, perhaps because they believe it may weaken their authority. The problem with this attitude is that people lose respect for individuals who cannot admit that they were wrong or made a mistake.

In one community hospital undergoing a major organizational culture change, employees showed significant distrust of administration. Five years previous, a layoff had occurred during a time of significant financial difficulty, and several very visible and devastating mistakes were made in the way the process had been handled. Although the executives talked about these mistakes behind closed doors, employees talked about them openly. The executives closed ranks and never talked with employees about the mistakes. The result was an antagonistic workforce that did not trust the executives to manage the new challenge because employees did not believe the executives had learned anything from the experiences of the layoff. How different the environment would have been if open dialogue and a sharing of ideas had taken place about what had been learned since the layoff.

Step 3: Make Amends

The last step in repairing broken trust is to make amends. Correcting mistakes and avoiding similar behavior in the future are ways to make amends. Sometimes the easiest thing to do is to ask, "How can I make this right? How can I make amends?" In many instances, an apology is enough. However, if behavior is to be changed and a commitment is made to do so, the leader must follow through on this commitment. It may take longer to re-establish trust than expected. People will be watching closely to determine whether they can believe the leader's promises.

Making amends also implies some reciprocal behavior from the follower. When the leader changes his or her behavior and maintains it, others at some point need to let go of past wrongs. A manager in one organization found that his behavior when he was first appointed to his position resulted in a reputation that still haunted him ten years later. Such trust problems need to be addressed; this manager can ask employees directly to let go of the hard feelings and harsh judgments in order to rebuild a trusting relationship.

Mutual Respect

The second essential element in forming a healthy relationship is mutual respect between the manager and the employee, which means having esteem for or valuing the other person for his or her skills, talents, and abilities. "Respect is listening to others with generosity rather than suspicion and valuing different views" (Gilbert 2008, p. 14). In a leadership relationship, respect can be offered in two ways. In the first, respect is offered unconditionally to all. Respect is not contingent on superficial attributes such as position, education, or socioeconomic status but is based on the contributions, both actual and potential, of the individual. Relating to followers as colleagues is a characteristic of a transformational leader (Burns 1978). This does not mean that a person would not respect another's achievement in terms of education or position, but that respect would not be withheld from an individual because he or she does not have a particular level of education or positional authority. Leebov (2006, lines 3–4) says that "the pecking order makes a lot of wonderful, contributing people feel inferior. The people on the downside too often feel discounted and invisible. It's hard to do your best under those conditions."

In health care, because patients and families are extended unconditional respect regardless of their situation, it is often assumed that this same respect exists among and between health care workers. All too often, however, respect is offered solely on the status or authority inherent in a title. Just as a person leaving a position becomes a nonentity because he or she no longer has a title, certain employees are not recognized as leaders because they have no formal title. Individuals with particular educational qualifications are believed to be most capable or the only ones with the ability to solve certain problems. These are all examples of respect based on superficial attributes. A leader understands fully that in another situation, positions may be reversed, placing the leader in a follower position.

Respect extended to followers is a result of a sincere belief that followers are partners and that they have ideas, abilities, solutions, and a keen interest in the situation. Max DePree (1989) says that the excellent leader begins with understanding the diversity and breadth of people's gifts, talents, and skills. "Understanding and accepting diversity enables us to see that each of us is needed. It also enables us to begin to think about being abandoned to the strengths of others, of admitting that we cannot know or do everything" (DePree 1989, p. 9). Extending respect to others includes seeking input, soliciting opinions and ideas, and using this information in making decisions. It also means providing freedom within the relationship and allowing a give-and-take process to occur.

A second way respect is offered is based on performance. In other words, the leader observes a person's skills or abilities and sees that he or she obtains desirable outcomes. This type of respect may be differential; in other words, the same level of respect is not guaranteed among people but is based on their individual performance. In this case, respect is withdrawn when appropriate or desirable outcomes are not achieved. The individual who makes repeated mistakes and does not learn from them may lose the respect of others and may even be removed from his or her position.

Communication

The third essential element of healthy relationships is open and honest communication. The paradox today is that leaders and managers spend more time than ever communicating with people, and yet the most common complaint of most employees is that no one tells them anything and they never know what is going on.

No leader is effective without the ability to communicate with others. This element involves excellent communication skills and a willingness to talk through issues. (Communication skills have been discussed extensively elsewhere and thus will not be examined closely here. Refer to *From Management to Leadership: Practical Strategies for Health Care Leaders* [Manion 2005] for an entire chapter on communication.) A leader may be highly skilled but unwilling to take the necessary time to do the work of communicating. In chapter 5, the research found that effective communication skills were a key factor for managers in creating a positive work environment. Not only were the skills important but also the manager's philosophy about communication was key. Most of the successful managers in the research clearly said that they subscribed to a philosophy of no secrets and open sharing. They believed not only that employees have the right to extensive information about what is happening in the organization but also that employees want to know the truth about things.

Another characteristic of healthy communication is that it is predominantly positive. Too often, employees only hear from the manager when there are problems, and this habit sets up a negative relationship between the manager and the employees. "Most managers acknowledge that they should give more positive feedback. Yet a recent Gallup Poll revealed that 65 percent of Americans haven't received recognition in the past year" (Wall 2007, p. 66). Wall notes that the number one reason people leave their organizations is that they do not feel appreciated. So, positive communication between leader and follower is not just nice to have, it is essential.

Creation of a Trust-Based Organizational Climate

The emotionally intelligent employee and manager know how to form healthy relationships with other people, they are able to assess and control their own emotions, and they can accurately assess the emotions of other people. The basic components of a healthy relationship are trust, respect, and open, positive communication. Healthy relationships among people in the workplace are more likely to lead to a culture of engagement and retention.

Healthy relationships are the foundation of a trust-based organizational climate. Effective leaders continually scan their environment and the reactions of the organization's members to assess levels of trust. Increasingly, leaders are becoming aware of the direct correlation between a positive, trust-based work environment and the competitive advantage of the organization.

> We are a society in search of trust. The less we find it, the more precious it becomes. An organization in which people earn one another's trust, and that commands trust from the public, has a competitive advantage. It can draw the best people, inspire customer loyalty, reach out successfully to new markets, and provide more innovative products and services. (Ciancutti and Steding 2000, p. ix)

This message is echoed in earlier work done by Reina and Reina (1999), who examined closely the issues of trust and betrayal in today's workplaces. According to their findings, "Unmet expectations, disappointments, broken trust, and betrayals aren't restricted to big events like restructurings and downsizings. They crop up every day on the job. Leaders are beginning to realize that people's trust and commitment to the organization affect their performance" (Reina and Reina 1999, p. ix). Reina and Reina offer a model for understanding the complex and emotional issue of trust and betrayal in today's organization. They believe that it is possible to create an organizational climate in which transformative trust exists. The four core characteristics that produce transformative trust are conviction, courage, compassion, and community.

In their book *Built on Trust*, Ciancutti and Steding (2000) talk about intentionally creating trust in the organization. They offer a model for deliberately and systematically establishing and maintaining high levels of trust. This model can be used by everyone in the organization to create a more trusting environment. The six stages in the model include:

1. **Closure:** coming to a specific agreement with every communication about what will be done, by whom, and with a specific date of completion.
2. **Commitment:** expressing a positive intention to complete what was agreed to with no conditions. If one is unable to follow through or fulfill the commitment as agreed to for any reason, then the person speaks up immediately.
3. **Communication:** disseminating information in a direct, open, and honest way that replaces dysfunctional forms of communication such as talking behind people's back, withholding information, engaging in hallway conversations, and so on.
4. **Speedy resolution:** clearing up unresolved issues as soon as they become apparent, as soon as possible.
5. **Respect:** using tact and respect in communications.
6. **Responsibility:** owning problems and helping others when needed. (Ciancutti and Steding 2000; used with permission)

In addition to these stages, Ciancutti and Steding include discussion of other principles such as being responsive to each other, telling the truth, agreeing to a "no surprise practice," handling issues at the lowest possible level in the organization, and having managers who serve as daily role models in each of these aspects.

Importance of Collaboration and Partnership

Unfortunately, the healthy relationships discussed here rarely exist throughout health care organizations. Many departments may have worked hard to create and maintain healthy relationships, but it is not the norm. Instead, relationships are characterized by conflict-aversive behavior and indirect or dishonest communication among co-workers. In some groups, individuals may be too accommodating to the needs of others and never consider their own needs. These individuals do not behave assertively or ask for what they need and want, and some display passive-aggressive behavior. A major role of every manager and leader is to clarify the expectation that employees will develop healthy relationships and to coach them as they work to improve the quality of their relationships. Holding people accountable for the quality of their relationships is essential if behavior is to change. (Performance management is addressed more fully in chapter 10.)

For leaders, establishing and cultivating healthy relationships with followers is the first essential step in developing the ability to influence others. This step can be accomplished by ensuring that the three elements of a healthy relationship—trust, mutual respect, and communication—are in place. But understanding the concepts of collaboration and partnership is also important, because these forms of relationship are healthier than the traditional command-and-control approach to leadership or "mama or papa" management styles characterized by unhealthy co-dependent relationships between employees and managers. As seen in the research findings in chapter 5, successful managers work in partnership with employees.

The concepts of collaboration and partnership also apply to relationships between departments. Leebov (2006, lines 1–4) says, "There is not nearly enough healthy respect flowing through health care organizations. This fact adversely affects not only the people who work for us but also the people we serve." This environment makes it more difficult for people to do their best. Strengthening these relationships among individuals and between departments is vital for creating a positive work environment.

The terms *collaboration* and *partnership* have similar meanings. Collaboration refers to work or labor accomplished by two or more persons working together. The word *partnership* is derived from the verb *partake*, which means to share. The essence of a successful manager's relationship with employees, peers, and key stakeholders is a combination of collaboration and partnership. Collaboration became a buzzword in the last decade, serving as a topic in many journal articles and workshop titles. But like most buzzwords, it was often overused and misused without a true understanding of the concept. A good leader may not need to know the actual definition but certainly needs to live the concept in relation with followers and colleagues.

Collaboration

Collaboration has multiple meanings, but the most useful addresses the concept of working together, especially in joint intellectual efforts. In the context of the manager–employee relationship, collaboration includes interactions between manager and employees that enable the knowledge and skills of both to work synergistically to influence the decision being made or the work being accomplished (Manion 1989). *Synergy* is a biochemical term that means that the whole is greater than the sum of its parts. In the leadership context, it means that when the leader and follower work together, they are likely to generate more and better solutions and alternatives than either would by working alone. To more completely understand collaboration, the relationship among coordination, cooperation, and mutual work is helpful to examine (Baggs and Schmitt 1988). These three ingredients comprise the whole of collaboration.

Coordination occurs when two or more people come together and share their points of view and their experiences to ensure a harmonious combination or interaction. One executive team meets regularly on Monday mornings for a short time, sharing plans for the week, discussing major issues, and briefly reviewing the members' calendars. Their intent is to coordinate efforts. Another example is a patient care conference in a rehabilitation department that is held for a similar purpose. Individuals from the different disciplines or shifts come together to compare their assessments of patients and to coordinate their efforts. Coordination is based on shared information.

Cooperation implies planning and working together in an actively helpful manner, more than being passively cooperative or simply accommodating. Cooperation as it relates to collaboration means meeting the other person's needs and yet being assertive in meeting one's own needs at the same time. Being aggressive and uncooperative is being competitive.

Sharing mutual work in collaboration means sharing goals, planning, problem solving, decision making, and responsibility. Contrast this with consultation, where sharing occurs during the planning phase but the individual proceeds alone in implementation.

Working relationships often show one or two of these elements, but not all three. In other words, people in a working relationship may come together to coordinate and cooperate with each other, but not necessarily to do mutual work. Other relationships may have high levels of cooperation but no focus on coordination. True collaboration requires all three elements—coordination, cooperation, and mutual work—in healthy amounts. Too often, a manager or an administrator makes a decision and then expects others to coordinate and cooperate in its implementation. The manager may honestly feel as though he or she is being collaborative because there is a general feeling of cooperation. However, unless the decision was mutually made, it is not collaboration in the true sense of the word. The basis of any partnering relationship is collaboration.

Partnership

People and organizations or companies that are capable of forming successful partnerships are more likely to enjoy future success. Partnerships are being seen at all levels of society today. Communities are forming partnerships with businesses and industries. Former competitors, such as Apple and IBM, are creating business partnerships. In a community in the Midwest, two hospitals from competing systems are considering partnering to build the third facility needed in their community. Strategic partnerships are appearing with more regularity in health care between health care systems as well as between individual organizations (Blouin and Brent 1997). Managerial partnerships are found at the executive and managerial levels (Manion, Sieg, and Watson 1998; Heenan and Bennis 1999). Today, leaders need to work in partnership with others. This effort is the very essence of the leader–follower relationship. "In a world of increasing interdependence and ceaseless technological change, even the greatest of Great Men or Women simply can't get the job done alone. As a result, we need to rethink our most basic concepts of leadership" (Heenan and Bennis 1999, p. 5).

The philosophy and approach of "every man for himself" in organizational life is gradually going by the wayside. In the past, managers were often rewarded for the size of their turf. The larger their budget, the more direct reports, and the greater number of people in their departments, the greater their status. Organizational environments were competitive and predominantly unhealthy. When one manager's request was met, another's had to be denied. In today's world, the manager who is a leader understands the importance of forming alliances and partnerships with employees, colleagues, and peers with the goal of accomplishing shared outcomes. The effective leader of tomorrow will be one who is able to form collaborative associations with others to fulfill the organization's mission. The concept of partnership is much more complex than it first appears because an individual, a group, or an organization may at one time be a competitor, a partner, a distributor, and/or a supplier. It takes a high level of maturity to balance such complex relationships.

Although successful leaders are willing and able to work in partnership with others, true partnership is not easy. Partnership may well be the highest level of interpersonal development, and some people are simply incapable of forming effective partner relationships.

Development Continuum

Stephen Covey, author of *The Seven Habits of Highly Effective People* (1989), has identified the stages of development and their ramifications in the professional world. (See figure 6-5.) As individuals develop, they progress from a state of dependence to a state of independence and finally to interdependence. Each stage of development represents significant and substantial progress.

In the stage of dependence, individuals rely on others. In the stage of independence, individuals rely more heavily on themselves and take responsibility for their own behavior, emotions, and accomplishments. Independent individuals are capable of moving to the higher interdependence level of development to work effectively with others and share responsibility and recognition.

Covey (1989) points out that only independent people can make the choice to become interdependent. Highly dependent people have little chance of moving into true interdependence. Independent people may choose not to become interdependent and, in fact, may see it as a weakness to relinquish control to others or share decision making. Executives and senior leaders in health care systems across the country are learning to balance a mixture of independence and interdependence as they partner with employees, colleagues, and peers in a variety of ways.

This development continuum is significant in understanding healthy relationships. Both Bennis (1989) and DePree (1989), when discussing leaders, describe seasoned, mature people who have recognized the need for—and have consciously chosen—interdependence with their followers. The excellent leader does not go it alone but derives energy and ideas from

Figure 6-5.   Development Continuum

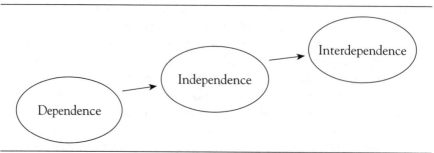

colleagues. Healthy leader–follower relationships are characterized by true synergy. Neither leaders nor followers exist in a vacuum but function in a reciprocal relationship that yields outcomes that exceed what either could have accomplished working alone.

Interestingly, the concept of partnership has been with us since the earliest times. However, many of our societies have lost this concept. In *The Chalice and the Blade*, Eisler (1987) describes the shift from a societal model of partnership in earliest human history to a dominator model. It is clear from her research that "war and the 'war of the sexes' are neither divinely nor biologically ordained" (Eisler 1987, p. xv). Based on her understanding and interpretation of historical artifacts and findings, in the earliest human societies, "difference is not necessarily equated with inferiority or superiority" (Eisler 1987, p. xvii), and neither gender is subrogated to the other. The application of this concept in today's organizations is clear: Many people are involved in organizations that are "working to create more mutual relationships, democratic institutions, and equitable societies . . . [and] they want personal and social power to be used with and for others, not over or against them. They believe that conflict can be resolved collaboratively and peacefully" (Eisler and Loye 1998, p. viii).

Collective Responsibility and Accountability

In any partnership, the members must retain a sense of personal responsibility and accountability. But a new dimension is added in the leader–follower relationship: the sharing of collective responsibility and accountability. For the relationship to thrive and continue to flourish, all of the elements in a healthy relationship must exist on both sides of the partnering agreement. Both manager and employee must be trustworthy. Respect is mutual and communication is two-way. Without these attributes, the partnership withers and dies.

Summary

The quality of relationships in the organization is a critical element of positive work environments. Healthy working relationships consist of those characterized by high levels of trust; mutual respect; and open, positive, and honest communication. These qualities describe relationships at all levels and among all people in the organization. Especially important is the relationship between employees and their manager. A manager/leader with strong emotional intelligence and a relationship based on trust and confidence, mutual respect, and honest communication creates a vital association. The nature of the relationship is one of collaboration and partnership, neither of which is easy to attain, but a healthy relationship is worth every ounce of effort it takes to build. Relationships in today's world are "parallel and simultaneous, connected, murky, multiple, and interdependent" (Bennis 1989, p. 101). Forming healthy relationships is complex and challenging, but it is an essential component of a positive workplace.

Conversation Points

Organizational Perspective

1. Are there clearly articulated behavioral expectations of all employees that relate to responsibilities for forming healthy working relationships?
2. What are the consequences for individuals who do not build healthy working relationships with others?
3. Are issues of trust openly discussed, even when it is difficult to do so?
4. Have there been issues of trust at the organizational level? How were they handled? How were employee pride and morale affected?
5. What is the span of control for the typical manager in the organization? Is it forty or fewer direct reports per manager?
6. Do members of the executive staff model healthy working relationships?

Leader Perspective

1. Use the three essential ingredients of a healthy relationship presented here (trust, respect, and communication) to assess the quality of your working relationships with employees.
2. Are there issues of trust among the people in your department? In your organization?
3. As a leader, what behavioral actions demonstrate your trust of other people?
4. Think of a time when you felt betrayed by someone or something that happened in your workplace. How did you handle it? Do you carry the sense of betrayal with you, or were you able to resolve it?
5. How do you demonstrate respect for others? What behaviors do you think let people know that you respect them?

Employee Perspective

1. How much do you trust your manager? The administration? Your co-workers? If there are issues of trust, to what are they related?
2. Are employees treated with respect in your organization? What are the behaviors you see that lead you to believe you are or are not treated with respect?
3. What do you do that shows you respect others? How do you show your support of others?
4. Do people in your department feel as though they have open, flowing, positive communication with your manager and other leaders in the organization?
5. Overall, what do you think is the quality of relationships in your department or work team? What could you do to strengthen them?

7

Creating Community at Work

Jo Manion

*The community exists to support its members while they fulfill
their purpose. . . . When partnerships, management teams, and
organizations build communities, they tap into a greater and deeper
reservoir of courage, wisdom and productivity.*
—Peter Gibb

HEALTHY INTERPERSONAL relationships in the workplace are a strong measure of a positive working environment. Relationships are important in all aspects of our work lives. Chapter 6 explores the relationships among individuals such as managers, executives, and employees in the immediate work group as well as co-workers and colleagues from other departments in the organization. This chapter examines the relationships that occur in a collective entity, such as an effective team, or when there is a sense of community in the workplace.

The importance of effective group relationships has been the focus of many research studies on job satisfaction. The presence of healthy teams enhances affective commitment, the type of organizational commitment that develops when people feel good about their relationships with others. This chapter carries the discussion of emotional intelligence further and examines how it applies to work teams. Capitalizing further on group relationships in the work environment relates to the creation of a sense of community among people who work closely together. A sense of community increases the sense of connection people feel with each other and builds affective commitment. Effective teams and a sense of community are factors that increase the emotional ties that bind employees to each other, to the leaders with whom they work, and to the team or community they form. The positive effect of community on retention has been demonstrated (Advisory Board Company 2000; Iverson and Buttigieg 1999; Kalisch, Begeny, and Anderson 2008).

Building Effective Teams

In today's work world, organizations and departments that are based on highly performing work teams have a distinct advantage over those that are undeveloped as a cohesive work group and lack a clear, concise, and collective purpose. As our work becomes increasingly complex and requires a broader range of knowledge and skills to complete, the need for well-defined, high-functioning teams is growing more apparent. Creating teams has been extensively covered in other publications (Manion, Lorimer, and Leander 1996; Manion 1997; Manion and Watson 1995), and the process for designing and developing teams is considered basic knowledge for managers and employees alike in our contemporary health care organizations. A brief review of the process is included in this chapter because the success with which a team is created often affects the development of positive relationships within the team. A special emphasis on team emotional intelligence is included.

Teamwork Defined

Team and *teamwork* are two distinct terms that are often confused and used synonymously by people who do not understand that there is a difference between the two concepts. The word *team* is overused in today's world, and it is loosely applied to exhort others to perform in a particular manner, usually through teamwork. Teamwork is a way of working together, and it may mean different things to different people. For most, it implies cooperation, open communication, and pitching in to help each other out. A team, in contrast, is a structural unit, a group of people designed and drawn together to complete certain prescribed work. How they carry out the work can be described as teamwork. As adapted from Katzenbach and Smith's (1993) definition in *The Wisdom of Teams*, a team is "a small number of consistent people with a relevant, shared purpose, common performance goals, complementary and overlapping skills, and a common approach to its collective work. Team members hold themselves mutually accountable for the team's results and outcomes" (Manion 1997, p. 31).

Types of Teams

Several types of teams operate in organizations today, including primary work teams, ad hoc teams, and leadership teams. Primary work teams are permanent structures organized around the primary work of a department. For example, in a business office, the teams may be organized around business functions, such as credit verification, billings, and collections. Primary work teams in a patient care department are organized around patient care. In a laboratory, teams are often designed around specialized functions, such as microbiology, hematology, and chemistry. In an emergency services department, there may be a trauma team and an urgent care team.

Ad hoc teams are temporary teams created to perform a particular piece of work. When the work is completed, the team is dissolved. Quality or continuous process improvement and project teams are good examples of ad hoc teams, which can last for years and yet not be considered part of the permanent structure of an organization. The third type of team is leadership teams. These are formed to provide collective leadership for a project or an initiative, a department, a service, or an organization. Some leadership teams are of a permanent nature, while some are ad hoc.

Managers today may create a team for a specific purpose (such as sharing the leadership function for the department), may actually redesign their department into teams, or may share responsibility for guiding or participating in the conversion of a bureaucracy to a team-based structure. The implementation of teams in health care is discussed extensively in other publications (Manion, Lorimer, and Leander 1996; Manion 1997; Lorimer and Manion 1996; Leander, Shortridge, and Watson 1996). Exemplary leaders who understand the concepts and language of systems thinking often form diverse teams that use systems thinking to focus on critical issues. These teams are capable of outperforming individuals because systems issues require multiple approaches, a variety of experiences, and diverse thinking patterns.

Process of Team Building

Regardless of the type of team, six concrete steps should be followed in creating an effective team. (See figure 7-1. The key questions to be addressed in each step are summarized in figure 7-2.)

Step 1: Define the Work

Before the team's members can be selected, the work of the team must be defined. The individual initiating the team delineates what the team is expected to do by considering several questions:

- What is the primary work to be accomplished by this team?
- Is this a problem-solving team focused on a specific issue or a project team formed to design and implement a new service or system?
- Is this team providing collective leadership for the department or within the organization?
- What will be required of this team? Is systems thinking required to challenge mental models and initiate breakthrough thinking?
- What are the general goals and objectives of this group?

Figure 7-1. Steps for Creating an Effective Team

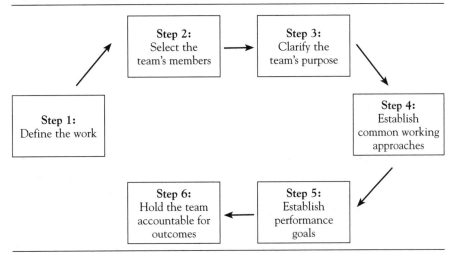

Figure 7-2.   Key Questions to Be Addressed during Each Step

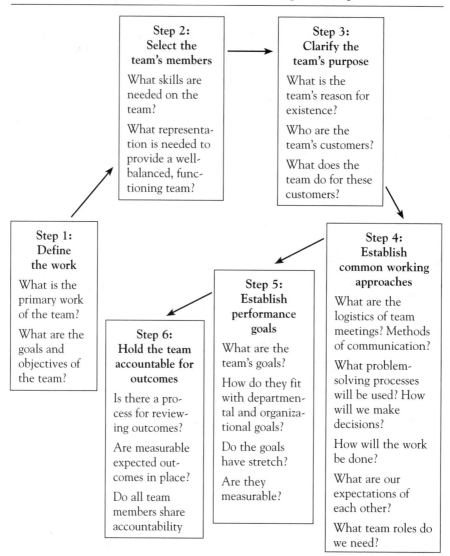

This step can be difficult, but it forces the leader to be clear about his or her reasons for initiating a team. If the leader is unable to clearly define the work of the team, confusion and chaos will be the result as the team flounders in its work.

Step 2: Select the Team's Members

Potential members are identified in step 2. The members are selected on the basis of their potential contribution to the team's work, as delineated in step 1. A team member may represent a particular part of the system or bring certain skills needed by the team. In some cases, it is impossible to obtain all of the skills needed by the team, and members may be selected for their skill potential, in which case the development of those skills is paramount.

Perhaps no one in the organization has exactly the skills needed, but the team, through its work, can develop those skills.

The most effective teams are those that have a small number of consistent team members. Teams of more than twelve members run into more logistical problems than do smaller teams. In larger groups, it is easier for members to disengage and remain anonymous. Finding a common time to meet is also a problem for large groups.

Consistency of membership is critical. Frequent changes in team membership directly affect the synergy of the group and the quality of the work completed. When team members leave and are replaced, the team usually regresses in its effectiveness until the new member is brought up to speed and is fully assimilated into the group as new relationships are forged. Consistency of membership also refers to consistent attendance at team meetings. Frequent absenteeism directly affects the team's ability to produce high-quality outcomes.

Step 3: Clarify the Team's Purpose

Once team members have been identified and the team comes together for the first time, the initial work of the team is to define its purpose. Although the leader may have given some preliminary direction to the group (based on his or her thoughts from step 1), it is critical that the team actually develops its own mission or purpose statement. This statement describes what the team does and for whom it does it. In other words, the statement clarifies the reason for the team's existence. Teams that are handed a completed purpose statement or are simply told by the leader why they exist never develop the same level of ownership as those teams that actually engage in this work. If the team is given a mission statement describing its work, one way to ensure relevancy and identification with this purpose is to have the team modify it to fit its beliefs and understandings. Even small modifications increase the team members' feeling of ownership. Team members simply do not engage with the work when they find the team's purpose irrelevant.

It is important for the leader to stay involved with the team during the development of the mission statement in order to prevent the team from heading in the wrong direction. The team's purpose must also be in alignment with the organization's or department's purpose. When the two are incongruent, the team is headed for trouble. An actively participating leader does not mandate the team's purpose but is involved in guiding and setting the team's general direction.

Step 4: Establish Common Working Approaches

Once the team is clear about its mission and reason for existence, the next step is to determine and agree upon the approaches it plans to use in doing its work. "A common approach means that team members discuss, delineate, and agree on [the] ways they are going to work together to accomplish their purpose. Common refers to the collective effort that is required, not an approach that is ordinary or average. There is nothing common or ordinary about a highly effective team" (Manion, Lorimer, and Leander 1996, p. 64).

Some examples of early decisions related to common working approaches include the following:

- **Logistics of team meetings**: How often will the team meet? When will it meet? Where will it meet? Will an agenda be circulated? How is the agenda developed? Who facilitates the meeting? Will minutes be needed, and if so, who will take them?
- **Methods of formal and informal communication**: Is there a need for frequent team huddles? Are team members readily accessible to each other? Do they need to be? How will they communicate between meetings? Is everyone on e-mail or available by texting?
- **Methods of problem solving**: How will the team tackle problems? Is there a specific quality improvement process to be followed?
- **Steps in decision making**: What types of decisions will be made by the team? What are the boundaries in regard to the team's work? Which can be individual decisions, and which should be made by the entire team? Will majority decision making or consensus be used? When would minority decision making be appropriate?
- **Work processes**: Do certain processes and approaches need to be done in a certain way? Does there need to be consistency in practices?

Roles and responsibilities within the team also need to be discussed. The team should decide whether specific roles need to be filled by team members to ensure that work is completed. The specific responsibilities of each role need to be defined clearly. Examples of special roles include meeting coordinator or facilitator and process person. The process person observes and gives the group feedback on its processes. For instance, the process person might note that no decision has been made and that only ten minutes remain in a meeting. Or, if the group has not heard from Sam, the process person will take note and may ask him for his input. The process person shares feedback with the group about its effectiveness, as well. In this capacity, the process person might note that during the meeting more quiet members of the group were ignored several times when they tried to speak, or that little attempt was made to understand a particular group member's point of view.

There are a variety of other roles besides the coordinator and process person. Some teams identify a celebrations role to ensure that key events and accomplishments are recognized and cheered. Some teams also identify the role of challenger. The challenger is "the team member who openly questions the goals, methods, and the ethics of the team, who is willing to disagree with the team leader, and who encourages the team to take well-considered risks" (Parker 1997, p. 8). This role is critical for most teams because the challenger is honest in reporting the team's progress and identifying problems. This individual, however, does back off when his or her views are not accepted and actively supports consensus within the team. In other words, this person does not always play an adversarial role. Another common role is the team recorder, who generates the minutes of meetings and circulates them to the rest of the team. This role is often a rotating one.

The final components of establishing common working approaches are the discussion of and agreement on team members' expectations of one another. Identifying and articulating behavioral expectations are key steps in early team formation for several reasons. These expectations lay the foundation for development of trust within the team. In addition, being clear about the expectations one holds of others is instrumental in preventing unnecessary conflict. Too often, people do not meet each other's expectations because they did not realize that the expectations even existed. The members of the group discuss what they expect or need from one another in order to do a good job. Expectations for appropriate meeting participation, communication techniques, and acceptable team behavior are commonly spelled out. The following partial list of examples from real teams demonstrates expectations related to these areas.

- We expect each other to be on time and prepared for meetings and to fully participate as evidenced by an attentive attitude, clarifying questions, and open-mindedness about the contributions of other team members.
- We expect each other to communicate openly, honestly, and directly, especially when we fail to meet each other's expectations.
- We expect each other to work toward the goals of the team and support the success of the team first and individual work second.
- We expect each other to stay focused on our goals and complete tasks and projects within agreed-upon time frames (and to communicate any unavoidable delays to other team members as soon as possible).

Clear expectations constitute formalization of the team's norms, and this is one of the first steps in building and creating team emotional intelligence (Cherniss and Goleman 2001). Being willing to address another team member's failure to live up to established norms and expectations is a critical sign of the team's emotional intelligence. Fear of conflict and confrontation is a common dysfunction in ineffective teams. Seen as accountability, the willingness of team members to call their peers on performance or behaviors that might hurt the team and its performance is essential for effective functioning (Lencioni 2002). The team's emotional intelligence is discussed more fully in the next section of this chapter.

Step 5: Establish Performance Goals

The team's performance goals are closely related to the team's mission. Larson and LaFasta (1989) examined high-performing teams and found, without exception, that high-performing teams have clearly identified performance objectives and goals. The team's performance objectives and goals can also serve as a way to measure the team's outcomes; that is, they give the team a mechanism for holding itself accountable. Porter-O'Grady, Alexander, and Minkara (2006) identify the establishment of goals as a key process factor for a successful team.

Team goals should be distinguished from system, organization, or department goals. "Teams take broad objectives or directives from the organization's management and shape them into specific, measurable goals for the team. Specific goals are stated in concrete terms so that it is unequivocally possible to tell whether or not they have been met" (Manion, Lorimer, and Leander 1996, p. 63). The most powerful goals provide for small wins along the way, and these intermediate victories serve to motivate and reinforce the team's progress along its chosen path.

Motivating goals are often those with stretch, that is, goals that force the team to extend itself and reach beyond its original targets. Ambitious goals produce momentum, growth, and commitment within the team. "Teams that face a significant challenge, or that develop their own ambitious goals, have a greater sense of urgency that forces them to focus their efforts in a unified direction. . . . The true strength of a team is realized when it faces and overcomes seemingly unbreachable obstacles to attain a worthy goal" (Manion, Lorimer, and Leander 1996, p. 63).

Step 6: Hold the Team Accountable for Outcomes

A final and essential step involves holding the team accountable for the outcomes of its work. This step represents a continual process of reviewing outcomes and determining whether established standards have been met and expected outcomes obtained. When its desired outcomes have not been attained, the team evaluates its process and its work to determine what went wrong, and then it takes corrective action.

The team reviews its decisions for their effectiveness and its processes for their beneficial outcomes. All team members are equally accountable for the outcomes of the team.

> Mutual accountability differentiates a real team from a working group. In both teams and working groups, individuals hold themselves accountable for the outcomes of their assignments. A team, however, takes the next step—members hold themselves mutually accountable for the team's outcomes or results. They continuously measure themselves against their established goals and objectives. (Manion, Lorimer, and Leander 1996, p. 77)

Group Emotional Intelligence

The primary role of the manager in developing teams, once these six steps have been achieved, is to guide the team as it builds and develops its own emotional intelligence. Group or team emotional intelligence is defined as "the ability of a group to generate a shared set of norms that manage the emotional process in a way that builds trust, group identity, and group efficacy" (Cherniss and Goleman 2001, p. 138). Team emotional intelligence emerges primarily through relationships, and it also directly affects the quality of the relationships experienced in the workplace. The relationships within the team can help the team become more emotionally intelligent, but dysfunctional relationships within the team can be destructive.

Group emotional intelligence operates in three distinct areas of interaction: individual, group, and cross-boundary. As a reminder, the two dimensions of emotional intelligence include self-awareness and self-regulation. As noted earlier, the most important action the manager or leader can take to help build group emotional intelligence is to guide the development of the norms. The norms must be consciously directed from the very beginning of the team, or their formation will be left to chance. Norms must be established for all three levels of interaction. The norms are summarized in figure 7-3.

Individual Level of Interaction

By looking at the dimensions of the group's emotional intelligence it becomes clear that norms are related to whether the interaction is at the personal, group, or cross-group level. For example, the group's awareness of its individual members is an important aspect of its emotional intelligence. At the individual level of interaction, norms relate to perspective taking and interpersonal understanding. Perspective taking refers to a willingness to consider matters from another person's point of view. Perspective taking is especially important when one does not agree with the other's point of view. An emotionally intelligent team, then, considers all points of view, regardless of who is contributing or whether or not the new perspective is in

Figure 7-3. Group Emotional Intelligence (Cherniss and Goleman 2001)

Group Emotional Intelligence Norms	→	Dimensions of Group Emotional Intelligence	→	Collective Beliefs
Perspective taking Interpersonal understanding	}	**INDIVIDUAL FOCUS** Group awareness of members		
Confronting members who break norms Caring orientation	}	Group regulation of members		
Team self-evaluation Seeking feedback	}	**GROUP FOCUS** Group self-awareness		Trust

Creating resources for
  working with emotion
Creating an affirmative
  environment
Proactive problem solving
	}	Group self-regulation		Group identity
				Group efficacy

Organizational awareness Intergroup awareness	}	**CROSS-BOUNDARY FOCUS** Group social awareness		
Building external relationships	}	Group social skills		

Reprinted from *The Emotionally Intelligent Workplace*, edited by Cary Cherniss and Daniel Goleman. Copyright © 2001 Jossey-Bass Publishers. This material is used by permission of John Wiley & Sons, Inc.

agreement with others. For example, the physical therapist assistant is not discounted because he is "only" an assistant, not a physical therapist; nor is the admissions clerk discounted because she could not possibly understand what it is like to be an emergency department nurse who is flooded with critically ill patients. People's opinions are sought, respected, and considered as the team completes its work. Differences of opinion are seen as opportunities for deeper understanding of an issue or situation.

The second norm emerging from the team's awareness of members is the interpersonal understanding team members have of each other. This means all the members have an accurate understanding of both spoken and unspoken emotions and feelings, interests and concerns, and strengths and weaknesses of the individual team members. This deep understanding exists in a close-knit work group that allows members to predict and cope with one another's day-to-day behavior. Research in this area has demonstrated that self-managing work teams show significantly higher levels of understanding of each other, they interpret each other's behavior more accurately, and they can tell whether a team member is having work-related problems or is just tired and needs a break.

The team members' expectations of each other in relation to this norm are often developed when the team members are agreeing on their processes. Several examples from real teams include the following:

- We expect each other to value the diverse contributions of all members as evidenced by our willingness to hear new ideas, confront issues that arise, and consider situations from a new and different perspective.
- We expect each other to be trustworthy as evidenced by honoring and meeting commitments made, by being loyal to absent team members, and by presenting each other in the best light to others.
- We expect each other to keep sensitive information about team members private and confidential.
- We expect each other to pitch in and help when one of us is having a bad day.
- We expect each other to ask for what we need.

Effective teams are those that can bring people with diverse and different skills and strengths together, maximizing the best of all team members. Cohen (2008, p. 19) recommends, "Maximize people's strengths, minimize their weaknesses, and adjust to their imperfections." Bürkner (2007, p. 21) reports that the best advice he uses when putting together effective teams is to "make sure it's spiky. And when people complain that their differences will cause problems . . . disagree. Find out what he's best at and show his strength to the team."

The second dimension of group emotional intelligence has to do with the group regulation of its members. A key task for a successful group is to create a balance between ensuring predictable team behavior and allowing members a sense of control and individuality. When the team is successful, members are more willing to put their individual needs aside for the good of the group. The norms that follow from this dimension include confronting members who break team norms and using a caring orientation. Confronting team members who break the norms means that when people are out of line, other team members speak up. It has been found that members of poorly performing work teams do not speak up for fear of confrontation or concern that it may make the problem worse or damage their relationships within the team. It is clear, however, that when the team member addressing the out-of-line colleague uses a caring orientation, this feedback is much better received. Using a caring orientation means communicating positive regard, respect, and appreciation for the other person. A study of seventy-six work groups found that a caring orientation in their relationships contributed to group effectiveness by increasing each member's sense of safety, cohesion, and satisfaction, all of which increase a person's commitment to or sense of engagement in his or her work (Wolff 1998). Caring does not require a close, personal relationship, but it does require validation and respect for the other person.

Group Level of Interaction

Emotion in a group context creates a powerful force that actually overwhelms individual differences in emotion and can create a new collective group or team character. Self-awareness was identified as a crucial emotional competence in chapter 6. Group self-awareness means that members are aware of the group's emotional states, preferences, and resources for dealing with emotion. Group self-awareness requires a norm that involves the ability of the group to evaluate itself objectively and accurately, including its emotional states as well as its abilities and weaknesses in the way it interacts as a team.

For example, instead of blaming others when team decisions are repeatedly overturned and team recommendations are overlooked by the larger hospital system, an emotionally intelligent team begins to ask why this is happening in an attempt to identify the team's own shortcomings. The team takes a good look at its own problem-solving and decision-making abilities. Maybe it does a poor job of analyzing various alternatives and instead relies on the same old refrain of "we need more resources" when problems occur. An emotionally intelligent team also continually seeks honest feedback about its performance.

It bears repeating that self-awareness is not enough for emotional intelligence. The second key dimension of group emotional intelligence is self-regulation. For a collective entity, it is group self-regulation. There are at least three norms in this area, including creating resources for working with emotion, creating an affirmative environment, and instituting proactive problem solving. In the case of a team, self-regulation means that the group accepts emotion as an important part of group life. It not only legitimizes the discussion of emotional issues but also develops a vocabulary for doing so. Members are comfortable talking about these issues. There is time for these discussions at meetings. Using a timed agenda has become popular in recent years, but when an agenda is enforced too rigidly, it can keep the group from addressing important issues fully. Most timed agendas, for example, take little or no account of the need to process emotions.

Creating an affirmative environment means cultivating and developing a positive self-image of the team's past, present, and future as well as comfortably using appreciative inquiry (a concept discussed in chapter 8) and positive expectations. As noted in chapter 4, an affirmative environment has been demonstrated to increase the team's effectiveness.

The third norm relates to proactive problem solving, or taking the initiative to resolve issues that get in the way of the group doing its work at the level of quality expected. Because problem solving is such an important skill, it is discussed thoroughly in chapter 8. Examples of expectations from a real team that are related to these norms include the following:

- We expect each other to give constructive, helpful, and private feedback regarding performance.
- We expect each other to accept constructive feedback about the team with an open mind.
- We expect each other to stay focused on the goal and to complete tasks and projects within agreed-upon time frames (and to communicate immediately with all team members if there is a delay).
- We expect each other to participate proactively in solving problems faced by the team and work together until a win-win solution is developed.

Cross-Boundary Interactions

The third area of interaction for a team is the cross-boundary focus. It is self-evident that group effectiveness requires networks of relationships with individuals and groups outside of the team's typical boundary. Thus, effective groups are outwardly directed as well as inwardly directed. As a result, they are able to obtain resources outside of their boundaries. In a health care organization, for example, laboratory employees and managers are able to get what they need from materials management, nursing employees are able to obtain the support and help of human resources specialists as they deal with difficult issues, and teams in the emergency department are able to work well with employees in admissions to get what they need.

Two important norms emerge in the area of group social awareness: organizational awareness and intergroup awareness. The team recognizes and understands the social and political systems within which it works, in other words, the organization. Teams are fully aware of the other groups operating in the organization.

The second dimension of group emotional intelligence relates to group social skills, and the key norm identified is building external relationships.

Research has found that the most effective teams are those that communicate frequently with the entities above them in the hierarchy, are capable of persuading others to support the team, and are willing to keep others actively informed about the team's activities and progress. Teams that are the least effective are those labeled as isolationist because they avoid engaging in boundary management and do not communicate with others to keep them informed about their activities. Examples of team expectations that are developed in this area include the following:

- We expect our team to work interdependently with other teams and departments in the organization, always seeking win-win solutions to problems.
- We expect our team to live up to the organization's mission, values, and goals when working across boundaries within the organization.
- We expect our team to stay informed of what is going on with other departments and the larger organization when it affects our work.
- We expect our team to address issues assertively and cooperatively with teams from other departments as well as with individuals outside of our team.
- We expect our team to represent itself positively throughout the organization.

Common Pitfalls in Team Development

There are many potential pitfalls in the development of teams. The most frequently observed are included here.

Often when a team is in trouble, the only solution involves the leader giving a pep talk or bringing in a dynamic, charismatic speaker who generates enthusiasm and excitement within the team. The results of this type of quick fix never seem to last long enough to get the team through its next crisis. Creating a sense of urgency is more effective in turning the team around. Giving the team a stiff work assignment that members see as important does more to mobilize stagnant energy and turn it into a productive force than any motivational speech could possibly do. This sense of urgent purpose can save a floundering team.

Another common error is not recognizing the special needs and unique challenges of the different types of teams (primary work teams, ad hoc teams, and leadership teams). Each of the three major types of teams has unique challenges, and to assume that they are all similar is to underestimate the difficulty a particular team may have.

For instance, most leadership teams find defining their work and purpose difficult. This difficulty may seem surprising because the team is composed of leaders—individuals who are usually self-directed and focused clearly on their work. However, most leadership teams confuse their work as a team with the work of the organization as a whole. The organization, for example, may have as its mission to ensure the delivery of safe, high-quality patient care to members of the community. The leaders may be used to working individually to ensure this care. But, as leadership team members, the leaders' mission is broader, for example, to focus on creating an empowering environment in which employees deliver safe, high-quality patient care. In a sense, the primary customer of the leadership team is the employee, while the primary customer of the employee is the patient. The directives are both similar and different enough to cause a leadership team in this position to have difficulty defining its work.

Another instance of the special needs of teams involves ad hoc teams formed to lead a change initiative. These teams often have difficulty in handing off the project to those who will actually implement it (usually managers from across the organization). The handoff is a primary issue in successful innovation. The people who implement a change are not as attached to the change as those who create it. The 1990s produced many examples of this issue in health care organizations. Quality improvement initiatives and work redesign projects in organizations were often designed by people on project teams who then handed off the implementation to managers who did not have the same investment or interest in the project. In many cases, full conversion and implementation failed. When this basic issue is understood, organizations with success in innovating do one of two things: They make implementation the responsibility of the innovator, or they ensure that those who will be responsible for the implementation are highly committed.

Primary work teams have special challenges as well. Probably the most common is that when work teams in a department are designed, any available staff are assigned to a team. This method of assignment can result in teams that have members who were not specifically selected because of their potential contribution. A way to increase the likelihood of a primary work team's success is to handpick members based on their skills and potential contributions. Understanding the unique challenges of each type of team alerts the leader to potential problems. A more complete discussion of the three types of teams can be found in *Team-Based Health Care Organizations: Blueprint for Success*, by Manion, Lorimer, and Leander (1996).

Ignoring any one of the key elements in creating teams is another major pitfall, but one that is relatively easy to correct. For example, one team that had frequent and recurring problems finally called in an external consultant to help. During this work, the consultant discovered that the team had never established its expectations of one another, nor had it agreed on common working approaches. Simply taking those two steps cleared up about 90 percent of the conflicts.

Another pitfall is minimizing the development time required to grow a team. This pitfall is very common. Too many managers and leaders today believe if they simply call a group a team, it will somehow become one. This misconception may also lead to the problem of everyone in a department believing he or she is on the new team simply by default. Not purposefully selecting team members or not taking the time to apply the proper steps of team development often creates a situation in which the group struggles needlessly, trying its best but being unable to determine why the team is floundering and struggling to succeed in its tasks.

It is vital that team members come together to accomplish their work collectively. Unless they do so, they do not become a team, no matter what they are called. Effective teams are those that are emotionally intelligent and are able to recognize and process emotion within the group and to regulate themselves in response to daily organizational events. The development of a team can be hampered or even sabotaged by a lack of emotional intelligence among its members. For a team to become emotionally intelligent, it is helpful, and perhaps even necessary, that at least some of the individual members have a high level of emotional intelligence (Cherniss and Goleman 2001). However, just because the team includes emotionally intelligent team members does not ensure that the team as an entity will be emotionally intelligent collectively or effective in its performance.

Being able to create high-performing teams is one of the most critical challenges facing leaders today. Virtually every future organizational structure (adhocracy, network, or clustered organization) is based on the premise that teams are to be a prevalent structure. Leaders must have the ability to tap into and release the potential of teams. Being part of a highly functioning team of people is likely to lead to strong affective organizational commitment and a positive work environment. It is also an effective way to soften the edges of the bureaucratic structure that defines most health care organizations.

Collective Leadership through the Development of Leadership Teams

The critical issue for any team is understanding and actualizing collective leadership. The benefit of collective leadership in a hospital is the creation of a forward-looking, mutually accountable organization. Every team needs to grasp the crucial difference between individual and team behavior and accountability. This is especially true when the main purpose of the team is to provide collective leadership.

The number of leadership teams required in any organization or department depends on the size and structure of the organization and the complexity of its functions. At the very least, managers should consider forming a leadership team for their areas of responsibility. In a department, this may mean a small group of assistant managers, supervisors, or selected employees who work closely with the manager to collectively perform the leadership function of the department. Each department will have its own unique composition for a leadership team. For example, in a hospital laboratory department, the leadership team might include the department manager, the supervisors of the different functions, the employee responsible for quality improvement processes, and the person who leads the employee governance council (if there is one). However, in an inpatient nursing department, the leadership team may consist of the assistant nurse managers or charge nurses, the department educator, the unit council chairperson, and the department manager.

Membership in a leadership team is determined by the team's purpose. In some leadership teams, selected employees may serve on the team to provide input from a particular segment of the staff, regardless of whether the employees play any specifically defined leadership role. In a specific situation, the manager may want someone from the night shift, a unit or department secretary, or a nursing assistant to serve on the team to bring a different point of view to the meetings.

Creating a leadership team within his or her scope of responsibility is one way for the manager to broaden and deepen the leadership strength within the department. It also serves as a tremendous source of support for the manager and improves leadership effectiveness. Commitment to the decisions that have been made for the department is stronger because there is group-level ownership and accountability. Collective leadership can also free up the manager to learn additional skills and take a more strategic approach that focuses on the issues and challenges of the department. And, perhaps most important, having solid leadership teams in place in the organization's departments creates a structure for a beginning succession plan. As emerging leaders work together in a leadership team, they are learning skills and developing capabilities that will serve them well as they progress in their careers.

Understanding the difference between a work group and a true collective leadership team is one of the most important hurdles for these teams. Too often these groups remain simply a collection of individuals who come together to coordinate and cooperate but rarely do any significant work that impels the organization to higher outcomes. Jim Collins wrote a monograph for the social sectors based on his seminal work that was reported in *From Good to Great* (2001). In the monograph he notes that leadership in business and industry is quite different from the leadership required in social-sector organizations such as hospitals and other health care organizations. Social-sector leaders face a diffuse and complex power map without concentrated decision-making power. He refers to this phenomenon as "legislative leadership," or leadership that is needed when no one has enough structural power to make the decisions alone (Collins 2005). Thus, in health care, it is almost impossible to lead effectively unless one can actualize collective leadership.

In a good work group there is a strong, clearly focused leader. Members of the group are responsible for their individual work products, and their implied contract is between the leader and each member of the group. In a leadership team, the leadership role rotates. Positional authority does not determine who the leader of the team is. An implied contract and responsibility exist between the members of the group, rather than resting solely on the leader with legitimate authority.

In an effective work group, the meetings are usually efficient and entail discussion, decisions, and delegation to others who do the work. The group measures its effectiveness based on the ability of the members to do their work more effectively as a result of having come together. A leadership team's meetings, on the other hand, are characterized by open-ended debate and active problem solving. The team discusses, decides, and does real work together. The team measures its effectiveness by directly assessing its collective work products. In other words, has the strategic vision and plan been achieved? Have resources been allocated appropriately? Is there cohesiveness in leadership approaches throughout the operational areas?

The most crucial difference between a work group and a true leadership team has to do with accountability. In a work group, each member is responsible for his or her particular assigned responsibility. In the laboratory, for instance, the supervisor of the blood bank has responsibility for service outcomes in the blood bank. If the supervisor of the phlebotomists is having difficulty, that is not the blood bank supervisor's problem. In nursing, the director for critical care is likely to feel no accountability for outcomes in the perioperative areas. In a leadership team, however, each member has individual accountability for his or her service area as well as shared accountability for the entire scope of services represented by the leadership team. There is both individual and joint, or mutual, accountability. One individual or area cannot be doing well if another area or individual is struggling or failing.

The leader's primary responsibility and loyalty is to the larger leadership team rather than to his or her individual area. This is a difficult concept to grasp for most health care leaders, and yet it is what makes the difference in their ability to achieve significant strategic and cultural initiatives in the organization. Collective leadership is what enables leaders to break down barriers between functions, destroy silo mentality, and chart ways to align and mobilize people on their path to a new future. It requires leaders to manage a polarity—individual accountability for their assignment and mutual accountability for the outcomes of the team.

Creating Community in the Workplace

Teams are vitally important to connecting people at the workplace and to the success of the workplace as a whole. A second aspect of creating a sense of connection among people at work relates to the concept of community in the workplace. Community resides in more than the individual relationships of people. A sense of community results in a collective entity or spirit within a work group, a department, or even an organization. Because a sense of community has the power to increase people's emotional ties to each other, establishing community is also a way to strengthen retention efforts and levels of organizational commitment (Manion and Bartholomew 2004; Manion 2004a). This strategy has been found to be effective regardless of the age cohort; in other words, it is as effective for Generation Xers as for Baby Boomers and may be increasingly important for those in the Millennial generational cohort.

Importance of Community*

Over the past two decades, the average American worker has added an extra month to his or her work year (Vogl 1997). Many people spend more of their waking hours in their workplace than with family or loved ones. Discretionary time is at an all-time low for many Americans, as longer hours are worked and more work is brought home to do after hours or over days off. Discretionary time is further reduced by the fact that in many families, all of the members who are able to work are contributing wage earners. Thus, the family's time away from work is often spent doing home maintenance, running errands, getting groceries, and completing tasks that were performed by an at-home partner in previous decades.

In today's world, a sense of community in the workplace has become increasingly important for many people because it may be the only source of community in which they participate. Decreasing involvement in family, church, and neighborhood activities; increased geographical distances from family members and childhood communities; and extremely harried and full work lives have all combined to escalate a general feeling of isolation and disconnectedness from the typical communities of the past.

Less discretionary time has led to a decline in our involvement in other communities over recent years. Working longer hours often leads to less inclination to get to know neighbors, and besides, those neighbors may move away in a few years anyway. Active membership in professional associations and religious organizations is at an all-time low (Putnam 2000). "Besides the broad decline in church affiliation and attendance, so, too, there has been a falloff in membership in other organizations—trade unions, parent-teacher associations, fraternal clubs like the Elks, Shriners, and JayCees—and volunteering for groups like the Boy Scouts and Red Cross" (Putnam 2000, p. 20).

Social scientists explain the yearning for community as a reaction to decades of individualism, which peaked near the end of the twentieth century. Americans have spent almost two centuries dismantling their roots and traditions in the pursuit of individual happiness only to find that happiness is more likely to come from community and a sense of connection to other people. All of these factors create a longing for a feeling of community in some aspect of our lives, and work is where many spend the majority of waking, alert time.

Many leadership scholars and experts believe creating community is an essential leadership skill. "The task for leadership in the coming century is to transform work organizations into viable, attractive communities capable of attracting workers with needed skills and talents. . . . A sense of community invigorates members' lives with a sense of purpose

---

*This section on the importance of community is adapted from Jo Manion and Kathleen Bartholomew, Community in the Workplace, *Journal of Nursing Administration* 34(1): 46–53. Copyright © 2004. Used by permission of Lippincott Williams & Wilkins.

and a feeling of belonging to an integrated group that is doing something worthwhile" (Fairholm 1998, p. 151). Understanding the definition of community helps increase understanding of the ramifications of the need for community in the workplace.

Community Defined

Community has become a buzzword over the past several years and, as such, can be overused and misused, which reduces its influential power. According to Rousseau (1991), community is a form of human association that binds people together. It is far more than simply a group of people living or working together who share common interests and projects. It is "a psychological reality, an act of will that constructs a tie that really binds" (Rousseau 1991, p. 45). And, Rousseau believes, the tie that binds is altruistic love. Altruistic love puts the other first; expects nothing in return; and loves generously, openly, and without reservation or expectation.

Rousseau further believes that contractual relationships are incapable of producing community because they are inherently egocentric. They exist for the good of one or more of the parties and thus can only link people together in this external aspect. "Those who love contractually are seeking their own fulfillment as their end, looking to other people as the means to their own pleasure or utility, they forge no existential bonds with each other" (Rousseau 1991, p. 49).

If this is true, according to Rousseau, it would be highly unlikely that community could exist in the workplace. How much altruistic love is experienced in business relationships? The primary nature of the relationship of employee to employer is a contractual one, as is, by extension, the relationship of employee to manager. Clearly, the organization requires certain work to be accomplished and compensates the employee in accordance with the completion of that work.

Although the initial and underlying nature of the relationship is contractual, however, that contractual agreement may not be the entire essence of the relationship. In other words, the employment relationship is not merely contractual. Many employees are committed and feel quite connected to their work and can feel in community, or in unity, with the co-workers to whom they feel close. Such connections are more likely in individuals who see their work as a calling rather than as just a job. People for whom benefits or financial compensation are the primary motivators for work are, by Rousseau's indicators, less likely to feel a sense of altruistic love that leads to a feeling of community.

"Community is a psychological reality, and our motives determine whether it happens or not" (Rousseau 1991, p. 51). In other words, it is important to look beyond the initial nature of the relationship (the contract) to try to determine the motivation of the people involved. Rousseau notes that motivation, or the subjective intention of the person who decides and acts in a certain way, is the key factor for building community. It is difficult or even impossible to truly know another's motivation or in some cases even one's own motivation. Rousseau suggests a way to think about this:

> It is seldom easy to achieve purity of intention, and it is never easy to know that we have. One test of our sincerity, though, is the price we are willing to pay in order to appropriate the community of being in altruistic love. If communal actions cost us significant money, time, energy, or physical pain, and we carry them out anyway, we have a reliable sign of that purity of heart. (Rousseau 1991, p. 148)

A simple example in a workplace community is evident when an individual willingly experiences the inconvenience of a scheduling change to help out a colleague who needs to change his or her schedule.

Scott Peck has studied and helped facilitate the formation of many communities. He believes that the lack of community is such a norm in our society that it is easy for us to believe that community is impossible to achieve. Community is more than simply the sum of its parts or its individual members. It is a group of individuals who have learned "to communicate honestly with each other, whose relationships go deeper than their masks of composure, and who have developed some significant commitment" to share life's deeper experiences (Peck 1987, p. 59). In this context, work lives can be considered potentially one of life's deeper experiences.

Elements of Community

The many facets of community are interconnected and interrelated. It is helpful to understand what various scholars of community have found when they closely examined the elements within a mature community. The aspects considered here are identified as essential; that is, if any of them were absent, it would be unlikely that the group could be a true community. These characteristics include inclusivity, commitment, consensus, realism, capacity for contemplation, safety, and a group of leaders (that is, the members all flow in and out of leadership roles). (See figure 7-4.) These characteristics are discussed briefly below to stimulate self-reflection and for use as an evaluation mechanism for assessing the current state of community in a department, a work team, or the organization as a whole.

Inclusivity

Community is inclusive in nature, which means that the group is continually seeking ways to extend itself and attract new members. Exclusivity is considered an enemy of community because it can turn the potential community into nothing more than a clique, a group organized to protect against a feeling of true community. However, inclusivity is not an absolute (Peck 1987). There may be valid reasons a particular member should be excluded, such as when the inclusion of the individual might damage the community as a whole. Excluding a potential member is considered with great care and concern. Community requires that diversity is welcomed and celebrated. A department with a strong sense of community

Figure 7-4. Elements of Community

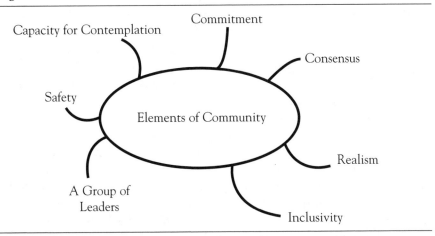

is effective at bringing in and incorporating new members into the established community. New members are welcomed, and rituals exist to help them assimilate into the group.

Commitment

Commitment is a second key aspect of community. Commitment has been defined as that which makes a person continue a particular course of action even when more positive alternatives or potentially negative consequences attempt to persuade the individual to abandon the chosen course of action (Brickman, Wortman, and Sorrentino 1987). This means that once committed to participation in the community, a person is obligated to follow through. One of the ways commitment is evidenced in a community is the accommodation of individual differences and the tendency of true community to actually encourage individualism (Peck 1987). The individual's commitment is to the community as a whole; in other words, individuals bind themselves to participation in the community. Commitment requires personal sacrifice, that is, giving up something that is valued (Kanter 1972; Rousseau 1991; Peck 1987; Brickman, Wortman, and Sorrentino 1987). For example, in a patient care department, many occasions arise when individuals might prefer to do things their own way but agree to subscribe to the team's approach of handling the situation, such as staffing coverage and requested time off. In every organization, standardized approaches and shared values and philosophies are in place that ensure consistency in the delivery of services.

Consensus

Consensus is a way of reaching a decision about an action to be taken whereby all members of the community agree to support the decision, even when they do not fully agree with the decision itself. Consensus is a process that works only in an open and trusting environment. It requires that all members have the opportunity to speak and be heard. In other words, ideas and opinions are shared openly, and even when disagreement occurs, members seek to understand each other's viewpoints. Peck (1987) shares examples of true community where consensus almost magically occurs. Consensus is not the absence of conflict, but the ability to work through conflict. In fact, he calls true community "a group that can fight gracefully" (Peck 1987, p. 70).

Many groups that suppress or deal with conflicts in a covert manner think the absence of conflict is a good sign, never realizing that they have only attained a level of pseudocommunity. "In pseudocommunity, a group attempts to purchase community cheaply by pretense. . . . It is an unconscious, gentle process whereby people who want to be loving attempt to be so by telling little white lies, by withholding some of the truth about themselves and their feelings in order to avoid conflict" (Peck 1987, p. 88).

Pseudocommunity is a significant problem in health care organizations because many health care workers tend to be conflict averse. True community is conflict resolving; pseudocommunity is conflict avoiding. Healthy conflict-resolution skills are essential for the development of emotionally intelligent employees and healthy teams (Cohen 2008).

Realism

Realism refers to the fact that issues considered by a true community are addressed more realistically because of a broader treatment of issues and ideas. "Because a community includes members with many different points of view and the freedom to express them, it comes to appreciate the whole of a situation far better than an individual, couple, or ordinary group can" (Peck 1987, p. 65). This is the power of synergy, or interdependent working relationships. The one-plus-one-equals-three phenomenon is at work in communities.

A classic example comes from the world of nature. The properties of hydrogen ions and oxygen ions can be studied in the laboratory, and these properties may all be described very scientifically. However, when these two elements are combined in a certain way, water is created and an entirely new characteristic called wetness exists. Neither the hydrogen nor the oxygen ions individually have this characteristic of wetness. Thus, together these ions are more than a simple collection of parts. Examples of this concept occur in the workplace on a daily basis. On any given day, staffing may be inadequate, perhaps due to the sickness of colleagues or an unanticipated high work volume. At the beginning of the day the situation looks hopeless. However, the combination of people is just right, everyone pulls together so that things just click, and everyone has a great work shift. This is one common example of synergy in action.

Capacity for Contemplation

True communities continually examine themselves. They are self-aware and recognize their abilities and strengths as well as their weak spots. Contemplation may start at the individual level, but it progresses to the collective level before long. No community can expect to be continually healthy and fully functioning. However, a genuine community, because of its contemplative nature, "recognizes its ill health when it occurs and quickly takes appropriate action to heal itself" (Peck 1987, p. 66).

In the work world, this characteristic is more often referred to as accountability. Accountability is the retrospective review of results to determine whether the group is working effectively. Is it achieving desired outcomes? Are the work and outcomes of high quality? Why are decisions being overturned? Why is the group dealing with the same problem it had last year at this time? A true community continually reviews and self-assesses, taking corrective action when needed.

Safety

Genuine community is a place where people feel safe to express themselves and to be themselves fully, without apology or explanation. The community offers acceptance. From sharing vulnerabilities, a sense of connection forms, and strength grows from this support. It takes a great deal of effort and energy for a group of people to reach the safety of true community. But it is essential for the honest expression of ideas and feelings. It is also crucial in setting a climate that acknowledges mistake making as sometimes inevitable and a source of learning. The concept of safety is one of the powerful benefits of community in the workplace. In times during which both the internal and external environments in health care organizations are increasingly turbulent and uncertain, the security experienced within a community can provide a haven of safety for people in the workplace.

Group of Leaders

Finally, a true community is a group of people who are all leaders. This concept is often described as a decentralization of authority (Peck 1987). Members who are accustomed to leading often feel comfortable and safe when they do not have to pick up the leadership reins. Members who are more reserved and not used to leading also feel more comfortable in picking up the reins, speaking out, and helping set a new direction. Peck (1987, p. 72) found that "one of the most beautiful characteristics of community is what I have come to call the 'flow of leadership.'" The flow of leadership results in decisions being made more quickly and an increased likelihood that each member's individual gifts will be brought forward at just the right time.

Stages in Community Building

Communities go through several specific stages during their development. Understanding these stages increases appreciation of both the dynamic and developmental nature of community. Instant community is an illusion. Using the concept of creating community as a retention buzzword is inappropriate. Building a sense of community must be based on an awareness that it is a developmental process, not the latest retention program. Although the stages in community building vary somewhat from author to author, Shaffer and Anundsen (1993) offer a model that is applicable and easy to understand. The stages are outlined in figure 7-5.

Stage 1: Excitement

Excitement is an enjoyable phase, much like the honeymoon phase of a marriage or an intimate relationship. The focus of the group is on its potential, with an emphasis on positive outcomes and a minimization of the problems that are likely to occur. The task for the group at this time is to create a shared purpose and vision. The purpose need not be a task to accomplish or a change to undertake. The purpose of the community may be simply to provide support to each other or to create a workplace where members enjoy each other. Alignment with this purpose, however, is important because it helps the members get over the rough spots ahead. It often takes strong leadership and someone willing to get the group started to move into and through this stage. This phase does not last, and, in fact, if it continues indefinitely, the group is probably a pseudocommunity, where community exists only in pretense.

Stage 2: Autonomy

Autonomy is the focus of the second phase of community building. Often, this stage can make or break a community. During this stage, the illusion of unity is shattered, and members often become disappointed with each other, feeling angry and disillusioned. This phase passes only when members give up the fantasy of harmony without struggle. Although unpleasant, struggle is a critical part of the community's developmental process, and this phase is considered successful when the group survives and remains whole. Members assert themselves as individuals, are able to differentiate their needs from the needs of others, and yet remain committed to the needs of the whole, the community. The members consciously choose to act and work interdependently. The need for safety is paramount

Figure 7-5.   Stages of Community Development

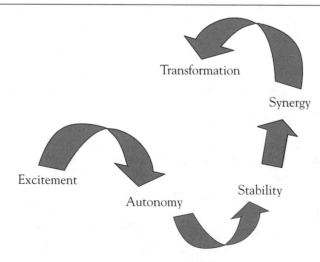

during this stage. When members do not feel safe within the community, its tasks are not accomplished.

Stage 3: Stability

During the third stage, community members settle into their roles and the community's structure. At this point, the fact that the community is still intact serves to reaffirm the members' caring for each other and their commitment to a shared purpose. Members know they are respected as individuals, and yet they understand the rules of the game (which they have helped establish). This understanding frees up energy to focus on the common tasks required.

A major pitfall in this stage is that members can become too settled in their roles, and the same member may continue to serve as the leader (developing agendas and leading meetings) or the resident critic (bringing up opposing viewpoints). Allowing one person or one small group to carry one role alone for too long can lead to burnout and stagnation. When one member is especially talented (or merely willing) in one area, a common tendency is to let that individual carry the load, which does nothing to develop the collective abilities of the community. This tendency can make it especially difficult for the community to embrace new leadership.

Stage 4: Synergy

Synergy is exciting and paradoxical. At this stage, members are acutely aware of their individualism and yet are more interconnected than ever before. Although aware of his or her own contributions and needs, each member is also very committed to the needs of the community. In fact, what is good for the individual is also good for the community. A characteristic of this stage is that roles reverse more comfortably, with leaders and followers flowing in and out of roles easily. Synergy, the excitement of combined abilities, talents, and strengths, is very apparent at this stage. The illusion here is that the work of community making is done. It is easy to believe that once synergy is achieved, it will remain and stay the same. However, all systems are continually in flux, and this community is no different.

Stage 5: Transformation

Transformation is the final stage of the cycle, when the community undergoes a death and possibly a rebirth of sorts. At this stage, the community may expand its boundaries or identity, break into smaller groups, or disband completely. Even the most successful communities reach a natural ending point, a time when members seem destined to move in new directions.

Leadership's Role in Creating Community

What can leaders do to develop a sense of community within their scope of responsibility? Unfortunately, it is not as easy as understanding the elements of community and the stages healthy communities experience as they mature. There is no guaranteed process a leader and employees can use that is certain to result in the development of a healthy community. Instead, the interventions are more general and foundational, and a sense of community develops only when the chemistry and efforts of the members determine it will be so. However, following are specific recommendations based on actual workplace experiences.

Hold a Clear Vision of the Possibility

Vision was such an overused buzzword of the last decade that many managers have become somewhat cynical about being told to have a vision. Yet vision is hope for the future. It is the ability to see something different from what currently exists. Vision is the ability to actively use the imagination. Using words and pictures to paint an image of community helps employees see and feel the direction in which they are heading. Few people jump onto a train unless they know where it is going. Creating and sharing a vision of community is the first and foremost task of the leader. It requires continually upholding what is possible: respecting the best of each individual and therefore the department as a whole.

When the leader holds a vision of possibility for the department that includes a strong sense of community, this vision can actually guide day-to-day decisions and actions. Coupled with an intellectual understanding of community, interventions can be deliberate and supportive of the future vision. For example, consider the inclusive nature of community. Thomas Moore (1994) believes that one of the greatest needs of the soul is for belonging. He contends that people must be welcomed into a group. Therefore, a new employee who has been hired or transferred into a department does not necessarily belong until invited. This invitation can be extended by the manager in the form of sharing his or her vision, making a strong initial connection during the interview process, and monitoring the new employee's progress closely to make sure that he or she is assimilating into the group. Invitation means looking for connections and creating opportunities for employees to connect on a personal rather than just a technical or professional level. For co-workers, this means reaching out and getting to know the new colleague and providing support as well as a gracious welcome.

Nurture Relationships

The second leadership intervention to encourage community is to nurture the development of healthy relationships. Rousseau (1991) firmly states that community is based on altruistic love. Altruistic love means authentically caring for and about the members of the community. It extends beyond the employees in the department to include physicians, patients, and other colleagues as well.

In chapter 6 it is noted that leaders can measure their effectiveness by the quality of their relationships. The strength of a community lies within these bonds. Forming strong, healthy relationships requires honesty, authenticity, and the capacity for intimacy. As in any relationship, it is important to realize that extending oneself to other people is taking a risk. However, the energy, support, and depth of meaning that come from working in a group of people who genuinely care for each other are profoundly rewarding. Only when each individual is seen as a gift and his or her unique contributions are valued are the elements of synergy and realism that characterize community developed. A nonjudgmental attitude fosters feelings of safety. This is perhaps the greatest gift that a leader can give to employees because it demonstrates the tolerance for differences that is unique to community.

Genuinely caring for others is at the heart of this authenticity. Pretense does not work. Although the focus in health care has shifted toward seeing the needs of the whole person, management sometimes lags behind in seeing the whole employee. A dichotomy between work and home no longer exists because lives are so much more complex than they were just twenty years ago. Instead, the relationship between these two aspects of life are interwoven and intricate. As noted in chapter 5, ten or twenty years ago, asking a personal question would have been considered intrusive, but today, asking about family and being aware of employees' personal challenges serve to enhance and build good relationships. A leader who arrives in the department (or at a meeting) and immediately begins asking rapid-fire questions about the project or tasks to be completed is often perceived by employees as caring more about work than about people.

Provide Support for Community Formation

Understanding the typical stages of community formation is essential for the effective leader. Knowing, for example, that in the early stages of community a stronger leadership presence may be required as opposed to the rotating leadership characteristic of later stages of community formation is crucial. Otherwise, a leader may inadvertently continue to exercise a strong, hands-on leadership role beyond the point at which it is healthy for the group.

Support may be needed in protecting the time community members have to spend together. The immense pressure to increase productivity in the workplace also decreases the amount of free time that employees spend together. For example, one physician remarked that ever since the hospital converted to bedside charting, he rarely talks with the nurses. The intention in this case was to streamline the documentation process, but precious time for human interactions was lost in the shuffle. In economics, this time together is called social capital, and it is considered vitally important because it produces "trust, cooperation, mutual support, bonding and . . . loyalty" (Putnam 2000). Balancing the need for productivity with the need for creating community and building social capital is a significant challenge for any health care manager today.

Seek Opportunities to Strengthen the Sense of Connection

There are endless opportunities for actions that strengthen the sense of connection people in the workplace feel toward each other. Simply being aware and looking for these opportunities are powerful leadership strategies.

Take the example of the new nurse manager, Katie, who was faced with the need to complete seventy performance evaluations shortly after her appointment. Although she could have treated the evaluations as a tremendous burden, she chose to look at them as an opportunity to hear from each of her employees and to begin building relationships. Through this process it became clear that a major problem existed in the relationship between physicians and nurses.

Katie went to the group of physicians with this message: "I had identified my major challenge as recruitment and retention. But after listening to the staff, I understand that we have another significant problem. Nurses who have worked here for fifteen years complain that you do not even know their names! How do you expect me to recruit and keep nurses if you make no attempt to even know their names?"

Katie decided to remedy this situation and made a commitment to attend the physician section meeting every month. She highlighted a different employee each month, which required extensive research on her part. She would present three interesting things about each individual; for example, one nurse loved to garden, was a ballroom dancer, and was a loyal Harley Davidson motorcycle owner. After sharing these unique characteristics, she would ask the physicians, "Who is this nurse?" Katie then proceeded to hold up a picture of the employee and announce his or her name. The physicians looked forward to these staff vignettes, and the special knowledge that they learned about the members of the nursing staff helped to bridge the professional gap that existed. In addition, the nurses were each given the task of learning something about each physician—hobby, children, interesting fact—and this goal was written into their performance evaluations. Relationships began to form in the spirit of community.

Katie took other actions in her department as well. She placed the community bulletin board at the front station to increase its visibility to physicians, nurses, and auxiliary staff. The bulletin board became a space where community members could post items that were of interest to others such as a flyer describing a bicycle or snow tires for sale or an announcement of a staff member's special achievement. The sharing of such information increased the department's sense of camaraderie and open communication.

At a holiday gathering, physicians, respiratory therapists, physical therapists, physical therapy assistants, unit secretaries, nursing assistants, and nurses were asked to write their favorite vacation spot or hobby on their name tag in place of their name. This simple idea elicited many conversations that staff would have never initiated under other circumstances. It helped everyone to step outside his or her comfort zone. Conversations are like threads that weave a group of people together and strengthen the bonds among individuals and thereby the group as a whole. Any activity that creates personal connections or stimulates conversation encourages the formation of community. The challenge for leaders is to constantly see and capitalize on the opportunities that exist.

When the atmosphere in the department is one of community, patients feel it. In Katie's department, even the patients began to feel as though they were members of the community. Ruth was eighty-two years old when she was admitted to the orthopedic unit with a hip fracture. Because she had no relatives and a legal guardian had not been established for her, her stay was extended from a week to two months. During this time, she became part of the community of the department. It was impossible not to fall in love with this pleasant and tender woman. She ate every meal at the nurses' station, and the staff eagerly devised recreational plans for her.

At the end of October, Ruth was finally discharged to an adult family home with three other residents. She was confused about the change of surroundings, but eventually she settled into her new home. Two days before Thanksgiving, the nurses received a phone call from the owner of the home. The owner said that all of the other residents were going home for Thanksgiving to their families, and Ruth wanted to come home, too. And so, on Thanksgiving Day, Ruth took her seat once again at the nurses' station so that she could eat her turkey dinner with her "family." The need for community is universal.

Benefits of Community Building

Do leaders need to develop a sense of community in the workplace? Arie de Geus of Royal Dutch/Shell argues that for "companies to endure they have to create a feeling of community, where workers think of themselves as members rather than employees. They belong to the organization" (Vogl 1997, p. 21). Paradoxically, although a sense of community can help create joy and connection in the work environment, community is difficult to attain in contemporary workplaces. Re-engineering, work redesign, downsizing, right sizing, layoffs, mergers, and acquisitions have become common, almost universal experiences in work lives. These initiatives are successful only when employees and employers work together in an atmosphere of trust and mutual collaboration. Yet trust and collaboration are the very elements that are often destroyed in these situations.

Other obstacles to community in the workplace arise as well. The increased use of per diem, contingency, or temporary employees creates continual change in the workplace. Another factor is the U.S. free enterprise system, which promotes individualism and results in subordinating the interests of community to those of the individual. Alienation, distrust, and competition are obviously major barriers to creating community. When the members' real agenda is increased personal power and fulfillment of personal needs rather than the well-being of the community, the group will not remain a community for very long (Naylor 1996).

It is precisely because of this experience in leaner and meaner workplaces that interest in a spirit of community in the organization has increased. "We humans hunger for genuine community and will work hard to maintain it precisely because it is the way to live most fully, most vibrantly" (Peck 1987, p. 137). The absence of community is keenly felt. Rather than rushing out to create community at work, it is important for managers to consider their interventions carefully and only after they have considered their own motivations. Otherwise, efforts to increase community in the workplace may backfire, leaving employees even more cynical. In his article "The Call of Community," Zemke (1996, p. 30) says that we have two options in the workplace:

> [First, community can be considered] nostalgic claptrap, a psychological retreat from what's happening in the real world. Or, as some proponents suggest, it may be an attempt to create a new, more civil code of workplace

conduct, a code that accepts the realities of the modern world but holds that we can both cope with the insecurities and create openness and closeness with one another that facilitates our work and our humanity. Which assessment is correct? Will we trivialize the notion of community, or will we use it as a springboard for changing our behavior and our outlook on the world of work?

Summary

Both the formation of effective teams and the creation of a sense of community in the workplace are proven workforce retention strategies, but workforce retention alone cannot be the motivation for their creation. The motivation, and accompanying commitment, must be the desire to create, support, and nurture a group of people who are genuinely valued. These initiatives are ways to create a positive workplace. Developing an emotionally competent team often leads to increased effectiveness in the workplace as well as a stronger sense of connection among co-workers. When a sense of community is present, people feel connected to something larger than themselves. Both approaches build on the ties of affective commitment.

Conversation Points

Organizational Perspective

1. Are defined, developed teams an essential part of the organization's structure? Or do they exist sporadically throughout the organization?
2. Are internal resources available for the development of teams? (Resources include experienced team facilitators from human resources or the education or organizational development departments as well as time available for the developmental work of becoming a team.)
3. Does the senior executive group work as a true team and provide a clear example and role model for other teams in the organization?
4. Is team activity reinforced throughout the organization? (Reinforcements include but are not limited to rewards and recognition programs based on both individual and team performance and organizational leaders who understand how to communicate with and develop collective entities.)
5. Is there a sense of community in the organization as a whole? What kinds of activities and specific interventions or initiatives help the people in the organization feel a sense of community?
6. How is conflict handled organizationally? Is there a conflict-averse culture, or is conflict handled directly and in a way that promotes the growth of people and the equitable resolution of issues?
7. How actively do employees participate in organizational community activities, such as summer picnics and holiday parties?

Leader Perspective

1. Do you have established teams within your area of responsibility? What is the purpose of these teams? How long have they been in place? Were they developed purposefully, or did they just emerge and evolve on their own?
2. If you do not have any formalized teams, are there functions or purposes that could be better met by a team? Where do you have an opportunity to improve your service by forming a team?
3. Do you have a leadership team that helps you lead in your areas of responsibility? Is it an informal work group or a true team? Could it be improved by becoming a true team?
4. Do your work groups demonstrate the essential elements of a team?
5. If you have teams, what is their level of maturity and effectiveness? Are they continuing to develop? Are they meeting their purpose?
6. Where in your areas of responsibility do employees experience a sense of community? Is there any place where you have deliberately tried to establish a sense of community, or has it evolved spontaneously?
7. If you see community in your areas, what stage of development is the community? Have you taken leadership action to assist in its development?
8. Are there places where you would like to see a true community form? What can you do as a leader to encourage this?
9. What are the benefits of creating a sense of community?

Employee Perspective

1. Do you function on a true team, or are you part of a work group? Would there be advantages to the work group becoming a team? What would need to be different?
2. Do you and your co-workers understand the difference between teams, work groups, and pseudo-teams? Or is the term *team* used loosely to describe any work group?
3. Are the expectations and norms within your team jointly established by team members, clearly understood by all, and lived up to by those involved? What happens when a team member does not abide by the established norms?
4. How emotionally intelligent is your team?
5. Do you and your co-workers feel a sense of community in the workplace? Where does community exist (for example, in a particular area of the department, on a certain shift, in a professional group, in the organization as a whole)? Are you certain you have a community and not a clique? (A clique is exclusive, with only certain people allowed to join, but a true community works diligently at being inclusive for others.)
6. Have you taken any action to help the formation of community? What is your role in helping with its formation?
7. What are the characteristics of community you see in your department or among people in your work area?
8. If you have a sense of community, in what stage of development is it?

8

Focusing on Results

Jo Manion and Sharon Cox

*Leaders are proactive—and able to make something happen
under conditions of extreme uncertainty and urgency.*
—James Kouzes and Barry Posner

SAVVY LEADERS and managers intent on creating a positive workplace where
people enjoy and are fully engaged in their work understand that one of
their responsibilities is to focus on and obtain needed results. They understand
that process for process's sake is not acceptable. How results are achieved is
important, but getting results, solving problems, and making improvements
are ways that effective leaders do their jobs and create commitment and
credibility among their followers (Manion 2004b). One proprietary study has
found that when managers help employees find solutions to problems at work,
employee initiative, productivity, and commitment all increase.

The ability to get needed results is strongly connected to the strategies
and interpersonal skills addressed in this and other publications. For example, in *Execution: The Discipline of Getting Things Done*, Bossidy and Charan
(2002) report that the first essential skill of getting things done is to know
your people and to continually expand people's capabilities through coaching. When the leader's relationship with employees is healthy and positive,
they communicate more easily with each other, negotiate difficult issues,
and work together to implement solutions.

The Failure to Get Results

Getting results and making improvements are much easier to talk about than
to do. Today's health care organizations are complex almost beyond comprehension. The scope of the many issues is often beyond what an individual
manager can influence alone. Some common examples of these types of issues
are sluggish patient throughput that results in lengthy emergency department
wait times and then backups in other departments; complex layers of managers and bureaucracy that miss vital information about emerging problems;

Portions of this chapter are excerpted from *From Management to Leadership: Practical
Strategies for Health Care Leaders*, second edition, by Jo Manion. Copyright © 2005
by Jossey-Bass Publishers. This material is used by permission of John Wiley &
Sons, Inc.

and work-arounds developed by employees to compensate for operational failures. All of these critical issues can be solved, but getting results takes exemplary managers to team with employees, peers, and leadership.

Failing to Learn from Mistakes

One common reason that managers fail to get results is that hospitals fail to learn from their mistakes. Tucker and Edmondson (2003) examined reasons that hospitals fail in this way. They concluded that "Hospitals historically have relied on a dedicated and highly skilled professional workforce to compensate for any operational failures that might occur during the patient delivery process. Great doctors and nurses, not great organization or management, have been seen as the means for ensuring that patients receive quality care" (Tucker and Edmondson 2003, p. 55). The increased scrutiny by the public regarding patient safety has led to a call for improved organizational effectiveness and responsibility for creating systems that ensure patient safety. A detailed study of patient care processes led these researchers to conclude that in spite of the increased emphasis on issues such as patient safety, hospitals "are not learning from the daily problems and errors encountered by their workers [and] . . . that process failures are not rare but rather are an integral part of working on the front lines of health care delivery" (Tucker and Edmondson 2003, p. 56). So why are hospitals failing to learn from the mistakes of these failures?

The study identified two kinds of failures. The first type of failure was errors. Errors were defined as "the execution of a task that is either unnecessary or incorrectly carried out and that could have been avoided with appropriate distribution of pre-existing information" (Tucker and Edmondson 2003, p. 57). The second type of failure was problems that were described as a disruption in the person's ability to complete a task because some item or element was not present that was needed (missing supplies, information, or medications) or some item or element was present that interfered with the task. Interestingly, 86 percent of the failures were related to disruption problems rather than errors. These reoccurring failures stonewall any attempts at getting results.

First-Order Problem Solving

Strikingly, when disruption problems occurred, the employee involved used first-order problem solving to deal with them. In other words, the person compensated for the problem by getting the supplies, the information, or whatever was missing. In these cases, the individual did not address underlying causes and, in fact, felt very positive about his or her ability to take initiative and work around the problem. This behavior is often valued by the manager, who is pleased that his or her staff are handling problems as they arise. Inadvertently, however, this type of problem solving is counterproductive behavior because the underlying issues never get resolved. The problem invariably reoccurs, sometimes on a daily basis.

This study found that thirty-three minutes were lost per eight-hour shift due to coping with system failures that could have been addressed and corrected once.

Although this study was done with nurses, it is highly likely that the same behaviors and practices occur with other hospital workers as well. The researchers found that two unspoken strategies predominated for these employees. The first rule of thumb was, "When you encounter a problem, do what it takes to continue the patient-care task—no more, no less" (Tucker and Edmondson 2003, p. 61). The second rule of thumb was to, when necessary for delivery of care, ask for help from peers rather than from the manager. Both of these very typical behaviors actually preclude addressing the underlying causes that might improve the system.

Second-Order Problem Solving

Second-order problem solving, the focus of the rest of this chapter, occurs when the individual, in addition to taking care of the immediate problem, takes steps to address the underlying causes. Because most first-line employees have little extra time, the presence or easy accessibility of the manager has a significant impact on whether this level of problem solving occurs. If the manager is present, he or she is more likely to observe the problems and become aware of them. The manager is also more likely to make the connection between the problem and the organizational steps that can be taken to help solve it.

Solving these disruptive problems increases the quality of work life for employees. No one likes dealing with the same problems over and over again. Seeing progress is an intrinsic motivator as well as a basic human need. Other studies have reported similar findings about the disruptive nature of these problems. Tucker and Spear (2006) found nurses spending from 10 to 25 percent of their time looking for other staff members. Forty-two minutes of each eight-hour shift was spent resolving operational failures, while at the same time, the employee was interrupted forty-three times during a ten-hour shift. Bear in mind that many of these interruptions are truly legitimate for meeting patient needs, such as responding to a family member who requests a dose of pain medication for the patient.

Despite the legitimacy of some of the interruptions, the workplace could be more conducive to better outcomes if, rather than repeatedly working around disruptions, the staff treated these occurrences as a trigger for potential process improvement. Process improvement is a key way for hospitals to begin learning from their mistakes. How much turnover is related to the frustration of first-line workers who experience this kind of a typical workday over and over again throughout the year?

The Danger of Common Occurrences

It is easy to become habituated to what are considered common occurrences. Just because something is common (like missing supplies, inadequate linen supplies, illegible handwriting) does not make it acceptable. Everything must be questioned. Managers also need to examine their own behavior. Common practices may lead to unintended consequences such as described in the behaviors identified in the Tucker and Edmondson (2003) study.

Another common practice that may lead to unintended consequences is the response managers have used for years with their employees: "If you come to me with a problem, also come with a solution." What the manager is asking for is active involvement on the part of the employee in helping to solve problems in the department. While involving the employee is good, this response can inadvertently lead to an unintended consequence.

Jack Gilbert, in *Strengthening Ethical Wisdom: Tools for Transforming Your Health Care Organization* (2007) points out that this rather typical admonition of manager to employee can lead to behavior that hides rather than reveals problems. He uses the example of medication errors to make the point. Based on examined data, for every sentinel event (where the error resulted in permanent patient harm, required intervention to sustain life, or resulted in patient death) there were about 24 harmful, nonsentinel events and another 1,900 nonharmful events that occurred as a result of the medication error. His point is that most quality improvement efforts will focus on the worst of the sentinel events in order to analyze and determine what needs to be fixed in the system.

However, focusing on the near misses and the nonharmful events can reveal problems waiting to escalate into larger issues. Often a first-line worker may have a sense that something is "off" or wrong in some way, an intuition that something just is not right. If the employee has been told to only come to the manager with a solution in mind, it may be easier for the employee to say nothing at all, and the chance to prevent an unfavorable outcome has been missed. Gilbert (2007) suggests that managers should have an open mind and actually encourage employees to speak up about their concerns, whether they have a solution or not. Otherwise, the manager may be inadvertently silencing the voice that could identify a potential problem early. The probing questions mentioned in chapter 5, "What takes you too long to do?" and "What keeps you up at night?" are good examples of ways to solicit employees' concerns and ideas.

Metrics Misinterpretation

Another typical leadership behavior that affects the ability of the organization to function at peak effectiveness involves the application of the organization's metrics. The measurement systems used by organizations must be applied with sound judgment and critical thinking. Too often the numbers and data collected may contradict key organizational values and make it more difficult to carry out the organizational mission. Turnover numbers are an example, as discussed in chapter 1. If a manager is held accountable for the turnover of employees in the department with no consideration of whether the turnover is expected or justified, punitive consequences may inadvertently be delivered to an excellent manager who is doing his or her job well. There may be employees who need to be separated from their job in order for the department to achieve its mission and goals. Some organizations that have certain goals for turnover rates in departments do not provide pay increases to those managers who exceed these levels, although they were doing exactly what they needed to do.

Another example comes from the long-term care sector. One very fine long-term care center has a stated value that residents are encouraged to be as active as possible. The homelike setting includes an atrium and inner courtyards where residents can walk and be outside. The encouragement of this activity has resulted in a higher number of falls. When balanced against the increased quality of life for its residents, a case can clearly be made for using judgment in evaluating this measure. If a manager or work group is penalized for this result, it could inadvertently lead to increased restraint use and a lower quality of life for residents.

Shared Responsibility, Shared Results

Second-order decision making and other techniques focused on getting results can be used to solve many of the systemic problems mentioned above. This chapter next explores models of shared decision making that are in use in health care organizations today. The section titled "Skills Needed for Shared Decision Making" then addresses several concrete process skills, such as problem solving, decision making, appreciative inquiry, and managing polarities that both managers and employees can use in getting results. An actively used continuous quality improvement process is closely linked to incremental improvements in our systems as well as to an individual organization's success in creating an innovative culture, as discussed in chapter 9. A basic problem-solving process is offered here that is congruent with the quality improvement processes practiced in many health care organizations today.

Models of Shared Decision Making

Perhaps one of the most important aspects of creating a positive workplace is related to the degree to which employees are actively involved in making decisions about their own work or giving valued input into decisions about their departments and organization. All of the models of shared decision making have at their core the intention of transferring responsibility to employees or empowering employees. Because empowerment was a common buzzword in the 1990s, many people are tired of hearing it. It was overused and often misunderstood. A brief review of the concept is offered here to serve as a basis for understanding shared decision making. (For a more complete discussion of the subject, see *From Management to Leadership: Practical Strategies for Health Care Leaders*, second edition, by Manion [2005].)

Empowerment

Empowering others by transferring increasing levels of responsibility to them is one of the most important processes managers and leaders need to master. The definition of *empowerment* is to be given the legal authority to take a particular action. The word *power* means the ability to act or to produce a result. These two definitions combined are "to be given the legal authority to act or produce a result." Gibson (1991, p. 359) defines *empowerment* as "a social process of recognizing, promoting, and enhancing people's abilities to meet their own needs, solve their own problems, and mobilize the necessary resources in order for them to feel in control of their lives."

The importance of empowering people in organizations cannot be overstated. Empowered employees are fully engaged in their work and contribute at a much higher level than their counterparts who see their work as simply a job. With the constantly shifting business climate and increasingly challenging external conditions facing health care, organizations need the ability to respond rapidly. Quick response is virtually impossible from a workforce that has to constantly be told what to do, that is basically uninformed and unaccustomed to making decisions, and that has never participated in collaborative planning. On the other hand, organizations that have dedicated resources to the continual development of their people and treat their employees as intelligent partners in the delivery of services are much more likely to have individuals who are able to respond quickly when external and internal conditions change. These employees are not dependent on the manager or leader for direction or decisions; they can function independently and interdependently when needed.

In many organizations, first-line managers, as well as employees, are not developed or empowered. This situation creates a tremendous ripple effect in the organization. Rosabeth Moss Kanter, professor at the Harvard Business School, has been on the frontier of management and leadership for nearly thirty years. She points out the dangers of not empowering managers in the organization:

> Managers with power accomplish more because they have greater access to information, resources, and support in the company. Being busy, they pass the information and resources to subordinates. Thus, powerful leaders are more likely to delegate responsibility and reward talent.
>
> Powerless managers who can't easily get access to resources and information are frustrated and weak. The result is often petty, dictatorial managers who wield the only power they can: oppression of subordinates. It is powerlessness, not power, that corrupts. (Kanter 1997, p. 6)

Empowerment does not occur simply because a leader says, "You are now empowered; go perform!" There is no Harry Potter magic wand to wave or incantation to pronounce so that people suddenly begin behaving differently. "Empowerment takes planning, patience, trust, and time. It's not something you can do overnight. If you want it to work, you have to commit to it. You must be willing to invest in it, support it with systems, and approach it in a logical, determined way" (McCarthy 1997, p. 7).

Process of Empowerment

As a process, empowerment begins with an understanding of four interrelated concepts: capability, responsibility, authority, and accountability. The sequential application of these four concepts leads to empowerment. (See figure 8-1.) First, the meaning of each of these terms is clarified.

Capability

Capability refers to the ability, knowledge, and willingness of an individual to carry out the task, assignment, or responsibility. Ability is not only personal competence comprising skill and experience but also the availability of needed resources. An individual may be willing to accept a particular responsibility but may simply not have the time, equipment, or resources necessary to do an adequate job, or the person may have ability in terms of both personal competence and resources but lack willingness. Without this element, empowerment fails.

Responsibility

Responsibility is the clear allocation or assignment of a task or piece of work that needs to be accomplished. Responsibility also implies acceptance of this allocation by the individual involved. The person to whom the task or assignment has been given must accept ownership before this responsibility has truly been transferred. For instance, a team accepts responsibility for carrying out its work, monitoring and controlling work flow, and making necessary decisions within its scope of responsibility and authority. It is responsible for maintaining an acceptable standard and for continually searching for ways to improve its processes and outcomes.

Figure 8-1. The Empowerment Sequence

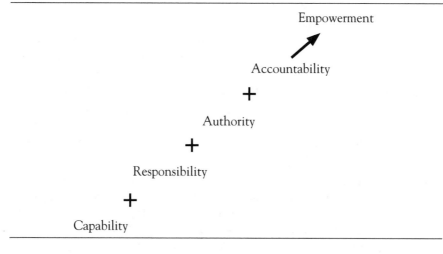

Authority

Authority is the right to act in an area for which one has accepted responsibility. For responsibility to be carried out, an individual must have a commensurate level of authority. Four commonly accepted levels of authority are summarized in table 8-1.

The first level of authority is the authority to collect data or gather information. No action is taken on the data or information, and decision making is retained by the person assigning the responsibility and granting the authority.

Once the data have been collected or the information gathered, the individual involved in the gathering also reviews it and makes a recommendation based on his or her assessment and previous experience. This is level-two authority. Decision making is retained by the person assigning the responsibility and granting the authority, but the gatherer's recommendation is considered in making the final decision.

At level three, the individual collects and reviews the information, makes a recommendation, and discusses it with the person assigning the responsibility. After their discussion and upon agreement, the individual proceeds to carry out the action.

Level four is the highest level of authority because it represents independent action. It includes the right to gather information, determine what needs to be done, and take necessary action. The person accepting the assignment is authorized to act in the place of the delegating individual.

Within these levels of authority, the individual's responsibility or authority may be limited by the constraints or parameters of a particular

Table 8-1.   Levels of Authority

Level	Description
Level 1	This is the authority to collect or gather data and information. No action is taken by the person who gathered the information; the decision is made by the person who granted the authority.
Level 2	The person or persons involved in collecting the information also review it and make a recommendation based on their assessment and previous experience. The decision is made by the person who granted the authority with consideration of the recommendation.
Level 3	The individual or individuals gather and review the information or data, make a recommendation, and discuss the recommendation with the person who assigned the responsibility originally. After discussion and mutual agreement, the individual or individuals proceed to take action or implement the decision.
Level 4	This level represents independent action. The individual has the right to gather information, consider it, determine a decision or course of action, and take the necessary steps to implement the decision. In some cases, it may be a courtesy to let the person who assigned the responsibility know the outcome, but in many instances this is not necessary.

situation. For instance, the individual is given responsibility for making a purchasing decision with level-four authority but within the constraints of an established dollar amount. Or a person may be given the responsibility to make a decision and determine necessary action but only after getting agreement from certain key stakeholders such as employees on the night shift, closely linked employees in another department, or physicians.

Accountability
Accountability is the retrospective review of decisions made or actions taken to determine whether they were appropriate. Were desired outcomes, in fact, achieved? If results were not satisfactory, what corrective action is needed to remedy the situation? This attitude of continual review is characteristic of a lifelong learner, a learning team, or a learning organization.

Application of Empowerment

When a leader applies the empowerment process sequentially, it goes something like this: Before the leader transfers a responsibility, he or she assesses the other person's ability and willingness to take over the responsibility. The leader asks the following questions:

- Does the person have the knowledge to carry out this responsibility?
- Are necessary resources, such as information and time, available?
- Has training or education been provided?
- Is the person willing to accept the responsibility?

Once the leader has determined that capability is present, the leader clearly defines and communicates the responsibility. Assumptions are not enough; the assignment must be clear to both the party accepting the responsibility and the other people who may be affected by this assignment. A discussion of applicable parameters is held, and agreement on the appropriate level of authority is reached. Finally, outcome measures are determined to monitor success. The same process applies to the transfer of responsibility to a group such as a team or a department council.

The significance of empowerment as a developmental process is now clear. As an individual becomes more capable and highly skilled, he or she can accept more responsibility. The level of authority is gradually increased following successful performance of a responsibility. Parameters and constraints may be expanded as comfort with an individual's performance increases. It would be highly foolish, and even dangerous, to give a novice performer level-four authority and no constraints the first time he or she takes on a responsibility.

Using this process appears simple, and yet the many pitfalls and potential missteps in any health care organization today may impede it. When situations arise in which people feel disempowered, the process presented here can be used to assess the source of the problem and to give guidance for correcting it. Following are some of the more common examples of pitfalls with each of these elements of empowerment as they relate specifically to shared decision making.

Common Pitfalls Affecting Capability

Job requirements change as a result of new needs in the organization, and yet people stay in their positions even when they are no longer able to do the work required. This situation leads to an environment of entitlement. New expectations in the workplace should be communicated, education and training provided, and employees given time to adjust and meet new standards. However, at some point, these individuals must be expected to develop the abilities required or face a change in roles or separation from the job.

Another problematic situation occurs when individuals take on or accept responsibility for an assignment they are not capable of carrying out. Perhaps they believe they have the skills, but in reality they do not. This situation creates frustration for both the employee and the manager. It also results in lengthy and potentially costly delays in completing the task.

Some people are simply unwilling to accept more responsibility. This development creates an admittedly difficult situation for a leader, manager, or co-worker. With reductions in staffing levels and downsizing of organizations, everybody simply has to pull his or her own weight. The highest levels of performance are needed from every individual, and shortfalls from those not contributing fully can simply no longer be absorbed by others. Although it is impossible to force someone else to accept responsibility, such acceptance can be made a requirement of the job, which, if not met, means job loss.

In addition, resources may be insufficient for people to capably accept certain responsibilities. Time, equipment, money, education, training, or coaching may not be available, although individuals may be willing to accept additional responsibility. Organizations that attempted to convert to team-based structures in the past are a good example. Redesign of work was accomplished and team structures were determined. Employees were assigned to teams and expected to carry out their work in a new way without preparation in the form of education or training; furthermore, they reported to managers who had little or no experience in coaching teams. In addition, no extra time was incorporated into work assignments for the collective work of the team. This approach created a no-win situation for all involved.

Common Pitfalls Affecting Responsibility

The most common pitfall with responsibility is that it is not clearly communicated but is instead assumed to be understood. For instance, both managers and employees make the mistake of assuming that the job description clearly and completely defines what the employee is expected to do. Instead, both parties need to realize that numerous other responsibilities are always involved for which an individual is held accountable, and these must be clearly articulated. For instance, as mentioned in chapter 6, employees should be told upon hire, "You are responsible for two things as an employee. The first is to do the work for which you were hired at an acceptable level of quality. The second is to form and maintain healthy working relationships with your co-workers as well as with your patients/customers." In other words, employees, not managers, are responsible for relationship issues in the workplace. Relationship issues range from resolving conflicts in a positive manner to having open, honest, and direct communication with co-workers. Managers are available for coaching in difficult situations, but it is clear that maintaining healthy relationships is everyone's responsibility. But how often is this responsibility discussed clearly among employees and managers? Most employees assume this is the manager's responsibility.

Another problem with the element of responsibility occurs when there is a significant overlap of responsibility. In one organization, the chief operating officer was a cautious individual with a bad habit of asking multiple managers to do the same task. A manager asked to investigate and follow up on a problem would discover that others had been asked to assume the same responsibility. It was irritating and demoralizing to the managers to find they were duplicating one another's efforts. In some rare instances, it makes sense for several people to share a task or responsibility. But in order to avoid a disempowering and discouraging situation, the involved parties need to clearly discuss who is doing what. Few people appreciate it when their time is wasted by having to do redundant work.

In some instances, individuals have an exaggerated sense of responsibility and take ownership beyond what is intended. This situation can also lead to frustration and discouragement for all involved. In one organization, a team of internal trainers was created to provide the education and training for a major organizational initiative in process improvement. In the beginning, the team mistakenly believed that its role was to lead this initiative. Its members felt responsible for the success or failure of the effort, and it did not help matters that managers in this organization abdicated their responsibility for leading the improvement process to the team of internal trainers. Conflict and difficulties were significant until the responsibility of each was clearly defined. This particular pitfall is especially important to avoid when working with department councils and other group decision-making entities.

Common Pitfalls Affecting Authority

The concept of authority is the one in which most confusion and problems occur for people. Many individuals believe empowerment only happens when they have level-four authority and that anything less than independent action is disempowering. Nothing could be farther from the truth. The level of authority has to be only high enough to carry out the responsibility, and when the authority level is commensurate with the responsibility, empowerment results. Even a chief executive officer or system president does not hold level-four authority for every aspect of his or her work. In any role, some responsibilities rightfully entail a lower level of authority.

A second source of confusion around authority comes from the mistaken but commonly held belief that the lower levels of authority are not as important as the higher levels. Many mistakes and poor decisions are made in today's organizations because of this misconception. Individuals are asked for their opinion or to gather information, but because they are not making the final decision, they do a halfhearted job of collecting or giving the requested information. The individual making the final decision is disadvantaged because of poor-quality input. Each level of authority is critical, and responsibilities with each level of authority must be taken seriously.

Levels of authority may be falsely assumed by both performers and leaders unless these levels are specifically discussed and agreed upon. Conflict occurs when it becomes apparent that there is disagreement. Quality or problem-solving teams often encounter this situation. In one organization this issue arose in the nursing department with a very visible employee team that had been asked to develop a clinical career ladder for the department. The team worked diligently for months and created an entire program based on extensive research from other hospitals. On the verge of implementation, they were stopped by the corporate human resources department because of compensation issues and a need for equity across the entire system. Home health and long-term care had not been included, nor had any of the other professional departments. This team had unwittingly exceeded its level of authority, and as a result, a significant amount of resentment and frustration developed between the hospital nursing department, corporate human resources, and the rest of the system. The team's level of authority had been assumed but never discussed.

Changing levels of authority in the middle of a project is sometimes necessary but should be avoided if possible. In some cases, a manager has given an individual a responsibility and an agreed-upon level of authority only to recall or decrease the level of authority when the individual or group does not carry out the work in the way the manager desires or expects. There are, however, multiple ways of achieving necessary outcomes, and a confident leader recognizes the need to relinquish control and let followers find their own way. When the project or assignment is snatched away midstream, the result leaves a feeling of resentment for participants and an unwillingness to accept further responsibility.

New authority-related problems are appearing today with the major structural changes in the workplace. In the past, managers were clearly delegated a certain level of authority, and reporting relationships were delineated and unambiguous. For many people in today's health care system, this framework has changed completely. Take, for example, the role of the nurse executive, who is responsible for the nursing function throughout the organization in hospitals. The responsibility has become increasingly difficult to carry out now that it is dispersed among a variety of managers, some of whom have no professional nursing background and may report directly to a different executive. Communicating the essence of nursing issues and ensuring quality standards in the absence of line authority require strong leadership skills.

A final problem related to authority is the reversal of authority. The authority is taken away or disregarded after it has been granted. This situation occurs when a manager undermines the work or simply shows a lack of respect for the final decision the individual or group has made. The most frequent cause of this behavior is the manager neglecting to identify key parameters up front and the decision made by the individual or group being based on incomplete information. Less frequently, however, the manager may have had no intention of relinquishing control at all but wanted others to feel as though they had participated.

In the early days of the quality movement, this lesson was frequently learned the hard way. One quality team worked for six months on a specific problem. Its recommendation would have cost $200,000 to implement and included the addition of several full-time-equivalent positions to the annual personnel budget. No one thought to tell the team that any recommendation could not exceed the current budget. Unfortunately, its experience led its members to conclude that administration was not serious about involving employees in decision making and that quality was not a primary concern. Although members of the team were selected because of their interest and commitment, they became unwilling after this experience to participate in any further projects. It is possible that the budget constraints might have been more acceptable if they had been identified during the initial stages of the project.

Sometimes, group members attempt to undermine decisions. A medical clinical affairs committee discovered this issue in one organization. The director of medical affairs was given the authority to solve a problem within the parameters of a certain dollar amount. Two weeks later he reported on his actions. Two physicians who had not been present at the previous meeting began questioning and second-guessing his decision. The chair of the committee firmly reminded them that the director of medical affairs had been given the authority to solve the problem and that his decision would be respected and supported. However, under other circumstances, this situation could have undermined the authority of the director of medical affairs.

Common Pitfalls Affecting Accountability

While problems with authority are the most common, issues concerning accountability are often the most serious. Accountability is potentially the weakest link in the empowerment sequence. If individuals are not held accountable for their behaviors and actions, whatever was accomplished through the first three steps can be quickly negated. One reason so many things go right in organizations today is because many employees and managers feel a high level of personal accountability, continually reviewing their outcomes and learning from them. People who are continual learners demonstrate a high level of internal accountability. Nevertheless, many problems are inherent in external accountability, or the formal, traceable lines of accountability in the organization.

Most organizations have only limited systems of accountability. It can sometimes be very difficult to ascertain what went wrong and why. Increasing numbers of part-time employees and per diem or temporary employees have made determining who is responsible when a problem occurs rather complicated. Assignments of employees are often inconsistent, and many handoffs from caregiver to caregiver and department to department increase the difficulty of tracking.

Another issue hampering accountability is the tendency of managers and leaders to protect employees. When individuals or teams make a mistake or a poor decision, the real role of the leader is to coach and support them in their efforts to correct the situation. Too often, however, the manager steps in and takes responsibility for correcting the problem. Take, for example, a situation in which a physician has a complaint about an employee or a team and goes to the manager. If the manager takes care of the problem, the employee or team has learned little except that it is not capable of resolving its customer service or relationship problems. On the other hand, if the manager coaches the individual or team to work directly with the physician to resolve the issue, both the team and the physician benefit. A manager's caretaking behavior is sometimes motivated by his or her satisfaction in solving problems or, in some cases, by expectations within the hierarchy. Many established bureaucracies have only limited tolerance for these situations and simply want them resolved in the quickest fashion possible.

The final major pitfall for accountability is that the consequences of mistakes or poor judgment are too often punitive rather than corrective. Many organizational climates today are characterized by blame and accusation when things go wrong. These negative, punitive responses are probably the fastest way to squelch the staff's willingness to accept responsibility in the future. People are quick learners, and they watch what happens to their colleagues and co-workers who make mistakes. Swift retribution designed at extinguishing poor performance may end up extinguishing all performance. People are not willing to take risks in a harsh and unforgiving environment. Extensive work in the area of patient safety initiatives has found that in a just culture, mistakes and errors are evaluated as learning opportunities, and each case is investigated thoroughly before interventions are determined.

Shared Decision-Making Models

Most leaders in health care organizations who are aware of empowerment issues and their pitfalls agree that capability, responsibility, authority, and accountability should be balanced and commensurate with each other if their organizations are to be effective and employees are to have any degree of job satisfaction. Clearly, employee empowerment is a valuable concept, especially in the effort to retain top-performing staff members. It is also generally understood that the closer decisions are made to the point of service, the better those decisions will be. "Those who have to make it work should be involved in the decisions about the work" is a generally accepted management principle that goes back to the formation of quality circles for process improvement efforts as long ago as the early 1980s. Shared decision making can span a continuum of formality. On the informal side of the continuum, it is simply the manager's philosophy and practice to include and engage employees in decision making. On the more formal end of the continuum, an actual structure may be designed to ensure that employees are involved in carefully identified issues.

Shared Decision Making in Nursing

Shared decision making was the major underlying principle in the development of shared governance in nursing almost thirty years ago. Although the description of the concept has expanded and changed somewhat over the years from shared governance to shared decision making or shared leadership, the principles hold true that professional nurses need to be making the decisions that affect their practice. As is the case with almost any major cultural change, a structure also needs to be in place to facilitate the process, which in this case is professional decision making. Dr. Timothy Porter-O'Grady (2001, p. 469) makes this point emphatically as he stresses the core principle for shared decision making and employee empowerment:

> Empowerment involves recognizing the power already present in a role and allowing that power to be expressed legitimately. Empowerment does not give anything to anyone. There is no transfer of the locus of control. It is more a recognition of the legitimate location for certain decisions and structuring the system to let those decisions be made where they legitimately belong.

Structuring the system to let those decisions be made where they belong has for many hospitals involved creating unit-based councils of staff nurses around key aspects of decision making such as clinical practice, management, education, and quality. (See figure 8-2.) Typically, the elected or appointed leaders of these councils represent their patient care units on housewide nursing councils to deal with practice, management, education, or quality issues that involve all similar departments across the organization or even the system. This approach helps promote consistency and standards

Figure 8-2.   Classic Model for Shared Governance

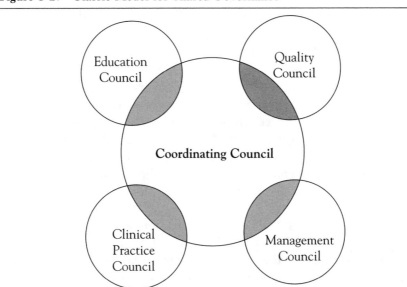

of practice and fosters a collaborative work environment. The leaders of the housewide councils form a coordinating council to act as a clearinghouse for projects or issues and to serve an oversight function of identifying and reducing any redundancy of effort or duplication among the councils. This model, or some variation of it, is in place in virtually all Magnet-designated hospitals across the country and in hundreds of other hospitals throughout the world (Porter-O'Grady 2001).

Shared Decision Making across Disciplines

Although the shared decision-making model has become a template for decentralizing decision making in nursing departments and is widely accepted as a framework for shared decision making among nurses and the management teams with whom they work, the same pervasive effort to develop similar models for employees has not been seen in other disciplines. Shared decision-making models that include all disciplines across the organization have not existed until recently. Any cross-disciplinary efforts that existed previously usually developed when members of other disciplines were invited to nurse-led councils for input and collaboration on relevant issues. Nothing more formal has been used on a widespread basis in health care. Efforts to involve all disciplines in shared decision making can be categorized in one of the three following ways:

1. The effort involved the formation of councils around strategic initiatives such as patient safety, customer service, or community involvement.
2. The effort was modeled after process improvement techniques that have demonstrated success in the business world. Some examples include Lean thinking, an approach to improve productivity pioneered by Toyota (Womack and Jones 1996), and Six Sigma, a methodology for statistical analysis and process improvement made popular by Jack Welch as he touted the $600 million addition to the bottom line experienced by General Electric in the late 1990s (Plotkin 1999). These ideas that were so successful in business have been adapted in any number of health care organizations with significant results and a marked increase in the involvement of managers and employees in a wider range of system changes and fiscal accountability.
3. The effort was apparent in other common organizational structures with goals similar to those of shared governance. For instance, organizations that implement a team-based design are accomplishing much the same end—placing responsibility for frontline decisions about the work to the people doing the work.

For organizations that have invested in the formation of councils across disciplines or in sophisticated training efforts like those just mentioned, there is no question that they have improved employee and management decision-making skills. The result is empowered frontline employees with more ownership for process improvement and productivity that ultimately results in a positive impact on patient and service outcomes as well as financial viability. These changes represent substantial improvements over the hierarchical, top-down decision making that has characterized health care workplaces for more than a hundred years.

Health care has finally begun, just in the last decade, to move toward sharing decisions with those who have to make them work. However, there is still much work to be done in fundamentally changing how decisions are made in the day-to-day operations of hospitals and other health care organizations. Too often, substantive decisions are made only at the top despite the fact that council members have been educated in the latest management techniques or that extensive time was taken to discuss issues. In the absence of a prevailing structure or infrastructure to share decision making and move decisions to the point of service, old patterns are unlikely to change (Porter-O'Grady 2001).

Lessons Learned from Shared Decision-Making Model Implementations

Significant gains due to shared decision making can be achieved by organizations that are invested and committed over the long term to increasing employee involvement. In difficult times, it is a challenge to not revert to the old patterns of hierarchical decision making. It is also essential that long-term commitment and support of the new culture must be hardwired into the organization from the board level through management levels in order to protect the fragile new structures and approaches from external events and internal changes.

Another significant challenge for organizations implementing shared decision-making structures is the increased amount of time and involvement they require on the part of employees. If this factor is not anticipated and built into the system, it will likely fail. One faculty member who talked about "shared governance" being considered in her school of nursing said she just did not see how it could work. If faculty were going to be part of these decisions, it meant they needed to be more involved and prepared, be more knowledgeable about the big picture, and spend more time in meetings. None of this additional work would be counted as workload credit or toward merit points, but instead would be in addition to the current requirements for teaching, research, and working in service. Employee involvement is a terrific idea, but if an individual's involvement is ultimately punishing in some way, it will not likely be sustained by an organization.

A sad example from an acute care medical center illustrates this point. A long-tenured, highly valued clinical nurse was involved in the center's shared governance structure. She served as co-chair of the education council in addition to working the night shift on a part-time basis. As part of her responsibilities on the council she was expected to attend multiple meetings throughout the month. These meetings, held during the day, were in addition to her work schedule on the night shift. What made her council membership more frustrating was that she was responsible for securing speakers and setting up educational events for the staff, even though she had neither the experience in doing so nor the authority to make final decisions. As a result, her council duties took a longer time to complete than they otherwise could have. She became exhausted at what had ballooned into more than a full-time job on part-time expectations. When she expressed her concerns and discouragement about the many meetings, no one heard her complaints. Although committed and enthusiastic at the beginning, she resigned and left the organization both depleted and demoralized.

This example drives home two lessons. The first is that work time must be allotted for employees to be truly involved in shared decision making. In the beginning stages of being included in the decision-making process, individuals may be excited and enthusiastic about participating. But if their participation is punishing in any significant way, the energy and enthusiasm of these once committed champions will ultimately be squandered. A second lesson here is that some common sense must be applied to the situation. The concept of staff involvement in decision making does not mean these employees must do all of the work of implementation as well. In the case of the nurse, the design of the educational event is rightfully her responsibility and that of the education council. However, the centralized education department exists to provide specialists in education matters and support for carrying out the details of the educational events. Not everyone on the council needs to be an expert in how to secure a meeting room, establish dates, negotiate a contract with a speaker, make hotel reservations, and so on. And the work of the council should not be foisted on one person alone. The organization in question, although well-intentioned, failed to see the unintended consequences of their poor management of employee involvement.

In spite of problems and difficulties, the models shared here can serve as prototypes for organizations that want to invest in an ongoing effort toward creating a more collaborative workplace where long-overdue changes can be achieved. As leaders and executives struggle with ways to create positive workplaces, they become increasingly aware that the old hierarchical, patriarchal, bureaucratic structures increase employee dependency and have a potentially negative impact on the quality of work life for everyone. This situation translates into fewer positive organizational outcomes. There is no better time than the present for developing an infrastructure for shared decision making, considering the increased numbers of knowledge workers and members of the younger generational cohorts who want to be in the loop on decisions and recognized for their contributions. Contemporary workers know that they have a range of opportunities and that their services will be in demand for years to come as workforce shortages grow more significant. Health care organizations are under pressure to change the workplace in fundamental ways if they are to attract top-performing employees. Examining current formal approaches to shared decision making is a first step, and applying these principles throughout the organizations and systems is the second step. Building an infrastructure for shared decision making has clearly become a priority for forward-thinking organizations. While these changes will not be easy, they are necessary.

Porter-O'Grady, the respected innovator of nursing shared governance for thirty years, conveys a sense of urgency in making the argument for shared decision making:

> Whatever the process of changing structure, locus of control, decision processes, and team-based initiatives are called, they are essential to the future of doing health services business. From shared governance to shared leadership, shared decision making, empowerment, point of service accountability, or whatever other name might be attached to the dynamic, shared decision making is an essential element of the work of reconceptualizing and configuring health care for the future. . . . It is not possible to empower the consumer to make [the] right choices if providers who enable this empowerment are not empowered. Building a structure for empowerment is not only relevant it is essential. (Porter-O'Grady 2001, p. 473)

Skills Needed for Shared Decision Making

This section of the chapter explores several key skills necessary for successfully implementing shared decision-making models. Problem solving and decision making are discussed in some detail. Two additional and relatively new approaches to problem solving—appreciative inquiry and polarity management—are also discussed briefly as possible alternatives to more traditional approaches.

Problem-Solving Skills

In hierarchical, top-down organizations, problem solving is limited in terms of both who is involved and the kinds of problems around which groups meet. Group problem solving is a bottom-up process requiring a visionary leader, a manager or leader who can relinquish control sufficiently to create an environment for employee empowerment. When problem-solving groups are prevalent in an organization, it is a good sign of employee involvement. Knowledgeable leaders understand that it is difficult for individuals to feel empowered when they have no tools with which to solve pressing problems that directly affect their ability to do their work. Seeing improvement in their daily work life creates a sense of momentum and hopefulness for the future in the work group and ensures future participation in these activities. Many quality or process improvement groups are essentially problem-solving groups.

Process of Problem Solving

Often what passes for problem solving is some spontaneous, inconsistently applied brainstorming technique that follows no proven methodology and misses one or more important steps. Most effective problem-solving processes include some variation of the following five steps, as illustrated in figure 8-3. A skilled leader understands that this process must be both sequential and methodical. All of the steps must be included and performed in the appropriate sequence in order to obtain a quality outcome.

The following problem-solving process can be used effectively by either individuals or groups. Group problem solving is the format considered for purposes of this discussion.

Step 1: Identify and Analyze the Problem

In the first step of a problem-solving process, the group describes, analyzes, and, ultimately, defines the problem. The discussion typically begins with descriptions of symptoms or other evidence of a problem as it affects various members of the group. In many instances, initial statements of the problem are vague and confused. Sometimes additional information is needed before the problem can be defined and a problem statement can be written.

It is important to bring to the surface as many characteristics of the problem as possible at this point and to avoid jumping to hasty conclusions. Psychologists who have experimented with thinking for over the past seventy years have discovered that once a person offers an explanation, he or she has difficulty revising it or dropping it even in the face of contradictory information. In early experiments, subjects were shown an out-of-focus 35 millimeter slide of a fire hydrant. The psychologists found that when a person mistakenly identified the object when it was out of focus, he or she often could not identify it correctly when it was brought into greater focus, whereas another person who had not seen the blurry slide could easily recognize it. Their conclusion was significant: More evidence is required to

Figure 8-3.   Problem-Solving Process

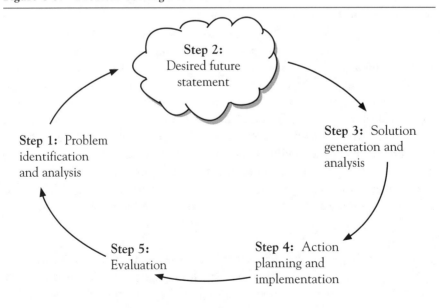

overcome an incorrect hypothesis than to establish a correct one. Individuals who jump to a hasty conclusion are less sensitive to new ideas and information (Adams 1986). This same concept is presented in chapter 3 with the exploration of commitment. It has been found that, to whatever extent a person is rational, he or she is less so after making a commitment.

Asking questions often helps to define the problem more fully, for example:

- What are the signs and symptoms of this problem?
- Whom does the problem affect?
- Is its effect direct or indirect?
- What is the frequency of occurrence?
- What are all of the possible causes or factors involved?

The group may determine that more information or data are required. Many of the techniques taught through quality improvement programs, such as using histograms, fishbone diagrams, Pareto charts, and process and scatter diagrams, can be helpful at this point in the decision-making process (Byers and White 2004).

During this first step, another important issue to consider is ownership. How have the group or individuals within the group contributed to or created the current problem? This factor is critical to consider because the group will have better success if it begins with alternatives over which it has control. Accepting some of the responsibility for the problem is difficult for many groups, which often begin by believing the cause and fault for the problem lie elsewhere. By pushing themselves, however, they usually begin to see how they have helped create the current situation.

Caregivers in one organization were angry because they often did not have enough clean linen in the morning to complete changing the patients' bed linens. They clearly attributed the problem to the linen services department. When forced to look at their own role in creating the problem, they were clueless. They continued to insist that it was the fault of linen services. But with persistent prodding, they gradually began to come up with ideas. "We stopped attending the liaison meeting with linen services because we didn't think they were listening to our concerns." They also recalled being told that over $200,000 in linens was replaced during the year because of employee theft. That money could have helped pay for a higher-capacity washing machine that would process linens faster. The final contributing factor to the missing linen that the caregivers identified was their common practice of hoarding linen and stashing it in all kinds of places so that it would be available when needed. This practice had made it impossible to get an accurate inventory count, which required linen services to plan inventory on the basis of inaccurate figures. Once these issues were identified, the group began to work more effectively on the problem.

Another situation in which individuals had to accept some ownership for a problem was in an imaging department where the problem was

incomplete requisitions for procedures. One way the radiology employees had contributed to the problem over the years was that they usually
accepted the patients and performed the procedures in spite of being
given incomplete or inaccurate requisition forms. As a result, the persons
responsible for the inaccurate requisitions never realized that they were
causing problems for radiology.

Once the problem is fully identified, the problem statement can be written. The problem statement is a concise description of the problem. Novice
problem-solving groups tend to put the solution into the problem statement.
One group, for example, came up with "the problem is inadequate staffing." So stated, this limits problem-solving creativity because the solution
automatically becomes getting more staff. When the problem statement is
changed to "there is more work than the current employees can handle,"
multiple possibilities become apparent, including eliminating some of the
work, changing the way the work is being done, obtaining time-saving technology, and making temporary adjustments in staffing levels.

Once the problem is clearly identified, the group determines its level
of authority in solving the problem. Determining the level of authority
at this point is critical because it ensures that everyone's expectations are
appropriate. Necessary communication and involvement with others in the
organization can be planned. Just because a group has a low level of authority does not preclude it from working on a particular problem; clarity about
authority levels prevents misunderstandings later, when it comes time to
implement the decisions.

Compare these two employee groups: Both chose to work on a problem
for which they had only level-one authority. The issue was employee benefits. The first group was very aware of its level of authority. The members
spent their time investigating the problem and gathering information, and
they made recommendations for the human resources department to consider based on their findings. Their work focused on a desired future that
included the successful presentation of their information and specific steps
aimed at their strategies for delivering the recommendations.

The second group had not clarified its level of authority. The members
proceeded with enthusiasm throughout the entire process, developing a
future vision that included employee benefits offered in a cafeteria-style
approach. Their action planning revolved around the implementation of
the new benefits. They were excited and eager when they finished the
problem-solving process only to become frustrated and angry when their
work was never acted upon. The members of the group cynically observed
that it was the last time they would volunteer for a problem-solving task
force, never realizing that the work they had done substantially exceeded
their level of authority.

Successful problem-solving groups require active involvement and
coaching from savvy managers who can ensure the methodical process is followed. A manager usually has more organizational understanding that can
prevent a group from spinning its wheels in ineffective effort.

Step 2: Focus on a Desired Future Statement

A common mistake problem-solving groups make is to focus almost exclusively on the problem and its causes rather than on what they would like to build or create for the future. Russell Ackoff, the creator of interactive planning, has demonstrated clearly that solutions are more creative if the focus remains on desired outcomes rather than on details of the current problem (Ackoff, Finnel, and Gharajedaghi 1984).

Just as important as the problem statement is the future statement. This step involves asking the question, What would this look like if there were no problem, if it were solved? The group then writes a future statement or a description of the ideal situation. For example, if the group's problem statement were, "Communication between hospital and home health personnel is poor, creating problems in delivery of quality patient care," a desired future statement might be, "Communication between hospital and home health personnel is free flowing, timely, and accurate." In another example, a group was working on coordinating community services for seniors. Its desired future statement read, "Community services for seniors are coordinated and easily accessible to participants, with information flowing freely and fluidly between agencies for the benefit of our program participants."

Focusing exclusively on the problem statement leads to more limited solutions. A clear, desirable future statement creates a picture for those involved and generates more imaginative and original ideas, as well as a broader scope of possibilities.

Step 3: Generate and Analyze Potential Solutions, Part 1

Step 3 is both creative and analytical, and it is helpful to separate the two phases of this step. The group first generates all possible solutions. The first part of step 3 concentrates on identifying all of the potential solutions to be considered. These solutions are not analyzed critically until the second part of the step. Nothing impairs creative flow faster than criticism or an analysis of the ideas as they are presented. Creativity techniques are important during the idea generation phase. Figures 8-4 through 8-8 (pp. 248–251) outline several examples of generating creative solutions, which can be reviewed in more detail in the many books available on the subject of innovation or creativity.

Step 3: Generate and Analyze Potential Solutions, Part 2

The second part of step 3 is to analyze all the solutions generated in the first phase. Once all of the possible alternatives have been identified, the group can begin to converge regarding the most viable options. A series of helpful questions for sorting and categorizing feasible alternatives includes the following:

- Are some alternatives very similar, or do they overlap?
- Can certain solutions be combined?
- Do any alternatives need to be rearranged?

- Can any be eliminated? If the answer is yes, should any worthwhile applications or characteristics of the eliminated options be considered?
- What is good about a solution?
- How would it solve the problem or help create the desired future?
- Are there any possible unexpected consequences of this option?
- If anything goes wrong, what would be the course of action?
- What is the group's degree of control or level of authority over this option?
- Are there key stakeholders who need to be involved to make this option a success? Are stakeholders likely to support it?
- What resources would be needed to implement this solution and are obtainable?
- Are more data and information needed?

Figure 8-4.   Nominal Group Technique

Description: The nominal group technique combines quiet, individual thinking time with a structured and yet free-flowing sharing of ideas. The nominal group technique follows a specific process that often yields successful outcomes (Delbecq and VandeVen 1971). This technique is especially useful when group members possess varied levels of verbal and expressive skills. (The nominal group technique is often mistakenly confused with brainstorming, a much looser process of generating ideas.)

Process:

1. The facilitator asks a question about the problem, and then group members individually respond in a way specified by the facilitator. For instance, if the desired future is for communication between two agencies to be free flowing, timely, and accurate, the facilitator may solicit responses regarding characteristics required to achieve this state. The group members then individually write down all responses that come to mind after the leader specifies either how many ideas (say, five to ten) each participant should list or the time frame in which the list should be completed (perhaps five minutes).

2. The facilitator provides these guidelines for sharing the ideas:
   - Take turns; every participant gives one idea at a time.
   - No one is to react in any way to the ideas as they are being presented, which means no clarification or discussion of any kind at this point.
   - If a group member runs out of ideas, he or she can pass until the next turn, when he or she may present another idea if one occurs.

3. The facilitator lists each idea on a flip chart or board, with no rewording of the idea, until all ideas from the group have been written for the group to see.

4. Once the ideas are gathered, the facilitator leads a discussion of the ideas to clarify, elaborate, defend, dispute, or add to the items.

5. The list is reviewed and categories are identified. Some items may be combined or eliminated.

Figure 8-5. Mind Mapping

Description: Mind mapping is similar to the nominal group process, but the recording of ideas is done in a circular fashion. Even totally unrelated ideas are captured because they may spark an idea for someone else. As Wycoff (1991, p. 48) explains, "Two things happen when you allow yourself to put the idea down—the first is that the mind is freed to go onto other ideas, and the second is that associations are made with this idea. This is where the best ideas come from."

Process:

1. In a box or oval drawn in the center of the chart or board, one or two words that capture the essence of the issue are printed. In the example described above in the text, it might be "communication between agencies."

2. As members contribute thoughts and ideas on the topic, the facilitator prints the key words describing those thoughts around the essence statement and then connects them to the box with lines. As ideas are generated that relate to one of those branches, the idea's key word is printed and then attached to the branch with a line.

Figure 8-6. List Making

Description: List making is a conceptualization technique. It uses the construction of lists as a method of forcing alternative thinking. A simple and effective approach, it starts with a question or an issue, and then the group members generate a list of ideas to address the subject. The value of list making lies in the fact that checklists require a person to consciously control his or her thinking in order to focus on alternatives that the unconscious mind might ignore in trying to simplify life (Adams 1986). For example, list making was used in a head injury rehabilitation center to discover ways of improving the environment for clients (Manion 1990).

Process:

1. The facilitator asks the group members to suggest items for the list. In the example above, the employees were asked to think about the things that they would miss or want if they were confined by a head injury to a rehabilitation facility for the months that recovery would require.

2. The facilitator creates a list of all of the ideas that were generated, for example:

Pictures of family and friends	Favorite television programs
The feel of sun or rain on my face	Favorite music
	My children staying overnight with me
The feel of sand between my toes	Surprises
The smell of coffee in the morning	Sleeping late in the morning
My hair and makeup done every day	Popcorn
	Ability to make my own decisions
Shopping trips	My pets

3. The list can then be used to guide changes, create solutions, or design new products or services.

Although this is a lengthy list of questions, each question is important. The group needs to think about the answers to each and get ready to move on to the next. There is no perfect solution for the problems in organizations today, and it is better to implement something than to be caught in a never-ending spiral of data collection. When the selected solution does not work, at least the group has more knowledge and information on which to base a new decision.

At the end of this step, the group should have identified at least two or three viable solutions. Stopping at only one solution is dangerous. If it is not accepted or cannot be implemented, the group members will feel demoralized,

Figure 8-7.   Attribute Analysis

Description: Attribute analysis involves breaking away from our common tendency to rely on generalization. When problem solvers consider the specific attributes of a situation, they come to different conclusions than they would have if they had applied generalized stereotyping.

Attribute analysis can be illustrated with a simple example: a standard lead pencil. The attributes of the pencil are that it is hexagonal in shape, pointed on one end, constructed of wood with a lead center, painted yellow, and topped with a rubber eraser. Each of these attributes could then be analyzed further. For instance, the properties of wood include its ability to burn, float, insulate against electricity, and provide structural support. Then each of the properties of wood could be used to create lists of things that burn, float, or provide insulation and structure.

Process:

1.   List the attributes of the situation.

2.   Below each attribute, list as many alternatives as possible.

3.   When completed, make many random runs through the alternatives, selecting a different one from each column and assembling combinations of entirely new forms of the original subject.

Example: This approach was used by employees of a new outpatient surgical center to design a user-friendly system with correspondingly friendlier processes. They began by listing attributes of a user-friendly system: easy access to the building, convenient parking, comfortable waiting facilities for family and friends, speedy admission processes, simplified discharge procedures, a pleasant atmosphere, and procedures scheduled for the convenience of the client. They then listed the specific attributes under each of these characteristics. Below convenient parking, for example, were listed "covered, inexpensive or free, safe, and not far from the door or shuttle service." By listing these various attributes and going through the lists several times in different ways, employees generated several unique (at the time) approaches that enabled the new center to quickly capture a large segment of the market. These approaches included valet parking, procedures scheduled for the convenience of clients (hours after work were in high demand), discharge prescriptions available prior to surgery to eliminate a stop at the pharmacy on the way home, comedy videos in the waiting room, beepers for family members so they can be called back to the waiting area, and snacks or meals for waiting family members.

Figure 8-8. Storyboarding

Description: The storyboard was created by Walt Disney as a planning method for his animators (Vance 1982). It is used to develop and record the creative thinking process. It is based on the premise that it is easier to see the interconnections among ideas when they are displayed visually. Storyboarding is a useful technique for stimulating and recording ideas between meetings of the problem-solving group.

Example: One executive team adopted this idea for use during strategic planning. In developing a group vision, members were each given a pad of sticky notes and asked to write down one idea per note that described an element of their vision. Individuals generated as many as twenty-five items each. These ideas were then shared and stuck on large pieces of paper around the room. As the notes were discussed, categories began emerging, and subsequent ideas were placed on appropriate pages.

Process:

1. Participants write their ideas on index cards or sticky notes and then attach them to a corkboard or wallboard accessible to everyone in the group.

2. Participants then are free to add cards with new ideas or expansions of other participants' ideas. They may also rearrange or remove the cards as needed.

---

as though they have wasted their time. Also, research has demonstrated that problem solvers are dominated by pressure to solve the problem and that adopting the first solution may reflect this pressure. Forcing the group to develop at least a second alternative results in more creative solutions because focus is on the desired future as opposed to the need to find an answer.

Deciding among the alternatives requires knowledge of decision-making approaches. There are several types of decision making, including voting and reaching consensus, which are explored later in this chapter.

Step 4: Develop and Implement Action Plans

Determining actions to be taken, the time frame within which they are to be completed, and responsibility assignments for each action must be specific and realistic. Once identified, the steps to be taken are prioritized. In many instances, they must be sequential because some are dependent on completion of others.

Once the plan is reasonably complete, costs for both current practice and recommended alternatives are estimated. Spending money or time in order to save a substantial amount of money or time can be a compelling incentive to adopt a new practice. In some instances, no more money is needed for an alternative, but quality of service is positively affected. At this stage, a communication strategy is developed based on who needs to know about this plan and who must be included in developing additional expectations. Questions of how and when to present the results of the problem-solving group are decided.

During implementation, the plan must be monitored closely to maintain momentum. This monitoring function is assigned to an individual who can also reinstitute the group if further work is necessary.

Step 5: Establish Evaluation Criteria

The final step in the problem-solving process is to establish criteria for evaluating success and to determine who will be responsible for the evaluations. The parties involved in implementation must know up front how success will be measured. Evaluation criteria should be as precise and objective as possible, which in some instances is fairly simple. A percentage error rate, the number of completed diagnostic tests, the number of patient falls, and employee productivity figures are a few examples of easily obtained objective measures. Other criteria are more difficult to quantify, such as improvement in relationships between teams or departments, satisfaction levels of key customers, or more subtle changes in the quality of service.

Specific review dates are established, and plans are made for celebration of the completion of this phase of the group's work. Results must be monitored and necessary corrections made. Divergence from expected outcomes means that the cause must be identified and another workable solution found. The second and third solution alternatives formulated earlier in the process are helpful in this case. At this point, the group may need to be encouraged and reminded that even if the first recommendation or solution did not work exactly as planned, the solution is now closer than it was before.

This problem-solving process was used effectively in a hospital in a Sunbelt state in the United States. An annually recurring problem of a lack of patient beds during the winter months with the influx of visitors from the northern states created conflict between employees and physicians, all scraping to come up with needed resources. Finally, during the summer months, the administration initiated a problem-solving team composed of employees, managers, executives, and physicians. The process took several months, but the result was a plan that increased the number of available beds during the winter months and clearly identified backup contingency plans. For the first time in years, the winter season was managed without key stakeholders coming to blows over beds for patients.

Common Pitfalls in the Problem-Solving Process

Two common pitfalls have already been discussed—the suggested solution in the problem statement and having an incongruous level of authority between the group and the action required. However, one of the most common pitfalls in the problem-solving process occurs when the group mistakenly chooses to use the process to solve an issue that would be better solved by another approach like appreciative inquiry or polarity management. Appreciative inquiry and polarity management are discussed later in this chapter. Some issues are simply treated more effectively with approaches like appreciative inquiry; others issues are not clear-cut problems but rather polarities to be managed. Determining early on which approach to use can prevent a great deal of unnecessary effort.

Hidden agendas and personal platforms are another pitfall. Some group members may have a personal strategy they want to promote, even if it has little to do with the issue at hand. These underlying issues cannot be allowed to interfere with a fully explored problem-solving process.

Yet another pitfall occurs when the time frames and the people responsible for each action step fail to be identified. These factors are critical to the implementation stage, at which point it is easy for the group to lose steam and neglect to carry out agreed-upon steps. Monitoring and follow-through are essential.

Following the problem-solving process sequentially is difficult for many groups. The process is a blend of both right- and left-brain activities, and some groups have trouble with one or the other or with switching between the two. Identifying and analyzing problems and developing action plans and evaluation measures are all examples of logical, left-brain thinking. Establishing a desired future and generating all possible options require creativity and spontaneity and involve right-brain thinking.

Moving from one stage to the next may be facilitated by taking a brief physical break between them or actually carrying out each step in separate meetings. This creates boundaries between the two types of thinking processes and helps members make the transition. If people in the group are characteristically logical and concrete thinkers, such as clinical laboratory professionals or operating room staff, the group leader may need to be very firm in keeping the group focused during the right-brain activities because there will be tremendous pressure to move to analysis and left-brain logical activities.

Not respecting the problem-solving process as a methodical, sequential process leads to several common problems. The most common is called the Band-Aid® approach, a knee-jerk reaction that occurs when the group moves straight from problem identification to action planning without taking the time to think through a desired future or develop a full range of creative options, as illustrated in figure 8-9.

Figure 8-9. The Band-Aid® Approach to Problem Solving

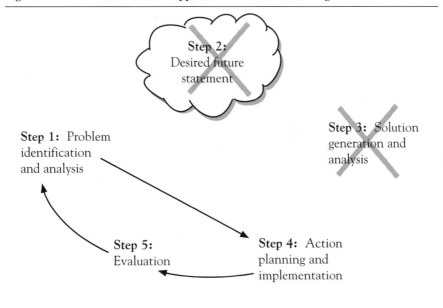

Another common problem, called analysis paralysis (figure 8-10), is experienced when the group stays in the problem-identification phase so long that paralysis sets in. It seems as though there are never enough data to make a decision, not all the facts have been collected, or there is not enough information with which to move ahead. The goal here is to reach a happy medium between gathering the information and coming to a decision. It is important to collect enough data to provide information for adequate analysis through a specific agreed-upon process and then to stick to an acceptable time frame for the problem at hand.

A final pitfall is the exaggerated sense of responsibility that some groups feel. They take on too much ownership for the problems. This situation can often be avoided by asking the important question, What is our level of authority for solving this problem? Groups may discover that they do not have an adequate level of authority for implementing a solution to the problem and can therefore accept that it is not their responsibility to do so. In some instances, they may realize that they are trying to solve a problem for a key group not represented and, as a result, they must modify the membership of their group.

Reasons Groups Fail in the Problem-Solving Process

It is imperative that both individuals and groups develop effective problem-solving skills. Most groups process problems rather than solve them, continually discussing the symptoms or effects, and anything but the root causes. In many instances, the problem itself escapes during the discussion without ever having been defined. Groups engage in unproductive processing for reasons including the following:

- The group uses voting to determine plans of action, which forces group members to pick sides. Once a person takes a side and another opposes it, the two opposing forces become even more adamant and continue to grow farther apart.

Figure 8-10.   Analysis Paralysis in Problem Solving

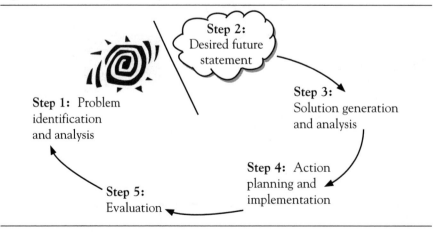

- Groups neglect monitoring their group process. Although members may observe unproductive process, they are too often unwilling to address it. For example, silent members are not asked to contribute, apathy is ignored, unprepared participants are not confronted, or disruptive behavior is tolerated.
- The group does not recognize or understand its patterns of behavior, which may include closing discussions prematurely or reaching decisions without fully analyzing the problem. Members may not recognize groupthink (see below) or behavior that is so polite and courteous that no one dares talk about the real issues. When the group's solutions or alternatives are not accepted, too often the group blames those with authority rather than reviewing their own process and truly evaluating the quality of their work.

Groupthink is a phenomenon "whereby team members become afraid of offering ideas that might conflict with the group's policies and actions. New ideas are often offered weakly and withdrawn quickly if opposed" (Chaleff 1997, p. 4). Groupthink can destroy creative initiative and even cause people with opposing views to be forced out. The remedy for groupthink is continual self-evaluation of the group's patterns and outcomes.

Managers and employees who understand problem solving also understand its relationship to decision making. The two are closely interwoven and highly interdependent. Good problem solvers make decisions, and good decision makers use a problem-solving approach.

Decision-Making Skills

In this context, a decision is a choice among alternative courses of action that may lead to the desired result. When no alternatives are available, no decision is made. Managers and employees alike assume responsibility for the consequences of their decisions. This notion can be frightening at times because many decisions are made under conditions of uncertainty.

Decisions are evaluated based on their results or consequences, which are often unpredictable. An individual or a group does not have to be right all the time, only most of the time. A sign in a printing shop provided this profound piece of wisdom: "Good decisions come from experience. Experience comes from wisdom. Wisdom comes from making bad decisions." If individuals or groups have difficulty dealing with uncertainty, they either postpone decisions until all of the uncertainties have been resolved or they make poor decisions because they are uncomfortable coping with the uncertainties.

"As important as sound decision-making is, many executives [and groups] neglect to use any formal decision-making process" (Clancy 2003, p. 343). Good decision makers combine a logical, systematic approach with their intuition. They sort and classify information; differentiate between the valuable, worthless, and redundant; prioritize; and integrate the whole into an accurate picture of reality. As the amount of information available increases, the complexity of decision making also increases. Managers and employees who are good decision makers evaluate and recognize what type of decision is called for from each new situation.

Types of Decisions

Five types of decisions are commonly made in health care organizations: individual, minority, majority, consensus, and unanimous. The type of decision that is appropriate depends on the specific situation.

Individual Decisions

Individual decisions are made by one person: a leader, a manager, or an individual with the responsibility and authority to decide. Others involved are expected to abide by this decision. This type of decision is most often used when the person with the decision-making authority perceives that there is no choice, the decision is not important, or the group does not want to make a decision. One example of this type of decision is called the "plop," a suggestion that gets accepted without any discussion. The plop can be offered by any member of the group.

Individual decisions are sometimes seen as an imposition or a mandated solution directed by someone with the authority or expertise to impose such a solution. Impositions are justified when the issue is truly nonnegotiable in terms of responsibility, when a group does not accept responsibility for the solution, or when the decision will have relatively little impact.

Minority Decisions

Minority decision making occurs when a few people, or a subgroup of the larger group involved in a situation, meet to consider the matter and make a decision. When a group decides that minority decisions are appropriate, expectations must be clearly articulated between the individual or group delegating the responsibility and the minority or subset of the group accepting the responsibility. The decision of the minority group is considered binding for everyone involved.

This approach is often used by teams and large employee groups. A subset of the team examines an issue and makes a decision for the team. This method can be effective in decision making when it is difficult for a larger group to come together and take the time to navigate the entire process together. It requires a high level of trust within the team or group. Team members with a vested interest in the decision are expected to be part of the subset and are not allowed to sabotage the decision later. This is often the type of decision making represented by a department or an employee council.

Majority Decisions

When more than half of the people involved in a situation make a decision, it is considered a majority decision and is often referred to as a majority rules vote. The resulting decision is binding on all. This type of decision is problematic because it often means that some of the members do not support the result.

Another significant disadvantage to majority decision making is that it forces people to take one side or the other. Often the best solutions are found somewhere in the middle. The more firmly one argues for a certain side or solution, the less likely he or she will be to support an opposing solution if it wins. This form of decision making can be useful when the decisions involve minor issues that do not require 100 percent support to implement or when large numbers of people are involved and no forum or structure is in place for resolving minority positions.

Consensus Decisions
A consensus decision results when the entire group or team addresses a problem with all group members, who fully present their views. It is, first and foremost, a group decision-making process. Consensus is said to exist when each group or team member can honestly make these three statements to every other member (Creative Healthcare Management 1994):

1. I believe I understand your point of view.
2. I believe you understand my point of view.
3. I believe the decision has been made in an open and fair manner, and I am willing to support the decision whether or not it is my first preference.

In true consensus, no majority rules voting, bargaining, or averaging of votes is allowed. The process takes more time to achieve but results in active support and prevents sabotage and undermining of decisions made. Consensus has been described as 70 percent agreement and 100 percent commitment. In other words, a group member may not agree 100 percent with the decision, but he or she feels comfortable with the process used and can honestly agree to support the decision 100 percent. Consensus is especially useful when full team or group commitment to the decision is essential for implementation. In an organization, for example, major decisions such as whether to embark upon a major cultural change initiative or to purchase another facility should be decided by consensus of the entire executive team. If the decision is made in any other manner, support may not be present during implementation, when it is required from the entire team.

Unanimous Decisions
A unanimous decision represents a higher level of commitment. In unanimous decision making, each group member fully agrees on the action to be taken. This type of decision may be needed when it significantly affects each member.

Process of Decision Making

Although group decision making generally results in a higher level of commitment to the decision than does individual decision making, the group decision-making process is also more complex, and arriving at a final decision can be more difficult. Managers and/or group leaders are usually responsible for deciding whether to use an individual or a group decision-making process. At a minimum, the following five factors should be considered:

1. **The nature of the problem or task:** Some problems are more easily solved by a group and others by an individual. In creating a new alternative or doing independent tasks, individuals often surpass groups. A project such as creating a new crossword puzzle is a good example. It is more effectively accomplished by an individual. When tasks are convergent or integrative and require that various pieces of information be brought together to produce a solution (such as solving that crossword puzzle), then a group is better. Most goal setting is also more effective in a group because it increases the variety of contributions and level of commitment.

2. **The importance of acceptance of a solution:** When people participate in the process of reaching a decision, they have more commitment to the decision. They work harder and have a greater interest in making the decision successful. When an individual solves a problem or makes a decision, two things must happen: Others must be persuaded that this decision is best, and others must agree to act on the decision to carry it out. Not all decisions require commitment, and such decisions can be made by an individual.

3. **The value placed on the quality of the decision:** If a manager is concerned with acceptance of a decision and with empowering others, he or she may adopt a decision of somewhat lesser quality because it has widespread acceptance. Decisions made by a group in the beginning of its skill development simply may not have the same level of quality as an experienced individual's decisions. If the quality of the decision is paramount, an individual expert in the field might be used. For example, if a group is having internal communication problems, it may produce and decide on the problem-solving alternatives to implement. If the outcomes are not beneficial, the group can then engage in additional problem solving. Getting it right the first time is not critical. However, if, for example, there are computer hardware problems with a particular application that could significantly affect the organization's information systems, a decision to bring in an external expert to solve the problem or make recommendations may be the prudent choice.

4. **The characteristics of individual group members:** Effective managers consider the expertise of the various group members, the stake each has in the outcome, and the role each is likely to play in implementing the decision.

5. **The operating effectiveness of the group:** It may be a better choice to ask an individual to solve a problem or make a decision than a group that is too new to make the decision or whose members cannot

seem to work together. The skills of the group facilitator have an impact as well.

On the upside, group decision making represents greater total knowledge and information. Each group member brings a different perspective, resulting in a greater variety of approaches. Group decisions may have better acceptance and fewer communication problems. Implementation is likely to be smoother and to require less monitoring.

On the downside, strong social pressure may be applied to conform in a group setting. Groups also tend to err on the side of quick convergence, perhaps settling prematurely on a decision that seems to have support. High-quality ideas introduced late in the discussion have a limited chance of serious consideration. A dominant individual can prevail because of status, verbal skills, or stubborn persistence. Hidden agendas create problems in group decision making. Unless these issues are brought to the surface, they may skew the decision-making process or result in unfair or poor decisions. A significant problem for group decision making is that it simply takes longer for a group to decide.

Common Pitfalls in the Decision-Making Process

One of the most significant pitfalls in the decision-making process is related to the paradox of choice. Author Barry Schwartz says that people today suffer from choice overload. Never before in human history have there been so many choices, and never before have people been more dissatisfied (Schwartz 2004). Rather than exhaustively examining every alternative and aspect of every alternative before making a decision, in order to arrive at the very best choice, Schwartz encourages people to be satisfied with a "good enough" decision.

In his experience, Schwartz found that there are "maximizers" and "satisficers" in terms of their decision making. Maximizers are those who expect the very best and search diligently and endlessly to find it. Satisficers, on the other hand, make a decision first about whether the issue is important enough to undertake such exhausting and endless research, and if it is not, they accept a good-enough choice and then relax and enjoy it. They save themselves a great deal of time, worry, and stress in the process of choosing. He found that maximizers often do get a little more of what they are seeking, but they are less happy than the satisficers. For example, consider a new graduate searching for a job. The maximizer often gets a higher-paying job but is never quite happy; he or she second-guesses the choice (e.g., If only I had waited, maybe I could have gotten more money, a better title, etc.) or harbors self-doubts (e.g., What would the next offer have brought?).

Another common decision-making pitfall is approaching decisions without due consideration of the various types of decision making. Without careful analysis of the situation or sufficient thought given to outcomes, a manager may miss opportunities for effectively engaging others in the decision. Employees can fall into the same trap. There are appropriate occasions for all types of decision making. If employees expect to participate and reach consensus but the manager is making an individual decision, the employees' expectations will not be met.

For example, in one urgent care business, Ellen, the chief executive officer (CEO), decided to reorganize and restructure the leadership and management ranks. Several managers were furious because they were not included in any discussion but were instead simply told what the new structure would be. Ellen elected to make an individual decision, which was her right as the CEO. Unfortunately, however, she had been preaching empowerment for some months, and her individual decision was seen as a slap in the face to those who were committed to building empowerment in the company. An open discussion about how decisions would be made and which were to be individual and which were to be group decisions may have prevented some of these hard feelings.

The third common pitfall is a lack of understanding of consensus. Consensus, like empowerment, has become an overused buzzword in recent years. Some people mistake participatory decision making (where the leader gets input from members, but then a small group or an individual actually makes the decision) as consensus. Consensus is, first and foremost, a group decision-making process. If a decision truly needs to be made by consensus, there can be no assumption that the conditions of mutual belief, understanding, and support have been met. Because reticent or disagreeing group members may not come forward or openly oppose the decision, the leader needs to ask each member of the group to openly state his or her commitment to the decision.

For example, a statewide ad hoc committee whose task it was to recommend a new organizational structure for the state association spent long hours debating this hot political issue. When the group finally settled on a recommendation, the leader asked for consensus. Every group member was individually asked, "Do you believe you understood everyone else's point of view? Do you believe your point of view was fully expressed and understood by the others? Can you support this decision?" Each participant stated his or her agreement. At the annual meeting, however, one of the committee members had second thoughts when he realized that representatives from a special interest group of which he was also a member were upset about the committee's final recommendation. This member began talking with key association members, trying to engender support for an alternative and basically undermining the committee's work. During a public discussion of the issue, the committee chairman reminded association members that the recommendation had been reached by consensus, and he reviewed exactly what consensus means. When reminded that he had agreed to support the decision of the committee, the individual ceased his efforts to overturn the recommendations.

Failing to carefully consider the various factors in group versus individual decision making can be another major pitfall for a manager. A healthy combination of the two is important. In some instances, it is also appropriate to explain why one or the other is used.

As alluded to above, decision making is closely related to problem solving but involves its own special issues. Exemplary leaders and managers are good decision makers, but they also are able to relinquish control and engage others in decision making when circumstances warrant. Shared decision making can strengthen any organization as long as it follows careful consideration. Understanding and applying the four key concepts of empowerment (capability, responsibility, authority, and accountability) can help ensure successful shared decision making.

Appreciative Inquiry Skills

An alternative approach to traditional problem solving or process improvement methodology is a form of action research referred to as appreciative inquiry. Appreciative inquiry is based on the belief that something is already working well in the organization. Finding and studying it can lead not only to a deeper understanding but also to insight into how to overcome the current difficulties and design a more desirable future.

It is well known in the research world that what a person dwells on increases in volume or capacity in his or her life. It follows, then, that focusing on problems is an approach that simply brings more problems or difficulties. Appreciating an issue or a function suggests that it is held as positive, that is, its positive traits or characteristics are seen. This perspective increases its value, much as real estate appreciates in value over the years. Appreciative inquiry is based on generative learning. It is

> [a]n ability to see radical possibilities beyond the boundaries of problems as they present themselves in conventional terms. High-performing organizations that engage in generative, innovative learning are competent at appreciating potential and possibility. They surpass the limitations of apparently "reasonable" solutions and consider rich possibilities not foreseeable within conventional analysis. (Barrett 1995, p. 37)

Traditional Problem Solving and Appreciative Inquiry

Traditional problem solving often involves looking closely at failures and trying to discover the causes. In contrast, appreciative inquiry involves inquiry into successes so one can discover his or her distinctive attributes and use them to build upon performance and create new strategic approaches. Traditional problem solving is a more mechanized approach based on the belief that problems can be isolated, broken down into separate parts, repaired, and then restored to wholeness. As an approach, it often totally misses the systems implications. And, in the same way that one can dissect the body and learn about it even at the smallest cellular level, no one has yet discovered the true essence of the person, the soul or the personality, that makes each person unique. Problem solving can miss the essence of a situation, or what it takes to make it work.

Problem solving is likely to be more effective in dealing with issues that are process improvement oriented, such as tackling the issue of inaccurate radiology requisitions or extended wait times for patients in the emergency department. Appreciative inquiry works well for issues related to less logical and methodical processes, such as changing the work culture or improving relationships. In some instances, a major issue might include both approaches. Improving extended patient wait times in the emergency department is an example of an issue that has both specific process improvement opportunities and needed cultural changes.

Proponents of appreciative inquiry point out that many consequences result from using a problem-solving approach, including the following:

- **Problem solving is a limiting approach to the issue.** Often, constraints of the status quo are accepted, which leads to coping with a problem rather than fixing it. Take, for example, the problem of a very high patient census and the potential need for diverting patients from the emergency department to another facility in town. Employees in one hospital were asked what they would do if the other emergency department in the city was also on diversion status. They were absolutely stymied and could come up with no solutions. When asked about setting a limit on elective admissions to ensure that beds were always available for emergency admissions, the employees found the idea inconceivable because they felt the administration would never consider such an approach. Yet it is a solution, albeit an unpopular one. And until action is taken to create a different scenario for these people, all of their planning is based on coping strategies for dealing with an untenable situation. At what point does it become riskier to continue to admit patients when inadequate resources are available to provide for their safe care?
- **Problem solving is based on an overlearned deficiency orientation.** The assumption is that there is something wrong somewhere. Managers develop self-worth as problem solvers, and so do executives. Thus, the more problems, the more important the person who solves them. This mind-set can lead to the dysfunctional behavior that occurs when individuals seem to be "stirring the pot" or creating problems because solving crises is what they do best.
- **Problem solving is based on a fragmented view of the world.** People in the organization become more and more expert in smaller parts of the system. Along the way it is easy to lose the ability to see the system as a whole and to understand the interdependencies and the intricate connections that exist.

Ludema, Cooperrider, and Barrett (2000, p. 8) sum up the consequences of an organizational focus on problem solving quite well: "As people in organizations inquire into their weaknesses and deficiencies, they gain an expert knowledge of what is 'wrong' with their organizations, and they may even become proficient problem-solvers, but they do not strengthen their collective capacity to imagine and build better futures."

In health care today one of the most important organizational tasks is the creation of learning cultures (Tichy and Cardwell 2002). An appreciative learning culture allows employees to explore and to extend their capabilities and experiment at the very margins of their expertise and knowledge. This culture improves the organization's ability to meet its mission: high-quality care for patients and clients.

Process of Appreciative Inquiry

Although there is no cookie-cutter approach to appreciative inquiry, several general principles and stages have been identified. One of the most important principles is that the leader or group needs to form a positive question or statement of the topic. This is the most critical part of the entire process because it serves as an intervention in and of itself (Zemke 1999). Although it sounds easy enough to accomplish, in truth, most people, when faced with a difficult issue or challenge, tend to focus on the negative and to create a problem-oriented question. Take, for example, the need to improve physician and employee interpersonal relationships and communication. The tendency is to identify this issue as a need to improve physician–employee working relationships. Inherent in this statement is the message that something is wrong at the current time, and it carries with it complex baggage such as the unequal positional power of physicians versus employees or the difference between employees and independent practitioners.

The challenge is to create questions that "inspire and encourage people to give . . . positive examples to use as models" (Zemke 1999, p. 29). So ask people in the organization a question such as, "What examples of positive working relationships between employees and physicians do you see in the organization?" and then further explore the characteristics of these relationships, asking, "What makes these relationships work so well?" Another approach is to ask people to "describe what it is like when you have a good working relationship with a physician (or with an employee)." If the first question is not answered in the affirmative, the initiative will fail.

The stages of appreciative inquiry are illustrated in figure 8-11. They include discovery, dreaming, design, and destiny.

Figure 8-11. Stages of Appreciative Inquiry

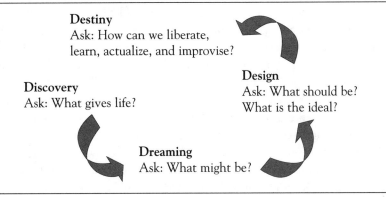

Stage 1: Discovery

The first stage in the process is often referred to as the appreciating phase, and it involves storytelling. It is a very collaborative stage. Participants think of and share examples of experiences that illustrate or answer the appreciative question. They focus on those moments of excellence and identify the factors and characteristics that made them possible. This stage basically answers the question, "What gives life?" From this work it is possible to build consensus around the strengths or basic principles inherent in the issue.

For example, one organization was concerned about creating a more positive work environment in order to attract and better retain employees. It used an appreciative inquiry approach. The questions from this first stage were, "Think of a time when you felt most energized and alive at work. What was happening? Who was there? Describe the workplace environment." Some of the answers included:

- I felt valued.
- I was learning a new skill.
- My manager coached me so I could build my expertise.
- I was involved in helping make the decision.
- There was progress as a result of our actions.
- What I did made a difference.
- I liked the people I was working with.
- We had a great team.
- I was asked my opinion, and it was used in making the final decision.
- I had a high level of autonomy.

From this first step, a list of positive attributes was developed to describe these environments. The current environment can be measured or evaluated against these criteria to determine opportunities for improvement.

Stage 2: Dreaming

The second stage is the dreaming stage, also known as the envisioning phase. The basic question is, "What might be?" This stage often starts off with an exercise such as the one posed by Zemke (1999, p. 30): "Let's assume that tonight we fall asleep and wake up five years from now. When you wake up, the hospital has become exactly the organization you would like it to be. What do you see that is different and how do you know it is different?" The result of this stage is that the group comes to some kind of coalescence around a vision for the group or the organization and drafts a statement of what it will look like in the future. Based on the previous example, a vision statement might be something like, "Our workplace environment is one in which there are healthy working relationships between people, there is a high level of employee involvement in decision making, and people are treated with respect and valued for their contributions."

This stage is similar to the visioning approach used by strong leaders (Manion 2005). However, it is not merely a dream, but a vision that is grounded in history, tradition, and facts. It is based on examples of what has worked.

Stage 3: Design

The third stage in appreciative inquiry is also referred to as the co-constructing phase because the work is to design the ideal. Questions include, "What will it look like? What are the principles that will help translate this vision into action? How can we make this happen?" Many successful books in the genre of business literature use this approach. Organizations or businesses that are successful are studied carefully to determine the principles that led to their success, and then the principles are shared with others, who attempt to emulate them.

A disadvantage of trying to duplicate another organization's successes is the resistance often encountered, because no other organization or business is exactly like yours. The differences are often used as explanations for why it cannot be done. One of the advantages of using an appreciative inquiry approach within the organization is that it takes away this rationalization. People do not resist their own ideas (Jaramillo et al. 2008). For example, if this positive environment can be created in the imaging department, why can it not be done in the laboratory? After all, similar financial constraints exist, the hospital administration is basically the same, community issues are shared, and so on.

Stage 4: Destiny

Destiny, the fourth stage in appreciative inquiry, is also known as the sustaining phase. The questions address how to liberate, learn, actualize, and improve. The work of the participants focuses on how to actualize, sustain, or create these characteristics through changes or projects that build internal capacity. Zemke (1999) notes that originally this stage stood for delivery and the work was focused on developing action plans, building implementation strategies, and monitoring outcomes. This concrete structured process has since been greatly deemphasized by supporters of appreciative inquiry in favor of more spontaneous, free-form sorts of activities. In other words, simply preparing people in the organization with the process of the first three steps and then letting them apply those steps on their own in the organization has been successful in many different types of businesses around the world.

Application

The end result of an appreciative inquiry process depends on the topic that started the cycle. This approach can be used in a very formal manner to identify needed cultural changes (Stefaniak 2007; Havens, Wood, and Leeman 2006) and guide needed improvements. A small hospital in rural Vermont experienced decreased staff morale when large salary hikes were announced at the large tertiary medical center an hour's drive away. Many employees were rumbling about leaving the small hospital and making the drive down the road every day. An appreciative inquiry approach was used with questions focused on what was good about working in the small community hospital. When the stories were told and the attributes identified, it became very clear that there were some possible improvements to be made, but overall, most employees recalled what they valued about the smaller organization.

As a philosophy, appreciative inquiry can also be used in a more informal manner to reverse negativity in the work group and return people to a more positive focus. One executive uses it for a Monday morning meeting with his direct reports. The first agenda item is, "What went right last week?" This is not the typical focus of most Monday morning management huddles.

Shendell-Falik (2008) reported on the use of appreciative inquiry as a method for creating a safer approach to handoffs, thus improving patient safety. The initiative examined the handoffs between the emergency department and other internal patient care units. Staff members were involved in the entire process, interviewing fellow staff members and determining the elements of a safe and effective handoff. They then designed processes that have since been implemented with significant improvements on a variety of measures.

Polarity Management Skills

Still another skill set is needed to deal with issues that arise in the workplace. In some instances, the issue or difficulty faced is not a problem as such, but rather what Barry Johnson calls a polarity. "Polarities are sets of opposites which can't function well independently. Because the two sides of a polarity are interdependent, you cannot choose one as a solution and neglect the other" (Johnson 1996, p. xviii). Believing that every issue or difficulty is a problem results in trying to solve some problems that are simply unsolvable, even if the person has all the necessary resources. By seeing polarities as problems to be solved, the leader greatly undermines results by wasting time in futile efforts. There are many examples of polarities in our health care organizations today:

- Which should be emphasized, leadership or management skills?
- When should individual effort versus team initiative be recognized and emphasized?
- When does the manager perform difficult tasks rather than coaching others on how to do them?
- When is a manager's accessibility and visibility more important than the manager's need for thinking time and privacy?
- When does the implementation of policies require rigidity, and when does it require flexibility?
- When should a priority be placed on the needs of employees versus the needs of patients?
- When does the organization emphasize service at any cost versus cost effectiveness and wise use of resources?
- When does an issue need employee commitment, and when is compliance adequate?

- When is specialization of employees and physicians more appropriate than generalization?
- When is centralization of services more appropriate than decentralization?
- In the face of workforce shortages, when does urgency to produce a supply of workers override the concern for professional standards and patient safety?

If any of these polarities are seen as problems to be solved, efforts are wasted. There are no clear-cut solutions to these issues.

Polarity Management versus Problem Solving

Polarity theory is a conceptual framework for dealing with some of these complex challenges. Johnson's (1996) approach involves identifying when the issue is actually a polarity and managing it as such rather than treating the situation as a problem to be solved. "The objective of polarity management is to get the best of both opposites while avoiding the limits of each" (Johnson 1996, p. xviii). In other words, the manager has the judgment to reward both individual and team effort and understands that in any modern organizational system, there is not only room for but also a need for both models. In some instances, the work is individually based, while in other situations, a team is much more effective. Overemphasis on either end of the polarity can result in problems. The earlier example of the nurse who resigned because of the unrealistic demands incurred as a result of participation in shared governance is an example. Attempts to completely decentralize highly specialized responsibilities in an organization create similar problems. A centralized department of education can be used to support the decentralized decision making of staff. Some elements of the function are carried out much more effectively and efficiently by people who do it more frequently and have experience and skill in doing so.

This approach to issues is very similar to a characteristic of effective leaders. It was addressed in a recent article by Roger Martin (2007), who spent 15 years studying how exemplary leaders think. He found that the leaders he studied all shared a somewhat unusual trait:

> They have the predisposition and the capacity to hold in their heads two opposing ideas at once. And then, without panicking or simply settling for one alternative or the other, they're able to creatively solve the tension between those two ideas by generating a new one that contains elements of the others but is superior to both. This process of consideration and synthesis can be termed integrative thinking. It is this discipline—not superior strategy or faultless execution—that is a defining characteristic of most successful businesses and the people who run them. (Martin 2007, p. 3)

Polarity Mapping

Johnson (1996) offers a concrete way to structure the management of a polarity. He suggests using a grid, or polarity map, with two poles. (See figure 8-12.) The left half represents one side of the polarity, and the right half represents the other side. The upper half represents the positive outcomes that focus on the particular pole, and the lower half represents the negative outcomes that come from focusing only on that pole. Before the individual can effectively manage a polarity, all four quadrants of the polarity grid need to be clearly seen. Johnson suggests filling out whichever quadrants are the easiest first and then working from there.

In figures 8-13 and 8-14, polarity maps are drawn to represent the four quadrants of an issue faced by a respiratory care department in a large tertiary medical center. The pediatric respiratory therapists included those respiratory therapists assigned to general pediatrics and those who were neonatal intensive care unit respiratory therapists. Conflict arose periodically about the issue of specialization versus generalization among these practitioners. The neonatologists and pediatricians were often in direct conflict with each other as well as with the manager and employees of the department about the issue. Over the years, the emphasis moved back and forth. When this conflict is examined as a polarity, the underlying issue is identified as determining whether patient needs or employee needs are paramount.

Mapping this polarity increases clarity of the whole picture or structure of the dilemma. To focus exclusively on patients' needs may result in important employees' needs not being met, which may then result in lower morale and productivity, indirectly affecting whether patients' needs are met. The clearest opposites in the polarity map are the downside of one polarity and

Figure 8-12.   The Polarity Map (Johnson 1996)

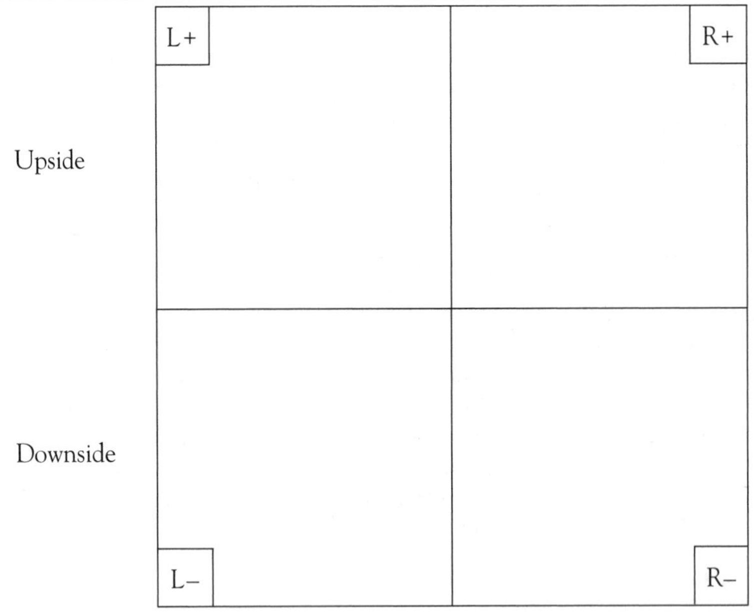

Reprinted from *Polarity Management* by Barry Johnson. Copyright © 1992, 1996. Reprinted by permission of the publisher, HRD Press, Amherst, Mass. (800) 822-2801. www.hrdpress.com.

Figure 8-13. Polarity Map: Patients' Needs versus Employees' Needs (Johnson 1996)

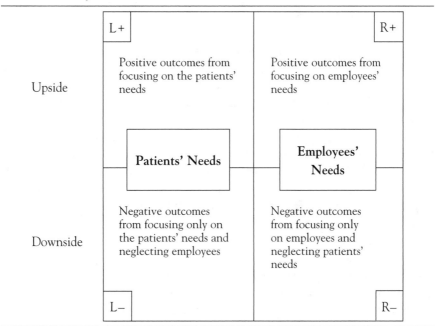

Reprinted and adapted from *Polarity Management* by Barry Johnson. Copyright © 1992, 1996. Reprinted by permission of the publisher, HRD Press, Amherst, Mass. (800) 822-2801. www.hrdpress.com.

Figure 8-14. Respiratory Therapist Example: Putting Patients' Needs First or Employees' Needs First

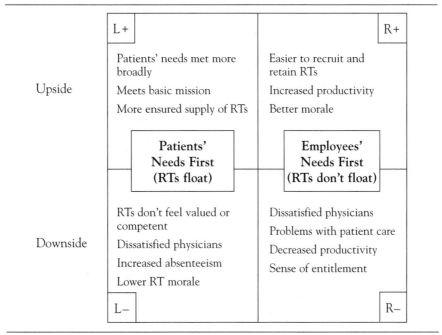

the upside of the other. Johnson (1996, p. 11) calls movement through the grid the "polarity two-step." The process starts in either lower quadrant and moves across, up, and down, and then it is repeated.

The difficulty in dealing with polarities occurs because the parties involved are convinced that they are right in their particular conviction and they basically see only their own perception. Working the group through the polarity map helps illustrate the whole picture. Instead of disagreeing parties contradicting each other's view, the task allows participants to supplement each other's view in order to see the entire picture. Parties on both sides of the polarity have key pieces to the puzzle; they just need this simple structure to help identify and share them. The opposition each side feels to the other actually becomes a key resource in dealing with the issue. No one is being challenged; instead the accuracy of each position is assumed. As a result, joint effort is used to combine two valid views of a situation so that a more complete picture is seen.

Johnson (1996, p. 45) says that "in most organizations there are often very serious and costly confrontations that take place because a 'both/and' polarity is treated like an 'either/or' problem to solve." In working out the polarity map together, the possibility of each participant seeing the other quadrants and more fully understanding the issue occurs because his or her own view of reality has not been contradicted but confirmed. "Successful management of polarities calls for intentional interventions that support both values [poles] simultaneously" (Wesorick 2002, p. 24).

One of the difficult challenges is knowing when there is a polarity to manage instead of a problem to solve. Johnson (1996) offers two questions to help distinguish between them: (1) Is the difficulty ongoing, and (2) are two interdependent poles involved?

If there is a solution that represents a definite endpoint in a process, the problem is solvable. Take, for example, the decision about where to have the holiday party. Once the decision is made, it is done. This is an either/or problem. The party will be held in either location A or location B. Once the decision is made, it is carried out. Problems of choice are solved the minute the choice is made. In contrast, people involved in polarities are continually engaged in dealing with them. Instead of reaching an endpoint, there is a never-ending change of emphasis or focus from one pole to another. For example, there are times to emphasize and reward individual performance, and there are times to focus on the team's effort.

The second question is whether there are two poles that are interdependent. "The solution in problems to solve can stand alone. Unlike a polarity to be managed, the solution to a problem to solve does not have the necessary opposite that is required for the solution to work over an extended period of time" (Johnson 1996, p. 82). Polarities, instead, require both poles. If the two opposing issues must be held in balance and if those problems are ongoing with no simple or definitive solution, they are polarities to be managed. The issue of manager accessibility to employees is an example. On the one hand, for the manager to be available to employees is an important aspect of the job, and yet there is also the need for the manager to have quiet, uninterrupted time in order to do work that requires concentrated thinking. Neither side of the pole is a complete answer to the issue.

Once the polarity map has been completed, the question is asked, "What do we need to do to stay in the upper two quadrants?" In the previous respiratory care example, how can we meet both the patients' and the employees' needs? How do we know when to shift the focus from one pole to another? The group then has identified actions to support each side of the polarity and is more likely to recognize when overemphasis on either pole occurs in the future. A perioperative director used this process to explore with the staff the two poles of using service-specific teams versus expecting staff to be generalists. They identified a blend of approaches that capitalized on both problem solving and appreciative inquiry. A director of education used it with her employees in the education department to deal with the issues of department-based educators versus a centralized education department.

Summary

This chapter examines the relationship between a positive work environment and the manager's focus on results. Models of shared decision making are discussed, as is the concept of empowerment. Several key processes that are used in obtaining results, specifically the skills of problem solving and decision making, are also presented. Two additional approaches are included to broaden the individual's results-oriented repertoire: the use of appreciative inquiry and polarity management. These skills, especially when combined with the interpersonal skills previously discussed, increase the quality of the work environment for all.

Conversation Points

Organizational Perspective

1. Is there an established continuous quality process in your organization? How widely is it used? What results does it produce?
2. Are problems actually being solved in the organization, or do you continue to recycle them (dealing with the same old problems year after year)?
3. Is there a formalized structure for shared decision making in the organization? What is it called, and how effective is it? What departments and employees are involved?
4. Do employees and managers feel empowered to make necessary decisions about their work? Is there an emphasis on hierarchical decision making? (That is, "I take it to my boss, who takes it to his boss, who takes it to her boss.")
5. Is decision making bogged down in the organization, or is it timely and conducted at the lowest levels possible?
6. Where have you used appreciative inquiry in the organization? Have there been any change initiatives undertaken or issues resolved using the underlying principles of appreciative inquiry?
7. What are key polarities you deal with on a regular basis?

Leader Perspective

1. What are typical system or department problems you deal with currently? Do you regularly use problem-solving groups in your department? How effective are they?
2. How many work-arounds do your employees use? Are employees engaging in first-order problem solving, or second-order problem solving?
3. Do employees from your department participate in organizational decision-making groups? What process do they use?
4. Think of the different types of decision making (majority vote, consensus, individual, and so on), and identify examples of each that you see in your work environment.
5. How could you use appreciative inquiry to deal with issues you are facing?
6. What are common polarities you see in your workplace?
7. Have polarities been mistaken for problems? How could you use the polarity grid for achieving more effective results?

Employee Perspective

1. Are you better with right-brain (spontaneous, creative, free-flowing) thinking or left-brain (logical, analytical, methodical) thinking? What about your work group? What is the impact on the effectiveness of your problem-solving efforts?
2. Do you serve on a department council, task force, or problem-solving group? How effective is the group? Do you follow a problem-solving process, or is your approach pretty loose and spontaneous?
3. Do you feel empowered in your decision making? What are examples of decisions you have a level-four authority to make? How about level-one authority?
4. How comfortable or familiar are you with the skills of appreciative inquiry and polarity management? Do you see any issues in your workplace for which these approaches might be helpful?
5. Does your manager know the number of times you have just taken care of a problem and worked around it? Is you manager readily accessible and visible in the department?

9

Creating an Innovative Work Culture

Jo Manion

Unimpeded on a daily basis by the concern for survival,
free from the generalized assumption of scarcity, a person stands
in the great space of possibility in a posture of openness,
with an unfettered imagination for what can be.
—Rosamund S. Zander and Benjamin Zander

A POSITIVE WORKING environment is one in which the people who work there are able to see results as an outcome of their efforts. As discussed in chapter 8, a focus on results requires a workplace in which employees enjoy a high level of autonomy and decision-making authority. Employees are skilled decision makers and problem solvers. The leadership philosophy is one characterized by managers who seek to understand the problems and difficulties employees face and who continually seek improvements in work processes. The creation of a workplace environment in which innovation is not only encouraged but expected is critical to achieving results.

Health care organizations characterized by encouragement and support of innovation are certainly more likely to have a strong, viable future. Creativity and innovation are hallmarks of the most successful health care organizations in the United States today. "Nothing is more risky than not innovating, with the possible exception of confusing innovation with something that fails to create value" (Hattori and Wycoff 2002, p. 25). To successfully navigate the chaos of today's business environment, the successful health care organization must be able to tap into the creative potential of its employees.

In health care today, organizations face a critical choice: innovate and change or expect to be replaced by those organizations that do. It becomes a choice between gradual decline and eventual demise or transformation. Because health care is a mature industry, transformation is more difficult than it seems. "Although the 20th century can be remembered as the most active age for health innovation, the 21st century promises even more technical creativity and service transformation" (Porter-O'Grady 2003, p. 31). In his essay on the consequences of innovation, Ellis (2004) notes that every

Portions of this chapter are adapted from Jo Manion, Chaos or Transformation, *Journal of Nursing Administration* 23(5): 41–48. Copyright © 1993 and used by permission of Lippincott Williams & Wilkins.

passing day brings innovations that seem almost more like science fiction than reality. Examples include the regeneration of limbs on and organs in human beings, the implantation of computer-assisted telepathy devices that help the disabled control their environments, the development of injectable DNA computers able to detect cancer and then produce custom drugs to treat it, and the development of gene therapies that may eliminate illnesses such as diabetes and Alzheimer's disease. Diabetes is an example of one disease that is being tackled on many fronts by multiple biotechnology companies (DeCovny 2007). The list goes on and on, but one conclusion is clear: Maintaining the status quo is simply not an option.

Successful innovation is not magic, and it does not happen spontaneously. Organizations with a track record of successful innovation understand that innovation must be managed. Innovation management requires the application of a developmental process that cannot be implemented overnight. To succeed in innovation management, employees as well as leaders need to have a clear idea of the relationship between creativity and innovation, and they also need to be skilled implementers of ideas.

The successful organizations establish an internal climate that supports entrepreneurial activity and goes beyond paying lip service to the idea of innovation and employee intrapreneurship (see discussion of this concept below). They recognize that innovation must be systematic, organized, and managed for it to have a significant and widespread impact on the organization's outcomes. Innovation is expected and encouraged in the organization, and it is assumed to be a part of the work to be done rather than something that happens in addition to the "real" work of employees (Manion 1990). Established mechanisms for disseminating innovations are in place, and people are expected to implement new ideas.

Employee innovation and empowerment are closely related. Individuals must be empowered before innovation can occur on a systematic basis. However, some individuals who are empowered in their daily work activities may not accept the responsibility for innovation. Some people simply are not interested in being innovators. In some cases, the individual may not have the specific skills needed. For others, a traditional, bureaucratic system may place so many barriers to innovation that the individuals do not even try to be innovative.

Innovation can be undertaken by anyone in the organization. Some of the most effective innovations are developed by people who know the organization at its core. First-line employees who form the base of any health care organization are in a position to be essential innovators. On the one hand, employees who are intimately connected with the work know it better than anyone else. On the other hand, being too close to the work or having done the same work over a long period of time sometimes makes it more difficult to find new and different ways to carry it out. In addition, the academic preparation and experience of most clinicians and support workers does not emphasize innovation, so the majority of health care employees lack innovation skills such as creativity, business planning, intrapreneurship, and change management.

Most health care workers have been socialized to their work roles in bureaucratic, hierarchical organizations whose structure alone intimidates the novice innovator. In addition, few health care organizations have had extensive experience in implementing successful and sustained innovations. Ray Stata, a co-founder of Analog Devices (the $2 billion semiconductor company) says, "I came to the conclusion long ago that limits to innovation have less to do with technology or creativity than organizational agility" (Govindarajan and Trimble 2005, p. 58). In other words, the emphasis must shift from ideas to solid execution of those ideas and from leadership excellence to organizational excellence.

Creativity and Innovation

Innovation is the key to transforming any health care organization and the U.S. health care system. Creativity involves thinking up new ideas or putting things together in a new way; innovation is the implementation of the new or creative idea. Innovation has been described as applied creativity, which implies that something has changed as a result of the creativity. Having a good idea is only the first step; actually converting the idea to a new reality that is useful is much more difficult. So, creativity involves thinking up new ideas, while innovation involves doing new things. If ideas are not implemented, they are useless. There is no shortage of creative ideas or creative people; there is, however, a shortage of successful innovators. Creativity does not automatically lead to innovation. It takes an individual or even several individuals with the know-how, energy, courage, and persistence to implement a creative idea. The old saying that creativity is 1 percent inspiration and 99 percent perspiration is true. Creativity is hard work more than it is genius.

More specifically, innovation is the transformation of ideas into something of value that can be used in some way. Innovations take a variety of shapes and sizes. The innovation may be as small as a simple change in the work processes of a department or team or as large as the development of a new service, such as a rapid response team, or the invention of a new product. Managers and executives experience more success in their roles when employees are skillful implementers of new ideas.

Many people mistakenly equate creativity with artistic talent, and so they conclude that they are not creative. Yet creativity has been defined as a process that results in a new combination of attributes, elements, or images, as something that gives rise to new patterns, arrangements, or products that better serve a need (Raudsepp 1981). Creativity is largely the result of putting together old ideas in a new way, a technique at which any one can become more skilled.

For those interested in learning more about creativity techniques, a wealth of resources are available for purchase. Including such resources as part of the organization's or department's library creates immediate accessibility to the wide variety of possibilities. Chapter 8 describes several creativity techniques in the context of problem solving. In addition, some health care organizations are looking outside the industry for assistance in managing innovation and creativity, and consulting firms can bring refreshing new ways of approaching opportunities. One example is IDEO, a product design and innovation strategy firm that is teaching the art of innovation to major hospital systems (Weber 2003).

In *Weird Ideas That Work: 11½ Practices for Promoting, Managing, and Sustaining Innovation*, Stanford University professor Robert Sutton (2002) offers suggestions for how to generate and capitalize on new ideas. Several of his suggestions may sound a bit strange, but his underlying message is clear: Innovation is not a process that is comfortable in most hierarchical, traditional bureaucracies. He says that the first step to filling the organization with good ideas is to fill it with good people. Following are some of Sutton's (2002) additional suggestions:

1. Hire slow learners of the organizational code, that is, people who ignore the way things are usually done and find their own way of doing things.
2. Hire people who make you uncomfortable, even those you dislike, and then take special care to listen to their ideas.
3. Hire people who are probably not needed. Sutton's point here is to hire people with skills that the organization may not need at the moment and then ask these people how they can help.
4. Use job interviews to get new ideas, not just to screen candidates. Give job applicants problems you have not been able to solve, and then listen as much as you can and talk as little as possible.
5. Encourage people to ignore their boss and peers. Hire defiant outsiders and encourage people to drive you crazy by doing what they think is right rather than what they are told to do.
6. Find happy people and let them fight. LaBarre (2002, p. 72) further recommends, "If you want innovation, you need upbeat people who know the right way to battle. Avoid conflict during the earliest stages of the creative process, but encourage people to fight over ideas in the intermediate stages."

These recommendations are echoed by Berwick (2003, p. 1973), who points out that "innovators will not be the easiest individuals to deal with in their organization; they may be abrasive, not invested in local networks, and demanding of latitude." All of this advice sounds straightforward enough, but consider what it is like to have one or two employees with these traits in the work group—it can cause a great deal of angst for the manager. Abrasive, disruptive people (even if they are creative) are not tolerated in most organizations and are seen as troublemakers who need to be controlled or eliminated. If health care organizations want to support innovation to any great extent, however, the organizational cultures will need to change to accommodate people who would otherwise be considered troublemakers in traditional organizations. Jaramillo and colleagues (2008) differentiate between a troubling disruptor and a positive deviant. The desired individual is one who exhibits the characteristics of a deviant but whose exceptional behaviors bring exceptional results. In fact, Jaramillo and colleagues go on to point out that most innovative cultures are deviant cultures.

Innovation Management

A specific process for creating a culture of innovation is useful for leaders in health care organizations who are attempting to encourage or beginning to demand more innovation from employees and colleagues. This innovation management process is helpful whether the scope includes the whole organization or just one department. John Kao, quoted in Flower (1999), reports that he often hears people in health care organizations say that innovation is of great importance and yet they admit that they are not sure where to start or how to do it.

> The issue is not whether people are creative but what happens when you try to organize creativity, to weave creativity into the daily life of a system, a team, or an organization. In the traditional industrial model of efficiency and operational excellence, organizations are especially good at taking the risk and uncertainty out of people's work, so that they can perform in a predictable and quantitatively comparable way. (Flower 1999, p. 15)

A process for creating a culture of innovation is also useful for giving guidance to organizational leaders who manage the process of unfolding and implementing specific innovations.

A Five-Stage Innovation Process

The following five-stage process for managing innovation is based on an energy model adapted for organizations by Nancy Post, an organizational development consultant (Post 1989, 1993). The framework has also been used for guidance in managing energy in an organization (Manion 1993; Cox, Manion, and Miller 2005).

The five stages of innovation management are preparation, movement, synergy, the new reality, and integration. In each stage, specific functions must be fulfilled and/or specific issues considered. During preparation, the issues to be managed are clarity and relevancy of mission or purpose and adequacy and allocation of resources. During the second stage, movement, structural issues such as decision making, authority levels, planning, and organizational structure are considerations. Synergy, the third stage, involves the issues of overall coordination and cooperation, priority setting, networking, climate setting, and internal communications. During the fourth stage, the new reality, productivity, and the maintenance of the change are key considerations. Integration, the final phase, requires attention to quality and evaluative efforts. (See figure 9-1.)

The five stages can be used as a model for balance as well as a developmental model. This means the key elements in each stage must be considered fully. When any of the issues of the stage are not addressed fully, the work of that stage is deficient or weak, and an imbalance in the system results. Imbalances have an impact on the effectiveness of innovation management in the organization and can impair the implementation of a specific innovation.

Figure 9-1.   Five-Stage Innovation Management Model (Manion 1993)

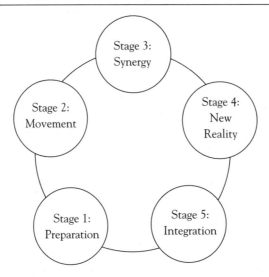

Reprinted from Jo Manion, Chaos or Transformation, *Journal of Nursing Administration* 23(5).
Copyright © 1993. Used by permission of Lippincott Wilkins & Williams.

Similarly, an overemphasis on the characteristics or issues of any single stage
also results in a system imbalance. For example, in stage 1, the mission of the
department as it relates to innovation and expectations for innovation from
employees must match the level of resources available, or dissonance and
disruption result. If the mission clearly states that innovation is an important
organizational value, then it follows that employees and leaders are given the
resource of time in order to focus on innovation.

As noted earlier, this model is also a developmental model, and as such,
it is sequential in nature. Following these stages in sequence can aid the
leader in managing the process of innovation. However, the model is also
interactive and dynamic. The primary issues in each stage are identified and
considered sequentially, although the issues of one stage can also appear
and are appropriate to consider throughout the entire cycle. For example,
although evaluation is a key element of the final stage, it must also occur
during the entire process, not just at the end, when it is of primary importance. Figure 9-2 shows the five stages of the process with a summary of the
key issues in each stage.

Stage 1: Preparation

In the first stage, preparation, purpose and allocation of resources must be
considered and managed. This stage is the foundation for the rest of the
process. It is primarily leader driven and is the responsibility of executives
and teams of internal leaders. Allocation of resources often requires management's involvement, especially if the organization is experiencing a reduction in available resources and budgets are tight.

Simply stated, innovation must be an important element of the organization's and department's mission and a part of the everyday language before it

Figure 9-2. Innovation Stages with Key Functions (Manion 1993)

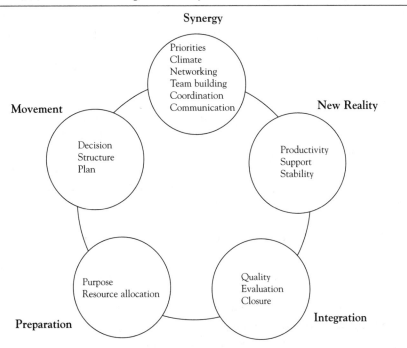

Reprinted from Jo Manion, Chaos or Transformation, *Journal of Nursing Administration* 23(5). Copyright © 1993. Used by permission of Lippincott Wilkins & Williams.

can be accepted as a value. The organization's leaders need to believe, and act on the belief, that innovation is a priority before employees will behave as though innovation is a desirable achievement. The relationship of innovation to patient care and customer service must be clearly stated and demonstrated. Not only is it important for members of the leadership team to speak the language of innovation but leadership must also communicate the expectation for innovation to employees. This can be further emphasized by inclusion of the goal for innovation in the organization's and department's annual goals, performance appraisal process, and position descriptions. The challenge for organizational leaders, says John Kao, is "to create a context in which people understand exactly why innovation is important, and how important it is to balance the creative and the operational imperatives" (Flower 1999, p. 15).

In this first stage, the complementary issue to purpose is the adequacy and allocation of resources, including human and material resources. Adequate resources must be available when innovation is an expected part of the work of the organization. Resources include far more than financial investment. The first stage must consider, in addition to funding, the amount of time available, access to other stakeholders, and personal development time. It is difficult to expect people to work on innovative projects wholeheartedly in addition to carrying a full work schedule. Although enthusiastic employees are often committed enough to do so, it is an abuse of the human resources of the organization to expect this additional commitment on a long-term or continual basis. People will be used up and worn out quickly.

Mentors and sponsors must also be readily accessible in the organization or department as support for the innovator. Sharing resources among departments and work groups increases the environmental support for innovation.

In some instances, the organization's human resources need further development. The skills of leaders and clinical and support staff should be carefully assessed to determine the need for educational opportunities. Managers must be prepared for their roles as innovation managers. Individual innovators need educational programs or opportunities that focus on innovation and the skills needed by a successful innovator. All of the members of the organization benefit from general programs that focus on the need for innovation, essential skills, and their role in supporting co-workers who are innovators. Another important aspect of preparing people for innovation is helping them to keep up to date with trends and developments in the health care sector as well as other businesses.

People need to hear the innovation message repeatedly and observe actual behaviors and structural changes that support innovation before they can internalize the message that innovation is desirable and expected. The stated values and mission related to innovation and creativity, as well as the day-to-day language used by leaders, must be congruent with the behavior of leaders. In some instances, changes in the structure of the organization may be needed. Dissonance is created when executives, managers, and leaders continually espouse the need for innovation and yet allow employees little to no access to funding for innovative ideas, when new ideas can only be implemented after a tedious and difficult approval process, or when the creative individual who is always searching for a new and better way is treated as a troublemaker who must be controlled.

In terms of an actual innovation, the first stage is the time when the proposed new service, new product, or change is evaluated against the mission of the department or organization. A decision must be made on whether the innovation does indeed support the primary mission and increase effectiveness in meeting the basic purpose. Take, for example, electronic medical record (EMR) systems. Ostensibly, the main goals of implementing such a system are to increase the accuracy of clinical documentation and improve the accessibility of patient records. However, many of these systems have also been sold with the implied promise that they would reduce the amount of time clinical practitioners spend documenting the care given to their patients. Yet first-generation versions of automated documentation systems actually increased the amount of time caregivers and clinicians spent away from the patient.

The second issue to be decided involves an assessment of needed resources against the resources available. Questions include, Are resources adequate? Do people need additional skills or time to implement or use the innovation? If additional resources are needed, how can obtaining them best be accomplished? What is the level of support for the innovation?

For example, many issues of resource allocation are implicit in the development and implementation of EMR systems. First, does the organization have the capital to invest in the extensive and expensive hardware needed to implement such a system? Is there recognition that when these systems are implemented, productivity levels often worsen for a period of time, as people learn the new approaches? Has the additional support required been assessed accurately? Do employees have the necessary computer skills to use the new system? Are there internal trainers prepared to teach the basics to others?

Examples of the application of these principles abound as a result of the wave of re-engineering and work redesign projects in health care during the early to middle 1990s. For many organizations, these efforts were their initial attempt at major systemwide innovation. Where the effort was successful, creativity and innovation were clearly linked to the organization's mission and its very reason for existence. Creative ideas were expected from everyone in the organization, and resources were allocated to carry out this important work. Entire teams of individuals were organized to lead the initiative, often referred to as resource or development teams. These teams included reassigned managers and employees who had the specific skills required to complete the work of redesign. Massive amounts of organizational resources were allocated to develop needed skills internally in addition to using external consultants.

Unfortunately, many organizations climbed aboard the re-engineering bandwagon without paying attention to preparation issues. Their initiatives were approached as cost-cutting measures, and some organizations used re-engineering to justify major changes in skill-mix ratio of caregivers, cross-training of highly skilled practitioners in all disciplines, reduction of managerial positions, and elimination of specialized and centralized departments. A number of these organizations discovered that their innovations did not make it easier to carry out their original mission of serving patients, but instead made it more difficult. One chief executive officer summed it up by noting that when he eliminated his organization's centralized infusion therapy department, his board of directors was very impressed with the money he had saved in operating costs and gave him kudos. Within months, however, the infection rates climbed and complaints from patients increased. Two years later, when he reinstituted the centralized department, he was hailed as a hero for dealing effectively with these new problems.

If innovation is mishandled and change is not implemented effectively, the organization's resources will be depleted for a number of reasons. First, the process itself costs money. Second, when the process is mishandled, employee dissatisfaction levels increase and competent employees who are able to find employment elsewhere do. The remaining employees are often left more demoralized, detached, cynical, and less willing to commit to the future initiatives of the organization. The social capital of the organization is depleted, as are the financial resources.

Stage 2: Movement

Once the functions of the first stage have been addressed, an important part of the foundation is in place. People are clear about how innovation supports the purpose of the organization, and innovation is accepted as relevant by employees. The need and expectation for innovation have been consistently communicated, both verbally and through the leaders' behavior. Adequate resources are in place, and employees begin to experience actual support for innovation.

During the second stage, movement, the structural elements supporting innovation throughout the organization or department need to be established. A vision of how the innovation will be carried out and how it will result in change is critical. When the vision is clear, the structure needed to support that vision follows.

Stage 2 includes planning and decision making. Planning for a structure that supports innovation in the organization and its many departments is a vital step. "Organizational structures can, in fact, be put in place that provide for a more predictable occurrence of innovation—the successful implementation of a creative idea, or an idea that is both novel and useful" (Gryskiewicz 1999, p. 18). At the organizational level, executive leaders facilitate this planning with participation and input from all levels within the departments. A process for proposing and evaluating new ideas and gaining approval and funding is established. Two separate structures may be needed, one for larger projects that involve integral changes in the organization and substantial funding and a simpler process for ideas with less impact and more modest resource needs.

One approach being used today is the establishment of a center for innovation within the organization. The center provides a structure for building a financial support base that generates revenue and receives gifts. Establishing a specific process for seeking innovative ideas from employees and guidelines for approval and the funding of decisions is part of the work of such a center, which supports the work of innovation throughout the system.

Potential innovators often need skill development in the planning function. Some innovative projects are approved with very little planning because they involve a small number of people and do not require additional funding. Formal business planning, however, may be necessary for larger projects that have significant ramifications in the department and organization or require extensive resource commitment. Innovators need support and encouragement in learning how to develop a business plan. Support from other departments such as finance or marketing may be needed. Planning ways for employees to have access to these resources is important.

The complementary issue to planning in this stage of the process is decision making, which is closely intertwined with planning. Decisions must be made as planning is completed. In some organizations, planning and decision making are clearly out of balance. Much time is spent in planning, but the plans are never carried out because actual decisions are not made. Once innovation-supporting structural changes are determined, assignment of responsibility is necessary. How will the process be initiated? Who is responsible? How will levels of authority be decided? Realistic time frames need to be established for each element of the plan and for communicating the plan to all of the key stakeholders who are affected in any way by the plan. Clear lines of responsibility are identified, and decisions are made regarding appropriate levels of authority for those working on the project.

As the planning is completed, the need for further education and skill development for both managers and employees becomes obvious. Planning skills often need to be developed or strengthened. In addition, there must be recognition that innovation planning is a process, not an end. By its very nature, innovation does not unfold as planned, and there must be support, not just tolerance, for ambiguity, mistakes, and revisions. Visioning and strategizing are key skills for innovators in addition to the basic skills needed to lead groups, conduct effective meetings, and reach consensus-based decision making.

A potentially unexpected reaction from employees and managers sometimes surfaces during this state: anger. Although the anger may not be significant or widespread, it may be present. In establishing a structure and process that supports innovation in a department, the extremely creative individual may see it as stifling rather than liberating. Managers and leaders who have been supportive of the concept of innovation may feel irritated when they realize that its successful management takes time and skill. They may need to develop new and different skills. It is important to see beyond the initial resistance and evaluate whether the established structure supports innovators or stifles their work. Too much rigid structure can inhibit creativity.

The importance of an easy-to-navigate structure that supports innovation cannot be minimized. When the decision-making structure in the organization has what is called a "tendency to no," innovation is stifled. In such structures, every decision must make its way through the decision-making channels before an answer can be rendered. At each step of the way, the proposed idea is dissected and examined for potential risks and faults until the innovator is so frustrated that he or she gives up. The likelihood of support for the idea becomes increasingly slim, and by the time the idea reaches the chief executive officer, frontline employee-innovators have lost interest or are bored and demoralized.

Compare this process to how innovation is handled by an entrepreneur. The entrepreneur who has a great, innovative idea that requires a substantial outlay of capital seeks out venture capitalists who are willing to invest. The first one approached may decline the opportunity, sending the entrepreneur on to the next, and so on. Out of seven people approached, perhaps only one sees the same potential as the entrepreneur sees and is willing to invest in the idea. But all the entrepreneur needs is one yes. Contrast this to the intrapreneur (an entrepreneur who is employed by someone else). The intrapreneur may also have a potentially solid innovation that he pitches to his manager. The manager agrees and talks with her director to obtain approval. The director thinks it is a great idea and takes it forward, as does her vice president. In the end, six managers or senior leaders have given the idea their approval, but in the end the chief financial officer may refuse to approve the change because of the level of financial support it requires. The point here is that the entrepreneur deals with six negatives and one affirmative before the project becomes a go. The intrapreneur has six affirmatives and only one negative, but the project is dead in the water. This "tendency to no" is one of the true killers of organizational innovation.

This scenario is incredibly frustrating to creative employees, to the point that many of them simply leave the system to strike out on their own. When they stay, what they learn is that it is just too difficult to develop significant innovation in the system. Take, for example, a nurse, whom we call Jane, who had attended a continuing education program where people were encouraged to look for creative, innovative ways to improve their workplace environment to help increase retention.

On Jane's return trip she had what she considered a brilliant idea that was very simple. Instead of using expensive commercial art to line the corridors and conference rooms of the hospital, why not hang pictures of employees doing their work around the organization? Jane believed it would be appealing to patients and visitors and it would validate employees and communicate respect for their work. The photos might also increase the sense of community in the organization. Jane brought her digital camera to work one evening and took pictures of her co-workers, which she added to a simple but attractive proposal. To her dismay, although she has had wonderful response on the part of many people, she has been unable to get the project approved. It has been months since she submitted her proposal, and she is not even certain where the idea died.

Contrast this scenario to an organization with the "tendency to yes." Kirby and Stewart (2007) interviewed Jeff Bezos, founder of the Internet bookseller Amazon.com. Bezos outlined the history of Amazon and its ruthless focus on customer service. He also described times when a trial-and-error approach does not work. Instead, making the commitment and moving forward is the answer. "It's the institutional yes. People say, 'We're going to do this. We're going to figure out a way'" (Kirby and Steward 2007, p. 81). When faced with a multifaceted problem, he and the decision makers turn it into a straightforward problem by asking, "Well, what's better for the customer?" Alignment of decisions must be based on their primary mission of serving the customer.

Stage 3: Synergy

After the foundation and structural issues have been dealt with in stages 1 and 2, things begin to come together. The third stage, synergy, is described as exciting, dynamic, and seductive. The innovators within the organization actually begin using the structure that has been established to support the new approaches. At this point, it feels as though the change is finally on the way. Issues of priority setting, climate, coordination, cooperation, team building, networking, relationship building, and internal communications must be considered. Each of these issues is an important key, and lack of attention to any one results in a system out of balance.

Priority setting is easier when the structure for evaluating and approving projects is effective. A formal structure facilitates the identification of the projects to be supported in the organization or department during the year. In almost every department, however, many other changes and projects are being implemented simultaneously. A major concern most organizations are experiencing is the need to fix everything yesterday. Unfortunately, when a system is engaged in too many projects, it is less likely that any one project will be managed well. Determining the sequencing of major projects in the system can be difficult, especially when other important projects are added because of external demands. Priority setting is the difficult task of determining what is most important to accomplish with the resources available. It does not mean doing everything that needs to be done; it means making the difficult choices between all those things that could be done. Priority setting requires extreme honesty by executives and the leadership team and a willingness to refuse to implement projects for which there are inadequate resources.

This process, of course, is easier to describe than to do. Take, for example, a typical senior leadership team meeting whose leaders are exhausted from trying to handle a large number of projects that all demanded their time. In one actual team, the first step involved creating a list of current projects. These projects ranged from relatively small implementation projects to massive, systemwide initiatives such as merging another hospital into their system, establishing a new and extensive cardiovascular surgery service line, finishing two major construction projects, completing a housewide work redesign project, and implementing a major cultural change in the organization. To the team's surprise, the list of current projects totaled 109. When the leaders were asked to prioritize the projects, they reported that all of the projects were critical for the organization's future viability. It was no wonder that everyone in the organization was exhausted and depleted. Their ambitions and mission far exceeded the resources they had. In order to tackle this issue in another way, the team considered possibilities for increasing resources to enable them to deal with these projects more effectively. This approach relieved the pressure somewhat, as more resources were allocated to support the projects.

Establishing a climate conducive to innovation is a key managerial role. Managers must be prepared and educated about the different elements of climate and group culture and accept responsibility for the climate within their work groups. Managers must see their role as a catalyst (they release the energy of innovators within the staff). The response to mistakes is a major feature of an innovative climate. When the system or the individuals within the system have a punitive or blaming response to mistakes, the environment impedes and stifles innovation. Do employees feel comfortable about making mistakes, and do they understand that mistake making is inevitable, or do employees want an environment where they do not make mistakes? When making mistakes is accepted as part of work life as lessons to be learned, people are more likely to be risk takers and successful innovators.

Companies whose very survival depends on innovation create a climate that encourages people to come forward with good ideas and to be risk takers. People are not criticized when ideas do not work out as intended or hoped;

instead, ideas are celebrated for what is learned from them. "Nothing will extinguish the flames of innovation more rapidly than a punitive response to ideas that don't work. Nothing is more reinforcing to creative energy than organizational tolerance for and even support of mistakes. Leaders of innovative organizations understand that the price tag of success includes the misfires" (Beglinger 2003, p. 40). This opinion is echoed by other skilled innovators, who note that successful innovation is not so much about having one good idea as having lots of ideas, many of which fail. And to find "a few ideas that work, you need to try a lot that don't" (LaBarre 2002, p. 70).

During this stage, attention must be paid to the coordination of efforts to prevent duplication. Roles and responsibilities must be clearly identified and boundaries established. Levels of authority and access to resources must be discussed before the innovator receives approval and begins work on a project. Too often, the limits and boundaries are not discussed until conflicts or problems occur.

Cooperation must be obtained from co-workers and project team members and potentially, depending on the project, other departments. Executives and managers may need to pave the way or open the door for the innovator to obtain needed cooperation from other departments in the organization. Executives and managers who state expectations for cooperation and act as role models help innovators work interdepartmentally in finding others to cooperate with the project.

Working effectively with a group or a project team is an important skill for most innovators. Diversity within the work group or project team leads to increased potential for creativity. At the intersection between differences lies the opportunity for innovation. However, differences also can lead to increased conflict and strife. Although an individual innovator may need extensive coaching to be successful in this area, this effort is often more productive than pulling the project from the person who had the idea and assigning it to someone in the department with these already-developed skills. Understandably, innovators feel discouraged when they lose the responsibility for implementing one of their great ideas.

For example, a radiology employee at a hospital, Marjorie, had an idea for improving a process. She completed a successful trial project on the day shift. She was committed to the success of the idea and persevered through the initial glitches of implementation. Everyone agreed that the process improved their work flow and level of service. When it was time to implement the process on the evening shift, Marjorie volunteered to work evenings to be certain that the process was successful. However, the manager was unwilling to transfer Marjorie to the evening shift because of short staffing on the day shift. Instead, the project was assigned to an evening shift employee who expressed multiple reservations about the idea. The innovation failed on the evening shift, and Marjorie was disappointed and frustrated. Because it did not work out well on the evening shift, it was no longer used on the day shift because of the need for consistency within the department. Not long after this fiasco, Marjorie left for a position in another organization.

Each situation needs to be evaluated separately. In some instances, there are overriding reasons why the creators of the idea should hand off the project to the implementers. However, in many cases, such handoffs are problematic. Innovation simply cannot be assigned. The people responsible for implementation are not successful when they are not fully engaged and committed to the idea. This sounds like a simple concept, and yet it is violated frequently in organizations that are inexperienced in innovation. A design team works on the redesign of a department and then turns the result over to the manager and other employees to implement and make successful. When those who are responsible for implementing the idea have not had significant roles to play in the development of the design, they may limit their efforts or commit half-heartedly to its success. Another common example seen in organizations is when a committee takes on a problem and develops several workable solutions. Members are excited about the possibilities, but then the solutions are turned over to others for what is often a lackluster implementation.

This stage also requires employees to call on their skills in leading meetings, managing group process, and using consensus-based decision making. Many project teams are more effective when they have diverse membership from various disciplines and support departments throughout the organization. Access to specialists between departments is important. Members of the project team may need training in practical creativity techniques such as game playing, brainstorming, mind mapping, storyboarding, and attribute analysis. (These techniques were discussed briefly in chapter 8.)

Communication is another key function of this stage. Effective innovation requires employees to have access to information about the organization and trends in health care and in their particular field or discipline. Truly amazing innovations can occur when members of the department understand the big picture and the major challenges the organization is facing. Open communication among all layers of the organization is critical. Key messages often need to be repeated as many as eight to ten times through a variety of methods. Usually, the fewer layers of organizational structure, the more open the communication becomes.

Members of all departments need to learn and use direct communication skills with each other. People who manage their relationships in a healthy and productive manner are an asset in any organization. As noted in chapter 6, healthy relationships are not the rule in most health care organizations, and these behaviors must be continually modeled by the leaders before they are embraced by employees. Negotiation skills are critical human skills for innovators. Selling their ideas and concepts requires approaching the decision makers with a win-win attitude. The successful innovative idea is one that benefits the system, its customers, and the innovator.

Stage 4: The New Reality

The fourth stage in managing innovation is called the new reality. The key issues engaged at this stage include stabilizing the environment, maintaining and supporting the direction that has been established, and producing results from the innovative projects and changes that have been made. A common error made in innovation management is expecting productivity improvements or gains too early in the cycle. In projects where productivity gains are expected, it may be months before the gains are realized. Productivity measures should not be prematurely used as a measure or indicator of success.

One hospital, for example, halted an implementation project that involved a conversion to a team-based organization because it found teams took longer to do the work than individuals took to do the same work. If the organization had been patient and waited several months, teams would have settled into their work routines, other time gains would have become apparent, and a different decision may have been made. Certainly, if increased productivity was the criterion for judging the successful implementation of the electronic medical record, many EMR projects would have been scrapped in the early days of implementation.

Stabilizing the change brought on by innovation is an important step and should be considered carefully. Ways to anchor the change must be sought. This can be done by formalizing a structure or process that was used in trial or by formally communicating the improvement or new service to the entire organization. Disseminating innovation is a major challenge. The Veterans Administration Office of Special Projects has developed a systemwide, cross-functional program to diffuse innovations. Called *Lessons Learned*, it is basically a virtual learning center into which anyone in the system can enter or review innovations. In addition, electronic communities of practice, such as listservs and blogs, offer people the opportunity to connect with particular interest groups that may be posting innovations of interest (Charles 2000). Berwick (2003) offers several suggestions for dissemination of innovation in the overall health care system:

1. Find sound innovations. A formal mechanism can be established to assign responsibility to an individual to review key scientific or professional journals and even to attend conferences and meetings. The responsible individual reports back to the organization on ideas that should be spread.
2. Find and support innovators. Because new answers to chronic, local problems tend to come from outside the current system, specific people should be assigned to scout out these solutions.
3. Invest in early adopters. Organizations should invest heavily in the curiosity of a few early adopters who are willing to test the innovations. Implementing small-scale trials and ensuring the supply of adequate resources reduce the risk.
4. Make early adopter activity observable. Many people watch the early adopters; when these people are visible, word of successful innovation spreads quickly through social channels.
5. Trust and enable reinvention. In innovation, new processes come from taking outside ideas and putting them to work in the system. They have to be tweaked in order to fit the unique organization.

6. Create slack for change. Trying new things takes an enormous investment of energy. "No system trapped in the continuous throes of production, existing always at the margin of resources, innovates well,
   unless its survival is also imminently and vividly at stake" (Berwick
   2003, p. 1974).
7. Lead by example. If leaders are to be champions of the change, they
   must be prepared for resistance from others. Crucially important is
   their willingness to begin the change with themselves.

The importance of diffusion of innovation was explored by Crow
(2006). He reports that attempts to implement change in health care organizations fail about 90 percent of the time because leaders do not take into
account how the change will affect employees. He cites other researchers
who found that two of three organizational transformations fail and because
of poor planning and execution, only about 60 percent of potential benefit
is gained from innovation in health care.

To stabilize the change, establish methods of rewarding and recognizing the innovator and project team. Rewards may come through increased
learning and skill development opportunities; increased access to funding
for future projects; increased funding and time off for taking a class, participating in a webinar, or going to an educational program or a conference; and
sometimes even monetary rewards. Recognition can be provided through
sharing of successes at employee or organizational meetings, through
department or organization newsletters, or through specific celebration
ceremonies. External opportunities for recognition and applause are won-
derfully reinforcing for project team members. Supporting publishing projects or presentations at national conferences is another way of rewarding
and recognizing innovators.

For example, in one emergency department, employees were involved
in several creative projects. One involved a grow-your-own graduate nurse
internship program, and the second was a hospital-wide initiative to reduce
admission wait times for emergency patients. Both of these innovative projects achieved outstanding levels of success. A call for a poster session at the
annual meeting was received from the Emergency Nurses Association, and
several of these nurses wanted to submit an abstract. The manager coached
them on how to write the abstract, which was submitted and subsequently
accepted. Four people from the manager's department then requested permission to attend the national conference. Undaunted, the manager presented a proposal to the hospital foundation for funding to allow the nurses
to attend. This effort created a high level of energy in the department,
which spread elsewhere in the organization.

Productivity is highest when managers and employees are well centered
with a healthy balance of energy. During periods of intense change and
innovation in a department or an organization, people often overexpend
their reserves of energy, leading to overall decreases in productivity and
resiliency. Encouraging self-care and paying attention to the self-care needs

of managers and employees are critical in an organization that innovates successfully. Although innovation is hard work, it is energizing for many people. There is a tendency to ignore replenishment needs. Successful innovation managers recognize that work for real change takes a great deal of energy and that sometimes time frames need to be modified, the frequency of meetings decreased, or extended periods away from work encouraged. The result in the long run is increased productivity and creativity.

Stage 5: Integration

The final stage of the developmental cycle is integration, or closure. The key issues in this stage relate to evaluative functions, quality, and closure. This stage is often overlooked or undervalued, and yet it is critical for future successes in the system. Although evaluation is an important process throughout this developmental cycle, at this phase it is a key issue. During the planning stage, key indicators of success were developed. At this point the indicators are used to evaluate the innovation for its beneficence and effectiveness. The process used to develop or implement the innovation is evaluated. Key questions should include, What was learned? What would/could have been done differently? Is there anything that should be stopped? Cultivate an attitude within the entire system wherein these questions are a normal part of the process. Never let the evaluation process be construed as blame placing.

The quality of the innovation and the implementation process are critical issues at this stage. How would the process be changed the next time? What are the lessons learned? In addition, the relationship between the innovation and improved quality of patient care or customer service should be clear and used as an indicator of success. The innovation may be only indirectly related to patient care, but the implementation of creative ideas implies that something is better as a result of the new idea. What is it that is better?

An important leadership function during this phase is to take the time to go through closure. Too often a project or innovation is completed without formal closure. Closure can occur in the form of celebrations or events that can be held even when the project or intended innovation was a failure. There are lessons to be learned and successes in the most dismal of failures. In almost every instance, innovations occur as the result of the efforts of many people in the organization. It is important to focus on the success or the process rather than on the individual whose idea it was in the beginning. Recognizing and rewarding team effort communicates respect for everyone's participation. "Innovative organizations know that celebration is an important part of completing a project" (Hattori and Wycoff 2002, p. 30).

Closure also implies letting go. There may be a need for grief work, the dissolution of a tight-knit project team, letting go of the old way, or releasing an old mind-set. The need for grieving should not be underestimated. When grief can be expressed, the individuals involved are often ready to move on to the next project more quickly.

What's Your Innovation Quotient?

Assessing the effectiveness of innovation management processes is a helpful first step for any organization or department seeking to improve its skills. The assessment tool shown in figure 9-3 may be helpful. The items are organized in groups of ten, with each group relating to one stage of innovation management. Questions 1 through 10 relate to stage 1, questions 11 through 20 relate to stage 2, and so on. Scores of twelve or less for each cluster of ten items indicate areas that need additional work.

Figure 9-3.   What's Your IQ (Innovation Quotient)? (Manion 1993)

Directions: Answer with the same environment in mind for each question. For example, complete the questionnaire thinking of an entire organization, a department, or a specific work group. (That is, do not answer one question with a single department in mind and the next item with an entire organization in mind.) Answer by circling Y for yes, N for no, and S for sometimes.

Y S N   1. Does the mission statement or statement of purpose include any reference to employee creativity and innovation?

Y S N   2. Do job descriptions or role expectations include the expectation for individual innovation or support of innovation?

Y S N   3. Do the annual goals include implementation of innovative ideas or strategies that increase employee creativity or innovation?

Y S N   4. Are the people who are always questioning the status quo and looking for a better way encouraged and seen as "creative types"?

Y S N   5. Is there a lot of energy and enthusiasm for change?

Y S N   6. Do front-line employees have ready access to funding for innovative projects?

Y S N   7. Are mentors and sponsors for the novice innovator available in the organization?

Y S N   8. Do front-line employees and managers have time during their normal work week to work on innovations and creative projects?

Y S N   9. Are the boundaries and limits openly discussed with the innovator and clarified before problems occur?

Y S N   10. Are resources shared among departments and work groups?

Y S N   11. Is time taken to plan for innovation (as opposed to moving very quickly from identifying the need to actual implementation)?

Y S N   12. Is there an established process for managing change and innovation that internal leaders understand and are expected to utilize?

(Continued on next page)

Figure 9-3. (Continued)

Y	S	N	13.	Is a formal proposal format or business plan required before an innovative idea is considered for implementation? Do interested employees know what the expected format is?
Y	S	N	14.	Is there flexibility in how the plan unfolds? (Or are people held to the specifics of the plan, that is, the timeframes, expenditures projected, process used?)
Y	S	N	15.	Do front-line employees have easy access to the executive leadership team without having to go through multiple layers of management?
Y	S	N	16.	Are plans developed before decisions are made?
Y	S	N	17.	Do individual managers have control over funding so that low-cost projects can be funded without a lot of rigmarole?
Y	S	N	18.	Are there established, agreed-upon timeframes for completion of projects?
Y	S	N	19.	Are levels of authority clearly identified for project teams and committees?
Y	S	N	20.	Do problems get solved in the organization so that you are not dealing with the same problems you were dealing with three to five years ago?
Y	S	N	21.	Is there a spirit of cooperation in the organization? Can an innovator find others to cooperate in implementation?
Y	S	N	22.	Do individual innovators retain control over their innovation as it is implemented rather than the idea being passed over to a manager or project director to implement?
Y	S	N	23.	Does the general climate in the organization support, encourage, and seek out change and innovation?
Y	S	N	24.	Is there a high level of trust in the organization among work groups, units, departments, managers, and employees?
Y	S	N	25.	Are priorities established, resources assessed, and progress made on the important and major change projects under way rather than expending time and energy on an excessive number of projects at one time?
Y	S	N	26.	Do managers and leaders act as catalysts for change and innovation?
Y	S	N	27.	Is the majority of the management within the organization stable and effective rather than involved in crisis management, continually "putting out fires," feeling burned out?
Y	S	N	28.	Are employees and managers skilled in the application of creativity techniques such as storyboards, attribute analysis, brainstorming, and mind mapping?
Y	S	N	29.	Can an individual innovator easily pull together a team of people from other departments and work groups to work together on a project?

Figure 9-3.   (Continued)

Y	S	N	30.	Are people comfortable with making mistakes rather than seeing mistakes as something to be feared and avoided?
Y	S	N	31.	Do people in the work group, department, or organization support each other rather than engaging in a significant amount of blaming, bickering, and backbiting?
Y	S	N	32.	Are people in the organization encouraged to take care of themselves?
Y	S	N	33.	Do people in the organization feel like they can set limits, say no to assignments and requests, and decline involvement in particular change projects?
Y	S	N	34.	Are managers and leaders well-centered with a healthy balance of energy rather than feeling burned out and out of balance?
Y	S	N	35.	Is workaholic behavior and perfectionism discouraged?
Y	S	N	36.	Is the organization basically stable and secure rather than an environment of great anxiety, high flux, and chaos?
Y	S	N	37.	Are there mechanisms in place that give long-term support to the implementation of changes and innovations?
Y	S	N	38.	Is there recognition and support that productivity increases occur only after the change is well-established rather than immediately?
Y	S	N	39.	Do people talk openly about their feelings related to change? Is it okay to express negative feelings about change, or is this seen and dealt with as resistance?
Y	S	N	40.	Are specific interventions planned and implemented to nurture people during change and major innovation?
Y	S	N	41.	Are the values of the organization or work group clearly articulated with a clear connection between quality and innovation?
Y	S	N	42.	Can employees articulate the values of the organization, and are the values articulated consistent with what is being practiced? (For example, while innovation and creativity may be articulated as important, in practice there is no allocation of resources to support it.)
Y	S	N	43.	Are employees and leaders in the organization inspired to become involved as innovators rather than being exhausted with the day-to-day work demands?
Y	S	N	44.	When new responsibilities and tasks are accepted, are current responsibilities and tasks modified?
Y	S	N	45.	Are managers and leaders skilled at managing change and the emotions involved to reduce the chaos and turmoil that typically occur when something changes?

(Continued on next page)

Figure 9-3.   (Continued)

Y	S	N	46.	Are people in the organization receptive to and excited about change rather than "fed up" with change, the "promise that things will be better after this, but they never are"?
Y	S	N	47.	Is there a specific evaluation process to determine whether or not, or in what ways, the change has been beneficial?
Y	S	N	48.	Are mistakes freely shared and seen as opportunities for everyone to learn?
Y	S	N	49.	Do people feel comfortable about eliminating the unnecessary? Or is it difficult to let go of things from the past, including people or ways of doing things?
Y	S	N	50.	Do people look forward to the future and change rather than continually lamenting over the good old days, the way things were before the change?

Scoring Directions: Each Y is 2 points, each S is 1 point, and each N is zero. Total the number of points.

Interpretation: If your total score is between 80 and 100, your environment is supportive of innovation; if the total score is between 60 and 79, your environment is somewhat supportive of innovation; if the score is 59 or below, your environment is likely to be a barrier to innovation.

Reprinted from Jo Manion, Chaos or Transformation, *Journal of Nursing Administration* 23(5). Copyright © 1993. Used by permission of Lippincott Wilkins & Williams.

Summary

The challenges facing health care today are perhaps some of the toughest ever experienced. Meeting these challenges successfully requires all of the strength the organization and its people have to offer. Having innovative, empowered employees is not merely desirable; it is absolutely essential for survival.

Creating a climate and structure within a system that empower employees and managers alike takes a strong commitment and consistent effort by the executive and leadership teams. To make the leap from creative ideas to a new reality requires a process for managing innovation. It also requires the establishment of a supportive climate and individuals who have advanced skills in creativity, plan and idea development, and change management. Valuable transformation of the entire organization is the potential result.

Conversation Points

Organizational Perspective

1. Is innovation a highly held value in the organization?
2. Is the need for innovation emphasized anywhere in the organization's or department's mission statement? Do leaders talk about the need for innovation?

3. Is there a structure in place that supports innovators and makes it easy for them to be successful?

4. How innovative is the organization? How successful is it at creating and handling change?

5. When major changes or innovations are made, how well are they assimilated into the organization? How many past organizational efforts became a passing fad rather than the new reality?

6. Is there a "tendency to yes" or a "tendency to no" in the organization?

7. How are individuals with new ideas and the enthusiasm to push them treated in the organization?

Leader Perspective

1. Do you have any innovators within your work group? How do you support them?

2. Do employees frequently bring forth new ideas? Do they offer implementation suggestions or just expect others to do the work of making them happen?

3. Do you have adequate autonomy and leeway to make decisions about ideas employees bring that relate to your areas of responsibility? Or do you have to seek permission from others in the hierarchy?

4. How skilled are you at leading creativity groups and coaching employees in innovation?

5. What new ideas have been implemented in your department or area of responsibility in the past year? How did the implementation go?

Employee Perspective

1. If you have a great new idea that will help solve problems or create new processes, is it easy to get it heard?

2. Do you know how to get a new idea implemented?

3. How comfortable are you with creativity techniques such as attribute analysis, nominal group technique, or storyboarding?

4. If you yourself are not intrapreneurial, how do you support peers and colleagues who are?

5. Who do you think is responsible for innovation in your department?

6. Is time available to create new approaches and implement improvements?

7. What new ideas have been implemented in your department in the past year? What role did you play in the implementation? How did you support the implementation?

8. What is your department's IQ (innovation quotient)? What can you do to help improve it?

10

Influencing Performance

Jo Manion, Sharon Cox, and Mary Jenkins

*In today's organizational environment, there is little prospect
that any one will be "taken care of." Believing that
is another illusion that yields resistance to owning one's work.
We will each have to manage our own work and cherish the
responsibility of creating the organization where we work.*
—Dick Richards

A KEY ASPECT of a positive work environment is an organizational culture in which problems are solved, systems are improved, and innovation is encouraged. In addition, there is a need to influence people's performance in a positive direction by encouraging and coaching colleagues and employees to continually grow and develop their skills. In some instances, this culture may require the manager to respond to, and deal with, inadequate or unacceptable performance or behaviors on the part of others. Although the majority of effort in managing and influencing performance, likely around 95 percent, focuses on encouraging and recognizing good performance, it is often the remaining 5 percent that causes the most difficulty. It was clear from the findings of the research presented in chapter 5 that successful managers do not let the presence of workforce shortages frighten them away from dealing with unacceptable or inadequate performance. They deal with problems head on by actively coaching employees, and they are not afraid to take appropriate action even when it means ending the employment relationship with an individual.

This chapter discusses two of the most common approaches to influencing performance: formal performance appraisal systems and coaching. This chapter also discusses job fit and job sculpting to improve job alignment, feedback, and positive discipline. Finally, the chapter offers suggestions for dealing with negativity in the workplace and extreme behavioral disruptions.

Performance Appraisals and Performance Management Systems

Conversations about managing performance often bring to mind the annual performance appraisal, which, for many of people—managers and employees alike—causes a groan and an immediate tendency to tune out. Health care organizations have invested massive amounts of resources, both human and financial, to develop, implement, and maintain systems of formal performance appraisal because they believe such systems are beneficial for employees and the system. But do these appraisals really improve performance? Do they improve communication between employee and manager? Do they increase the alignment of the employee's goals with the department's or organization's goals? Do they motivate employees and help them with their career planning and progression? Are they an effective method of distributing pay increases and determining job promotions?

These questions are raised in a provocative book by Coens and Jenkins, *Abolishing Performance Appraisals: Why They Backfire and What to Do Instead* (2000). When the title of the Coens and Jenkins book is shared with managers, most of them perk up immediately and their interest becomes obvious. Some of them actually cheer. Perhaps it is because they know, if only on an intuitive level, that formal performance appraisal systems are not delivering on the promises made. As Coens and Jenkins suggest, it is time to acknowledge that improving the level of performance in organizations, including health care organizations, is not about building bigger, better, or different appraisal systems. They argue that it is time to question the underlying assumption that such an approach can actually accomplish the positive results being sought.

Even more disturbing than the above misconceptions is the realization that the appraisal systems in which organizations have invested so heavily not only have failed to bring the positive outcomes anticipated but also can actually result in serious negative consequences for the organization. A common experience is the sense of disappointment felt by the employee who leaves the annual appraisal session realizing that the manager or supervisor does not really recognize all of his or her accomplishments or even really understand everything that the job entails. Even worse, because the process is usually tied directly to the determination of pay increases, the process may actually impede deeply felt conversation and honest feedback. Ask most employees (as many research studies have), and they will tell you that these systems are ineffective.

Furthermore, the annual appraisal approach to performance management is solidly ingrained in unhealthy organizational assumptions such as:

- Employees need to be told what to do.
- The manager is better able to judge and evaluate the employee's performance than the employee is.
- Employees are not smart enough or insightful enough to evaluate their own performance.
- If given the opportunity, employees would inflate their ratings because they only see their positive traits.
- Employees are not capable of holding themselves accountable for their performance without the guidance of their managers.

It is past time that these assumptions were challenged. Noted author Peter Block uses the formal performance appraisal system as a key example for pointing out just how "patriarchal and demeaning institutional life can become" (Coens and Jenkins 2000, p. xiv).

Chapters 1 through 9 of this book emphasize the need to apply affirming principles and methods to the workplace. These chapters present new ways for both managers and employees to approach the issue of healthy work environments. The contention in this chapter is that formal performance appraisal systems are not the best approach for managing employee performance. And perhaps even more significantly, the entire concept of performance management ought to be engaged in a different way. Paramount to the idea of abolishing performance appraisals is the idea that "employees want to be and are fully capable of being responsible for themselves. With a supportive work culture and access to helpful resources and training, employees will take responsibility to get timely and useful feedback, grow their skills, and improve their performance in alignment with organizational needs" (Coens and Jenkins 2000, p. 9).

Rather than exploring the issue of performance appraisal systems more fully in this chapter, the reader is referred directly to Coens and Jenkins's book and encouraged to use it as a resource and a thought-provoking guide to considering the issue. This chapter concentrates on several other ways of influencing employee performance, including coaching, giving feedback, using positive discipline when needed, and dealing with specific challenges such as negativity in the workplace and disruptive employee behavior.

Coaching for Performance

When most people in health care organizations think about managing the performance of employees, the annual performance appraisal comes to mind. Coaching, however, takes a different approach. Coaching others for optimal performance is an ongoing process embedded in the everyday work of the manager or expert colleague. Coaching is a process engaged in by anyone in the workplace who has some responsibility for or interest in helping other workers to develop and improve their skills. Although the coach is often the individual's manager, educators and trusted colleagues with special expertise assume the role of coach at various times. Many health care providers also serve as coaches for the patients and clients they serve. For purposes of discussion, this section will focus on the coaching role involved in influencing or improving the performance of employees. The concept is presented briefly here, and the reader is referred to *From Management to Leadership* (Manion 2005) for a more complete exploration.

Coaching can be defined as "a process of facilitating an individual's or team's development through giving advice and instruction; encouraging discovery through guided discussions and hands-on experiences; observing performance; and giving honest, direct, and immediate feedback" (Manion

2005, p. 276). To be effective, the coaching relationship between two individuals must be based on a relationship characterized by trust, openness, mutual respect, positive and ongoing communication, and support. The effective coach is also familiar with the principles of both intrinsic and extrinsic motivation.

Briefly, a coaching process begins with some idea of what is to be accomplished. The desired outcome is identified as a goal that can be used to measure progress and achievement. Once the goal of the coaching has been identified and agreed upon, an assessment of the performer's current abilities is conducted. This assessment of the employee's previous experience and opportunities results in a conclusion about the person's current standing in relation to the goal. For example, perhaps the manager is coaching an employee who has just assumed responsibility for leading a key task force. It is helpful for the manager to know that the employee has had similar experiences with leading committee work before but that the previous work did not involve committees with systemwide membership that included physicians and community members as a part of the process. For a coach, this knowledge would be useful to key into the specific processes and concerns that the employee needs to understand in order to be successful.

Once the assessment is complete, the coach and performer work to develop a clear understanding of the task force members' roles and responsibilities. The coach and employee can also look for additional training opportunities when they are needed. In order to determine the effectiveness of the coaching, the next step is for the coach to observe the employee's performance. This step can be achieved through direct observation, progress reports, and/or outcomes analysis. Finally, the coach provides feedback to the individual on how well he or she performed, and the process is complete. The rest of this section examines several specific aspects of coaching for performance.

Feedback

Feedback is a critical element of coaching. Feedback validates or expands the performers' assessment of their achievement. Whether realized or not, each of us is giving other people feedback all of the time. The responses to a person's behavior lets him or her know whether one is pleased, excited, disappointed, dismayed, angry, or any other of myriad possibilities. Feedback can be given verbally or through simple nonverbal cues and facial expressions such as a frown, a look of confusion, or a smile. Body language communicates to others a reaction to what they have done or said.

Another source of feedback is offered by what is paid attention to and noticed. For example, a group of managers in an organization was responsible for organizing and providing leadership development programs for their peers. They not only arranged for the speaker but they also obtained the necessary facilities and notified participants in advance of the program. To add a special touch, they arrived early and expended a great deal of effort on decorating the conference room with a seasonal theme. When the chief executive officer (CEO) walked into the room, he took one look at the tables and asked in a critical tone of voice, "Where are the water pitchers for the tables?" The team felt let down and demoralized that he never noticed the hard work they had done and the effort they had made in preparation for the day but only noted what they had missed.

Interpersonal feedback is a crucial aspect of helping people improve their performance. Seashore, Seashore, and Weinberg (1999, p. 3) define feedback as "information about past behavior, delivered in the present, which may influence future behavior." They note that feedback gives us the ability to test our perceptions, reactions, and observations. It is a primary method for influencing someone to start, stop, or change his or her behavior in some way. "Feedback in the workplace is fundamental for helping those who wish to improve their performance reach an objective, or avoid unpleasant reactions to their efforts" (Seashore, Seashore, and Weinberg 1999, p. 7). Feedback is the final step in coaching. It closes the loop for the performer and lets him or her know the degree to which a goal has been successfully attained.

Giving Feedback

Those who share feedback with others need to be reminded that it is always the receiver of the feedback who, in reality, determines whether he or she internalizes the message and acts on the feedback given. Although it is possible to learn ways to improve one's skill in giving feedback, delivering the message effectively does not necessarily mean the receiver is going to change his or her behavior. When the person delivering the feedback is a credible source of information and has the best interests of the recipient at heart, willingness to accept the feedback increases. However, additional factors play into whether a person acts on the feedback. For example, perhaps the potential consequences of not changing the behavior are significant enough that it motivates the individual to make the necessary alterations. Or perhaps the recipient has heard the same message on previous occasions, and it is starting to make more of an impression. Sometimes the behavioral change requested is just too hard to make, or the suggested change is related to behavior that is an inherent and permanent part of the individual's personality.

Although giving feedback is an important step in the coaching process, many people find the process difficult. When the feedback is positive and consists of observations that the recipient is likely to want to hear, the process is usually less difficult. But it can be a different story when the information to be shared may be perceived by the receiver as negative criticism. Negative feedback often feels confrontational and uncomfortable to give. In some instances, the person may feel uneasy about his or her right to deliver the message. In situations where the individual needs feedback but there is significant reluctance to give it, Clarke-Epstein (2002) suggests consideration of these three questions:

1. If I were the person in this situation, would I want to be given this feedback? Would I want to be told about my behavior?
2. Can the person change his or her behavior, given the feedback?
3. Will I be embarrassed to give the feedback, or will it embarrass the other person to hear it? If the answer to either of these questions is yes, take the time to organize your thoughts and carefully craft your message rather than delivering a spontaneous remark.

As Clarke-Epstein suggests, when giving feedback is difficult because of the negative content or the potentially uncomfortable nature of the feedback, it is helpful to write a script to guide the interchange. It forces the person to think carefully about what the specific feedback is and provides time to allow strong emotions such as anger or disappointment to fade. When feedback is delivered during times when strong emotions are at a peak, the emotion often drives the response, and aggression is the result. Similarly, if a person is feeling fearful or intimidated, it is easy to come across as passive and unassertive. The challenge is to share the information with the other person clearly and assertively but in a manner that does not result in the individual feeling angry or demeaned.

Writing a script also allows the person to practice giving feedback when the situation promises to be especially difficult, as may be the case when it involves giving the boss feedback about his or her annoying or destructive behavior. Scripting helps prepare for what may be highly charged interpersonal interchanges. The basic elements and structure found in most feedback scripts include the following four elements:

When you _____,

I felt _____.

This causes a problem because_____.

In the future I would like you _____.

This basic model provides a framework that can be used to complete the sentences and form a script. Thus, giving an employee feedback about behavior may look like this:

When you responded to Susan's request for help negatively and with complaints about your own workload,

I felt angry because I have seen Susan help you several times when she also had a heavy workload.

This causes a problem because our patients won't receive the kind of care they need if we don't help each other.

In the future, I expect you to pitch in and help others and to be more positive about it.

There are several common difficulties with using this model. Some people feel that beginning with the phrase *When you* is too confrontational and that a softer approach would be more effective. However, the feedback giver's tone of voice and body language have more to do with expressing a confrontational, aggressive style than do the actual words used. If the interchange starts with *When you*, it cues the person that specific feedback is coming, and it says "this is about you." Most people are so inundated with massive amounts of information that messages are not fully heard or even cued into unless it is clear that the message is about them or is about something of value to them.

The second issue arises with the *I felt* portion of the structure. In initial efforts to develop a script, there is a tendency to describe observations rather than true emotions. For instance, a person might write, "I felt like you did not take the other person's needs into account." This statement does not describe an emotion; it is a factual statement. Writing this part of the message in a way that shares the emotion being felt would be something like, "I felt angry that you did not take your team member's needs into account." Or "I was disappointed in the way you handled the situation." Being willing to communicate feelings, although not appropriate in every instance, is a clear, positive sign of confidence and assertiveness. It is also a characteristic of high emotional intelligence.

Developing the *This causes a problem because* part of the script is probably the trickiest but most important part of the message. In this part of the message the reason for the receiver to change his or her behavior is being verbalized. The most common mistake made is giving the receiver a reason that is important to the sender but may not be important to the receiver. To make it more likely that the feedback will result in a desirable action, the receiver's values need to be considered. For instance, people and relationships are highly important to some of us though less important to others.

In addition to people and relationships, there are at least three other common value categories, including image, goals and achievements, and facts and information. People who highly value image tend to be more concerned about factors such as reputation and how the world sees them. Other people are more concerned with their ability to accomplish goals and reach achievements, and still others are more likely to be swayed by factual information such as data.

One of the reasons a person does not change behavior based on feedback received is that the reason given for changing does not seem important enough. When people are given a reason to change their behavior that is important to them, the feedback is more likely to influence their behavior. Take, for example, the manager giving an employee feedback on the effects of her response to a teammate who asked her for help. In the first example, the reason given was based on a value related to goals and accomplishments:

> *When you* responded to Susan's request for help negatively and with complaints about your own workload,
>
> *I felt* angry because I have seen Susan help you several times when she also had a heavy workload.
>
> *This causes a problem because* our patients won't receive the kind of care they need if we don't help each other.
>
> *In the future,* I expect you to pitch in and help others and to be more positive about it.

To deliver a message that has value for the receiver, it is important to make certain that the third element of the script fits something of value to the receiver. Examples of ways to change the third portion of the script on the basis of different values include:

> **People and relationships:** This creates a problem for you because others will be less willing to help you the next time you need it.
>
> **Image:** This creates a problem for you because your co-workers will see you as a whiner, complainer, and non–team player.
>
> **Facts and information:** This has created a problem because I've had to step in and deal with one of your irate co-workers four times in just the past week.

Finding the right approach to motivate different individuals may take some experimentation. If no improvement occurs after the first attempt at giving feedback on a problem, try another reason for the person to change when the behavior comes up the next time. Sometimes it is difficult to determine from cues in a person's language which of the four values is most important for that individual, especially if the manager does not know the person well. In such cases, start with what is believed to be the person's values but be willing to modify the message when a behavioral change is not apparent. When the feedback does not work, try recrafting the message, but remember that no matter how articulate and clear the sender is, there is also responsibility on the part of the receiver for responding to and using the feedback given. It is up to the receiver to decide whether to make use of the feedback offered or to ignore it. In some managerial–employee feedback situations, acting on the feedback in a positive manner may be a requirement for staying in the job.

Judith Briles (2008) recommends another variation of this feedback model and calls it "carefronting," based on a term first coined by Tom Augsburger, author of *Caring Enough to Confront*. It includes inserting the statement, "Was it your intent to _____?" after the third element. The sender pauses long enough to give the receiver time to respond. A reply by the receiver of, "No, this wasn't my intention" increases the likelihood that the receiver will act on the feedback. After the "In the future _____" statement, she suggests asking the person for commitment to the new course of action and then stating the consequences if the person does not follow through. The script would look like this:

> *When you* responded to Susan's request for help negatively and with complaints about your own workload,
>
> *I felt* angry because I have seen Susan help you several times when she also had a heavy workload.
>
> *This creates a problem because* our patients won't receive the kind of care they need if we don't help each other.
>
> *Was it your intent to* withhold help from Susan when she needed it? (Stop . . . do not respond until there is a response from the receiver.)
>
> *In the future*, I expect you to pitch in and help others and to be more positive about it.
>
> *Are you committed to* helping your co-workers? (Wait for the person's response.)
>
> *If there isn't a change*, we'll be talking about this again to determine whether you fit on this team.

The last statement, *If there isn't a change* _____, may not work in every case. It can sound threatening, and the consequences identified must be ones that the manager is willing to carry through. The intent is to convince the individual that there is a reason for him or her to change the behavior. This message can also be conveyed by changing the third element of the script: *This creates a problem because* _____. In some cases it is perfectly reasonable to let the person know the next steps you will take. For example, consider the following situation. The manager of an exceedingly busy inpatient department, Jane, has talked with Tom, the director of environmental services, on multiple occasions about the lengthy time it takes for empty patient rooms to be cleaned and prepared for the next patient. This lag causes a backlog of patients who are waiting to be admitted. Jane is getting tremendous pressure from the manager of the emergency department for not being more responsive. Tom has assured Jane on repeated occasions that his department staff will do better and uphold the standards they have established. But the situation keeps occurring. Consider this script:

> *When you* fail to follow through on your promise to deal with this problem,

I am frustrated and angry *because it* makes it harder for me to get these sick patients up to this department in a timely fashion so they can get the care they need.

Is it your intent to prevent these patients from being admitted on a timely basis? (Stop and wait for a response.)

In the future, I need the rooms to be cleaned within two hours after a patient's discharge, as we agreed is our standard.

Are you committed to ensuring that your employees meet this standard?

If there isn't a change, I'm going to talk with our vice president about the issue. You can come with me if you would like, but this level of service is not acceptable.

This final step is often referred to as escalating the assertion. It lets the other person know what action will be taken if the needed change does not occur. It does not have to be presented in an aggressive tone of voice, but it can be delivered in a matter-of-fact manner. This approach is much healthier than reporting these problems to the vice president without letting Tom know, or worse, sending off a blistering e-mail to both executives involved.

Whichever script is used, to be successful, the person using the script must always exercise his or her best judgment. No script will work exactly the same in different situations. Consider the intent of giving the feedback and be willing to try again if the message is not acted upon the first time it is received.

Receiving Feedback

Receiving feedback well is perhaps as important as being able to give feedback well. Coens and Jenkins (2000, p. 144) suggest that the receiver of feedback has "at least as much responsibility, and probably more, than the giver of feedback." Everyone is privileged to receive feedback from others at various times in their career. The immediate response, as well as how well the feedback is incorporated into future behavior, often determines whether the person who offered the feedback will do so again in the future. Furthermore, the receiver's reactions influence the comfort with which co-workers will approach future feedback opportunities.

Negative feedback is frequently uncomfortable for both the giver and the receiver. Clarke-Epstein (2002) suggests specific responses that can be used in such situations. Sometimes the initial response to negative or critical feedback is shock or surprise. When the listener has no idea how to respond, the best response may be simply to do nothing or to say, "I am completely surprised. I need some time to think about this. When can we talk about it again?" An angry response to negative feedback often elicits a similar reaction from the giver. To quell the possibility of a damaging encounter, Clarke-Epstein recommends that when the listener feels anger in response to feedback, the best recourse is to do nothing and realize that the initial feelings of anger will pass. Then, once the person has calmed down, he or she can offer a reasonable response instead of a biting, angry, or sarcastic retort.

Rationalization is a second typical response to negative feedback. Before the message is even complete, excuses and defenses are all called forth. However, before sharing such responses with anyone else, it is helpful to reflect and separate the purely defensive responses from the legitimate ones. When a person sounds defensive, much of what is offered may be disregarded when in fact the responses may be a worthy explanation. The person's tone of voice, if defensive or negative, reduces the effectiveness of the message.

Finally, in some instances, the reaction to negative feedback may simply be acceptance. Perhaps the receiver knows that the feedback is true and that the giver has shared this information in order to help improve performance or relationships in some way. Occasionally, negative feedback may concern behavior that the person has already recognized but is not certain that others had noticed. In this case, the person should respond assertively and ask questions about anything that is unclear, such as, "Can you give me another example to help me understand?" or "I want to be sure I understand what you are saying." Although a person need not accept all of the feedback, a useful response is to think it through and take what is helpful and put it to use.

Recognizing Problem Performers

Managing problem performers ranks right up at the top of the most difficult challenges a manager or leader must address. In fact, few issues trigger more angst or cause managers to feel more helpless than the daunting task of confronting poor performers. Why? The answer is often all too predictable and follows themes such as these:

- Addressing the problem is not worth the effort because the organization's performance appraisal system is so cumbersome that it is easier to work around the employee.
- The human resources department does not support managers in their efforts to remedy poor performance and instead works as the employees' advocate.
- The performance problem has existed for years, and no one has ever attempted to address it.
- The employee has a volatile personality, and the manager is afraid of the employee's reaction.

Although confronting employees with performance problems is never easy, demystifying the process of identifying and addressing the root causes of good and poor performance may help. The case studies described in figures 10-1 and 10-2 shed light on the process and increase understanding of how to coach people for improved outcomes.

Figure 10-1.   Case Study: Struggling to Perform

Mary was an exceptional obstetrics nurse and was often asked to help with com-plicated cases. She loved her position and the opportunity to touch the lives of so many people. There were some drawbacks, however, including salary and shift changes. So, when offered the opportunity to become a nurse manager, she quickly accepted the new position with only a passing thought about the super-visory skills that would be required in the new assignment. Mary knew she was a good learner and had always adapted well in the past; besides, she could really use the salary increase and was excited about spending more weekends and holidays with her family.

After a few months on the job, Mary was frustrated with her position and began feeling guilty about not effectively addressing the people problems in her depart-ment. She understood that her work would be easier if she could learn how to deal with difficult people without internalizing the conflict. She considered reading a book or attending a class to help her learn the new skills she needed.

Mary's boss was also concerned. Mary was not getting her schedules completed on time, and she seemed to be on edge most of the time. Her nursing staff was growing increasingly disgruntled with how Mary barked orders and spent most of her time in the office. It was clear that she was trying very hard and putting in unusually long hours to stay on top of the demands placed on her. Her co-workers reached out to try and support her, but she did not respond to their offers of help.

After a year as a manager, Mary felt burned out. Although her administrative skills had grown, the effort was leaving her exhausted. She felt distant from the patients, and rather than having more time with her family, she was spending even less time at home than before. When she was home, she felt distracted or tired. Mary knew the quality of her work had improved; however, she frequently felt that her work was no longer meaningful. Although Mary's boss was satisfied with her performance, she avoided involving Mary in any special assignments for fear that Mary would not be able to handle the additional workload.

Both of the individuals described in the case studies elected to take on a new position. Although both employees held demanding positions that required hard work, one was struggling and had lost the sense of joy she felt in her previous position, while the other was thriving.

To understand why one employee performs better and experiences less stress than another, it is useful to know exactly what factors drive perfor-mance. The most important factor in performance is the alignment of an individual's values, interests, and skills with those required by the position and the organization. How well matched the person is to the requirements of the job and the organization is the key to performance and certainly is related to the ability to experience joy at work. When any of the three ele-ments of values, interests, or skills is out of alignment, the level of stress increases and generally the level of performance decreases. Although Mary's performance (depicted in figure 10-1) was acceptable, she was putting tre-mendous stress on herself. This situation is not unlike driving an old Ford that is out of alignment. Although this car may be able to get the person to the desired destination, the attention and physical effort required to drive it is exhausting, and permanent damage to the car may occur if it is driven in this condition for too long. In contrast, Sharon (figure 10-2) fulfilled her goals with ease and enjoyed herself while doing it. Her situation is like driving a new Lexus with automatic steering, cruise control, and a concert-quality sound system.

The importance of alignment was profoundly illuminated in the 1980s, a period marked by extensive downsizing in many organizations. Outplacement firms were flourishing as major companies reduced staff by 10 to 20 percent. In many cases, organizations targeted individuals they believed they could most afford to lose—poor or marginal employees, those who performed their jobs poorly—even though their positions may have been essential to the organization. In droves, these individuals were informed of their separation and quickly sent off to the care of outplacement counselors, whose first job was to help them deal with the pain and

---

Figure 10-2. Case Study: Working in Alignment

Sharon's job as a marketing specialist for a health system foundation seemed to be an odd match to many of her friends. They had known her as a physical therapist, and her love of the field was evident in her interactions with others. In fact, when anyone in her family or circle of friends had health care questions, Sharon was called for advice before anyone else.

When Sharon first took the marketing position, she had strong reservations about her ability to handle the responsibilities. Her predecessor had a degree in marketing and had worked in several nonprofit organizations before joining the foundation. Sharon had neither a relevant degree nor the appropriate experience, but somehow Sharon's manager was confident in her passion and knowledge of health care along with her excellent interpersonal skills.

Sharon often felt up to her eyeballs with work and sometimes found it difficult to leave the office on time, but she rarely felt overwhelmed. At first, Sharon thought the contacts with potential donors would be awkward and uncomfortable. However, she quickly found that it was easy to enroll others with her vision of what was possible, and she thrived on the opportunity to talk with people about what she loved. Sharon also received positive feedback from community members for doing what came naturally to her: engaging people in dialogue about current health care issues and opportunities.

Sharon's manager was extremely pleased with Sharon's work and was confident that the department was going to overachieve its financial goals for the year. Sharon attended a couple of marketing courses to learn the technical side of the field, but it was her knowledge of health care and interpersonal skills that made her a real standout. She found it hard to believe a year had passed since she started her marketing position, and she was confident that she would soon secure enough donations to fund the opening of an adjacent building for the new residency program.

shock of losing their job. Once stabilized, these individuals were taken through a series of self-assessment instruments designed to increase their self-awareness. Armed with a greater knowledge of themselves, individuals then began the search for new positions that were deemed a better fit; that is, positions that were in better alignment with each individual's values, interests, and skills.

The outplacement counseling had an interesting result. The majority of individuals were perceived as strong performers in their new position. Most of them received significant increases in pay and reported greater satisfaction on the job (Brightman 2002). These employees were the same individuals who had been perceived as poor performers in their prior positions and organizations, but with better job alignment they seemed like different employees.

This lack of alignment, or fit problem, can be related to the skills or interests of the employee or to the fit between the employee's values or behaviors and the culture of the organization. In Mary's case, for example, the problem was a lack of alignment between the skills needed to perform the job effectively and the skills Mary possessed. As a result of trying to compensate for her skill shortcomings, Mary found that the effort required to stay afloat in her new position left her feeling exhausted at the end of the workday. In another situation, the employee may be able to apply the necessary skills but have no interest in the work to be done, or the employee may have the necessary skills, find the work interesting, but disagree with the predominant values underlying the organization's culture.

In other words, individuals thrive when they are placed in circumstances where the values of the organization feel right, the skills needed to perform are available, and the work itself is interesting. For the individuals studied after being downsized in the 1980s, finding the right fit in their new jobs made all the difference (Brightman 2002). Many of them said that they wished they had found self-understanding earlier in their careers. Since that time, some organizations have even begun to offer self-assessment courses to their employees.

Matching people to jobs is not as easy as it sounds due to the complexity of jobs and the diversity among people. In the sociological literature, many studies focus on this issue. Kallenberg (2008) suggests that other kinds of mismatches between the employee and the job include skill level (under- or over-qualified), geographic issues (the job's location prevents the person from being a fit), temporal aspects (the number of hours desired or needed), earnings, and work-family balance needs. The difficulty of finding a viable fit between individual and organization further highlights the need for self-understanding. Self-understanding gives an individual a "leg up" when assessing job fit.

Chris Oster, director of organizational development for General Motors, believes that self-understanding, once identified, can become a source of stability in an unstable world. "Identifying your enduring values, interests, and skills gives you a strong sense of control. You are able to more effectively direct your career rather than being at the mercy of someone else's view of what's right for you" (Oster 2004).

Too often, the attraction of making more money or having more prestige or some other external motivator clouds self-awareness and leads to misalignment. In some situations, the assumption may be made that no employment options are available that would better suit the unique needs of the person. Without the person pausing and taking personal stock of who she is and what attracts her, it is easy to go off track. Lots of Marys in the work world lack self-knowledge and operate by keeping their heads down, continuing to work hard, and continuing to feel miserable. Whether at the initiative of the employee or through the coaching and support of a supervisor, exploring issues of alignment or fit may very well be the key to engaging people more fully and facilitating higher levels of productivity. Fit is also one of the first areas to explore when performance is less than satisfactory, and exploring fit issues offers employees the opportunity to participate in identifying the root cause of their own poor performance. Imagine if Mary had recognized that her interests and skills were not well matched to her position, she might have been able to take the steps necessary to get her career and personal life back on track.

All too often, early opportunities to assess the roots of poor performance are missed. Even though a manager may be aware that an employee is performing at a level below what is required, the manager may choose to adopt a wait-and-see attitude rather than addressing the problem immediately. So, just how can it be determined whether a performance problem is serious enough to warrant significant action?

Defining Problem Performance

One of the hurdles to improving problem performance is deciding whether an individual's performance is unacceptable enough to warrant action beyond regular coaching. In other words, is the performance really that bad, or is it just marginal? Making this determination is a judgment call. Most managers have a gut sense of when a problem warrants significant action. However, having a working definition can be a useful tool. To identify exceptional performers (both at the top and the bottom of the performance spectrum), Coens and Jenkins (2000, p. 175) offer the following definition:

> An exceptional (or problem) employee has inarguably stood out from the rest of the work team for a sustained period of time in contribution as evidenced by the results achieved and/or the behaviors exhibited. [A problem employee] is easily declared by those that know him or her. . . . Exceptional, given its most elementary definition, is rare. To identify more than a few individuals as such negates the exceptional label and makes it [an] intolerable contradiction. It is more likely a given work team will have NONE rather than ONE exceptional team member.

By definition, problem performers are readily identifiable. But notice that the definition excerpted above includes an element of time, varying circumstances, and a consistent conclusion by multiple people who know and interact with the individual. Although judgment is required, in the case of performance it is a conclusion arrived at after carefully sorting out all possible factors that influence performance but are outside the control of the employee. Reacting too quickly may cause a manager to attribute the cause of problems to an individual simply because he or she was nearby when the problem occurred. ("Because of recent flash floods, we have fired our weatherman.") Of course, the opposite is also true. Credit may be given to individuals for making improvements and performing well when they had no control over the situation. They were just lucky. ("Congratulations, Ms. Tucker, on your award for most outstanding school nurse. During the past year, there were no reported cases of measles in your district.") These examples are extreme, but they point to common mistakes in judgment with regard to performance problems. Individual performance is highly interdependent with numerous complex variables in the work environment. As a result, variation in performance may occur but have nothing to do with individual effort and skill. A healthy dose of skepticism about using data combined with observation over time is the best way to determine whether special attention is warranted.

Assessing Individual Problem Performance

After ruling out various system- or environment-related causes of poor individual performance, managers may conclude that the problem is rooted in the individual's behavior and/or capabilities. At this point, the options fall into three categories:

1. Helping the individual improve to an acceptable level
2. Altering the job or finding a position that is better aligned with the individual's skills and potential
3. Taking measures to remove the employee from the organization in a manner that is respectful and caring

Choosing the correct course depends on the facts of the case as well as good judgment. The first option, helping the employee to address the performance problem, should always be the beginning point unless it is absolutely clear that any such efforts would be futile. The second option affirms the belief that performance is a function of fit and holds on to the possibility that the employee would be productive if he or she were placed in another, more appropriate position. (Cases such as Mary's fit this description.) Organizations that readily dismiss poor performers create a cloud of fear for the remaining employees and damage overall morale. (Although it is demoralizing to keep a nonproductive person in a job, co-workers still expect the organization and manager to treat that person fairly.) In cases where finding a better fit would not be wise, justifiable, or possible, then the third option, dismissing the employee, must be pursued.

As a guide for determining the best course of action, Coens and Jenkins (2000) offer several questions for managers to ask when facing a serious performance problem. The questions are listed in figure 10-3. When these questions do not lead to a solution and involuntary separation seems to be the only logical course, there is still another option: voluntary separation.

Figure 10-3. Questions to Ask When Facing a Serious Performance Problem (Coens and Jenkins 2000)

Checking for fit
- Is the performance a pattern or a recent development?
- Does the person have the necessary skills, knowledge, abilities, and temperament to do the job?
- Does the person like the work? [Does he or she] like the organization?

Checking for bias or inconsistent expectations
- Is this the first incident of this type, or have variations happened in the past?
- Can the observations of the supervisor be confirmed by others?
- Is there a personal, chemistry, or political issue that may have triggered the problem?
- Has the person received adequate training, guidance, and feedback?
- Has the job undergone significant change recently?
- Have management or performance expectations changed? Does the individual understand these changes?

Assessing the influence of systemic issues on individual performance
- Has the same performance deficiency/problem been observed with other people in the same job?
- How long has the person been in the job? Could subpar performance be explained by insufficient time on the learning curve, stagnation, or burnout?
- Has there been a change in the workload volume, increase in stressors, staffing shortages, or other changes that may be triggering the performance issue?
- Are there barriers or issues that are causing the performance problems that are not the fault of the individual (e.g., proper tools, equipment, training, support, etc.)?

Adapted and reprinted with permission of the publisher from *Abolishing Performance Appraisals: Why They Backfire and What to Do Instead,* copyright © 2000 by Tom Coens and Mary Jenkins, Berrett-Koehler Publishers, Inc., San Francisco. All rights reserved.

Sometimes open and honest dialogue about performance issues can lead individual employees to resign voluntarily. For legal reasons, certain safeguards must be taken in such cases. Working in partnership with the human resources department can be helpful and is required by many organizations. Human resources staff can also provide guidance on the process of dealing with unacceptable performance, should it be necessary.

Although taking steps that eventually lead to either voluntary separation or involuntary termination can be emotionally difficult, not taking them often leaves managers in a state of paralysis while the situation continues to deteriorate. It is all too common to observe two polarized approaches, neither of which is helpful to the individual employee, manager, department, or organization:

1. **Waiting until the situation becomes intolerable before making the decision to terminate the employee immediately:** Human resources professionals report that it is more common than not for them to be contacted only at the point of termination, which makes it difficult

at best to go through the necessary legal steps of intensive coaching and documentation.

2. **Deciding to do nothing:** At this point, facing the discomfort and conflict entailed in confronting the employee seems too difficult. Managers resort to a default strategy: They hope that the situation will go away, that the employee will leave or transfer, or that they will find ways to work around the problem individual.

Waiting too long to move into an intensive process makes a difficult situation almost impossible to deal with. Although doing nothing feels like the easier path to take, it exacts a heavy toll. Most obvious is the disillusioning effect on the immediate work group members, who often need to take on extra work to make up for the problem employee's poor performance.

Less obvious but even more destructive is the tendency of managers and organizations to create policies based on the actions of a few poor performers rather than addressing performance issues on an individual basis. For example, a manager may find that tardiness is an issue for a handful of employees. To address the problem, he may establish a policy that stipulates how many times each individual employee is allowed to be late during a specific time period, say, three times per year. The policy stipulates that the employees' pay will be docked and disciplinary action will be taken when they are late a fourth time, and so on. The policy seems objective and fair to everyone, but the problem is that it eliminates the element of judgment. Eventually, policy manuals become filled with policies meant to address the behavior of a few but affect everyone in the organization. Employees get the message that this organization does not trust its employees. Consider the following example from the "I am not making this up" department:

> The human resources vice president for a large health care system shared an example that demonstrates this tendency. Over the years, his organization had created many policies for all employees that were really designed to make it easier to correct the behaviors of a few. One of these policies dictated the number of times someone could be tardy in a year. When an employee was late more than the number of times allowed according to the policy, he or she was subject to disciplinary action. To emphasize the importance of coming to work on time, the organization also issued quarterly perfect attendance awards in the amount of $500 for those employees who were neither late nor absent during the preceding three months.
>
> During one unusually harsh winter, snowstorms left several inches of accumulation on the ground, and road conditions were sometimes treacherous. One day when snow had decreased the level of visibility on the roads, a multiple-car accident closed the main expressway for several hours. As might be expected, several employees on their way to work were delayed by the traffic jam and they were late for work. The tardiness of employees on this day was recorded, and disciplinary action was instituted for those who had exceeded the allowable level of tardiness.
>
> As might be expected with so much at stake, those who were stuck on the expressway because of the accident asked to have the tardiness for the

day removed from their records because they were late due to circumstances beyond their control. The organization's decision? The tardiness on that day was not removed from the record because "others who were not stuck in the accident arrived at work on time." Fairness, it was determined, had nothing to do with the circumstances. The policy was applied without exception.

When managers are confronted with inappropriate behavior or a pattern of unacceptable performance, the tendency is to create a solution and impose that solution on all employees. The cumulative effect of these actions unintentionally erodes motivation and the health of the work environment. The message to people is, "You are inferior and untrustworthy, even when the official rhetoric speaks of respect for people" (Scholtes 1998, p. 297).

With this broader view of the ramifications of avoiding the performance problem or waiting too long to seek assistance, the best course of action is to contact the human resources department to ask for support when it is suspected that a performance problem may lead to a separation or termination.

Taking Action to Address Problem Performance

Once it has been decided that a performance problem must be addressed, the next challenge is to determine the best course of action. Generally speaking, there are two distinct approaches:

1. **Performance improvement:** The performance improvement approach is a rigorous feedback and documentation process that generally spans sixty to ninety days, depending on the nature of the problem. It is designed to clearly specify the performance expectations, identify the gap, document what is expected in the future, and articulate how management will support the individual. This intensive process serves the dual purpose of providing rigorous support in the hope that the individual can improve his or her level of performance and documentation in the event the outcome results in involuntary termination.

2. **Corrective action:** The corrective action approach follows a path of progressive discipline. In some organizations, this approach takes the form of positive discipline, which will be discussed later in this chapter.

Broadly speaking, health care organizations tend to rely heavily on the use of the corrective action method, although a few organizations have implemented a positive discipline approach. However, exercising a corrective approach misses the mark when the root cause of the problem involves capability or skill deficiencies. The decision on which path to take should be based on an accurate assessment of the underlying cause of the problem and matching it to the process that is most likely to facilitate improvement.

Consider a similar situation in another context. The Harper family has two children, Bill and Sarah. Ironically, both brought home report cards one quarter with a class grade of a D—Bill's was in math and Sarah's was in French. Bill is an active child, plays sports, and has a very full social life. He rarely studies for math and often misses his homework assignments. Sarah, on the other hand, studies, asks for assistance from her teacher after school, and even sought out help from a tutor. Despite this effort, Sarah continues to perform poorly on her French tests.

Both children are performing at an unacceptable level. Should the action taken by Mr. and Mrs. Harper be the same for both? Should both Sarah and Bill be grounded? The action of grounding is the family equivalent of the corrective action path. Bill neglected his studies even though he knew that the consequences would be an unsatisfactory grade and trouble with his parents. Grounding may be an appropriate way to convey to Bill the need to make better decisions and choices about how he spends his time. It helps clarify his parents' expectations and demonstrates the consequences attached to the willful or intentional act of ignoring his homework. The result may very well be an improvement in his performance in math as he learns to rebalance his time.

But would grounding Sarah have the same result? Clearly, her performance was not the result of neglect but rather of a more fundamental comprehension or skill problem. Grounding Sarah would have no effect on her French grades, and it might actually make them worse. Sarah is likely to benefit more from targeted support. Perhaps putting together a study plan designed by her teacher and supported at home would be of greater value. This path would be akin to performance improvement planning. The plan may result in improvement, and that is certainly the hope. It may also help confirm that French is not the best language for Sarah to master, and other decisions might be considered. Perhaps learning Spanish, for example, would be easier for Sarah.

Performance Improvement Approach
The performance improvement planning (PIP) process is directed more toward the correction of unacceptable performance than toward unacceptable behavior. Performance improvement planning is typically exercised when regular feedback and coaching have not sufficiently raised the individual's level of performance. The purpose of performance improvement planning is to give the individual every possible chance to correct the deficiencies while at the same time creating a documented record of the actions taken by the manager. It is considered a serious process, and it may end in termination when performance does not meet improvement goals. Performance improvement plans vary considerably in format according to the type of work and the type of problems to be addressed, but every PIP should be designed to fulfill the following goals:

- Point out the difference between present performance and agreed-upon expectations.
- Describe the specific changes to be made.

- Document the actions that will be taken to support the employee, including periodic reviews of progress.
- Document the duration of the plan (usually thirty to ninety days, depending on the circumstances and results expected).
- Clarify the actions (that is, transfer, demotion, or termination) that may result if performance does not improve to an acceptable level by the end of the designated period of improvement.

The PIP process protects the employee from unfair treatment as well as the organization from potential litigation. In a performance-related discharge, a paper trail describing the performance problems and the remedial efforts to counsel and assist the employee before discharging should be continuous. Too often, managers think of compiling a paper trail only after they have decided that termination is the best course. They rush the improvement program and try to fire an employee who has years of tenure with only three months of documentation, because they did not document the actions during the long period of time earnestly spent trying to help the employee through informal coaching. The deficient paper trail leaves the impression of a very unfair or biased discharge and becomes the basic ingredient for a potential lawsuit.

Whenever serious performance problems arise, formal meetings must be held with the employee to provide the necessary guidance and counseling and to accumulate the needed documentation. Documentation of the performance improvement process can include appraisal forms, e-mails, memos, and formal notices of deficiency. After remedial measures have failed to lead to improved performance, involuntary termination may become necessary. The following facts need to be confirmed before the actual termination meeting can take place (Coens and Jenkins 2000, pp. 239–40):

- The employee clearly knew what was expected of him or her.
- The employee was given all of the information, training, and resources needed to perform adequately.
- The deficiencies were serious enough to warrant action, and specific examples of the deficiencies have been documented (for example, if the employee repeatedly failed to complete major projects on time, documentation needs to show exactly which projects were left incomplete or submitted late, how the employee knew that the projects were a priority, what the consequences of the employee's poor performance were, and so on).
- The details of how and when the employee was advised of the deficiencies have been documented (for example, the content and times of counseling and meetings with the employee, forewarning that the employee would be terminated for continued poor performance, and so on).
- The particulars on any special help, counseling, assistance, retraining, or other measures offered to help the employee have been documented.

Obviously, this description of how to handle and document performance deficiencies of a serious nature is a bare-bones overview of the process. For more details, a more complete treatment of the subject can be consulted, such as the *Supervisor's Guide to Documenting Employee Discipline* by Lee Patterson and Michael Deblieux (1993).

Corrective Action Approach

The choice of corrective action or positive discipline is pursued in cases where the incident or the performance issue is willful or intentional on the part of the employee. Making this distinction is important. Corrective action is appropriate only in cases of gross misconduct, improper behavior, insubordination, or violation of a clearly defined work rule. Although many organizations pursue a progressive path (increasing the duration of the time without pay with each additional infraction), the process can be stepped up when the seriousness of the infraction warrants immediate termination. Theft, harassment, abuse, and immoral or indecent conduct are all examples of acts that can result in immediate termination. The actions to be taken in response to such infractions depend on the circumstances surrounding the case, the nature and severity of the offense, the employee's past record, and the past practices of the organization. With all of these variables at play, it is advisable to seek counsel from the human resources department so a more systemic view of the circumstances can be considered.

Conventional wisdom in health care has been that when employees fail to meet performance standards or guidelines for attendance or personal conduct, managers should put them through a disciplinary process, or as one manager bluntly stated, "Get their name and write them up!" Traditionally, health care managers have seen discipline as something they have to do to the employee in order to bring him or her back in line. Inextricably woven in this punitive mind-set are the concepts of discipline and punishment. Paradoxically, this line of thinking leads managers to treat employees worse and worse while hoping that their behavior becomes better and better. Seldom does any employee come back from a suspension with a good attitude.

Despite the lack of evidence that this system for dealing with behavior problems engenders good outcomes, most health care facilities adhere to this 1930s human resources philosophy and euphemistically call their system "progressive discipline." In reality, very little about this approach is progressive. It is based on the belief that the failure to comply with standards or meet expectations should be met with punishment. Often, the only question asked by managers is, "Did the punishment fit the crime?"

Discipline and punishment are so intertwined in the culture of most health care organizations that the two terms are synonymous in the minds of many. Managers are expected to enforce compliance, which they often refer to as their law enforcement or policeman role, and most admit privately that they regret and dislike this role, especially when experienced and knowledgeable employees are involved. Regret and dislike are not the only side effects of this outdated approach. Managers also report that they are averse to taking on what feels like a controlling, parental role when they are trying to foster adult professional behaviors.

Sometimes, managers put off dealing with issues because they feel that too many stifling requirements are placed on them by the human resources department. Employees often complain that managers allow some individuals more leeway than others. Savvy employees learn how to manipulate the discipline system, and after a while, punishment loses power and being written up no longer carries any significance. Employees simply accept their warnings, and little discussion of taking ownership or committing to a personal plan for change in the future occurs. They know that no real consequences for their actions await them.

The entire concept of escalating punishments (verbal, then written, warnings followed by suspension and finally termination) as a means of bringing about behavioral change totally undermines the goal of progressive managers who want to work in partnership with their employees. It is increasingly obvious that "little of value comes out of the common belief that discipline and punishment go hand in hand" (Harvey 1986, p. 2). Clearly this age-old mind-set needs to be revisited if there are hopes of creating a culture of engagement and retention.

Positive Discipline Approach

In many areas of business and industry, the outdated punitive approach has already been replaced by a genuinely progressive system. Beginning in the mid-1980s, large corporations such as General Electric, Proctor and Gamble, Penzoil, and others opted to reorient their approach to discipline by moving away from punishment and toward building commitment. In his now classic article, "Discipline versus Punishment," Harvey states that:

> Successful organizations no longer look upon "discipline" as something that a manager does to a poor performer when he or she misbehaves. Instead these companies now approach discipline as something that must be created. They have abandoned traditional punitive measures, and in their place have developed systems that require acceptance of personal responsibility, individual decision making and true self discipline. They have made the transition from the concept of "doing discipline" to the more constructive perspective of "being disciplined" (Harvey 1986, p. 2).

Ironically, developing a system with the intent of encouraging commitment rather than executing punishment is not a difficult process. Such a process appears similar to the more traditional approach, but the premise on which this system rests is substantially different. (See figure 10-4.) The positive discipline approach is based on the basic belief that managers in an organization are responsible for leading the establishment of standards and expectations for performance. They are also responsible for letting individual employees know when those expectations and standards are not being met. The employee is the only one who can decide whether to adhere to the organization's standards and meet its expectations. In other words, the employee owns the choices regarding his or her behavior, not the manager.

Figure 10-4.   Model of the Positive Discipline Process

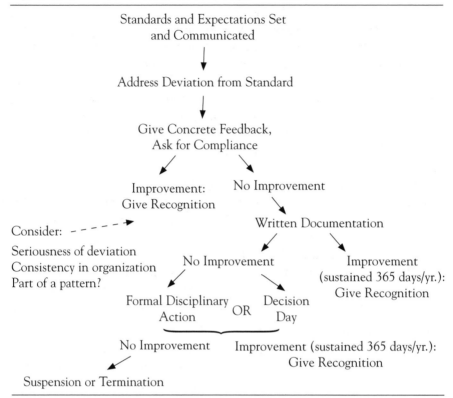

Changing how disciplinary issues are dealt with can create a more engaged and committed workforce, and it speaks volumes to employees about the organization's desire to help them be the best that they can be. The positive discipline process is not a panacea for every problem related to discipline, nor does it fit every situation that requires intervention on the part of the manager. It fits well, however, when managers are dealing with one of the following situations:

- The misconduct warrants a response other than formal discipline or termination.
- The problem is not a skill deficiency, but a behavioral issue.
- The use of this approach will most likely prevent further problem behavior.
- The employee takes ownership for the misconduct and expresses a willingness to change and sustain the needed changes (Murray 2003).

Managers in health care organizations must deal with such behavioral situations on a regular basis, and most managers would probably welcome a more workable solution that focuses on ownership and accountability for personal behavior instead of a system of escalated punishments. For example, one manager in Arizona said, "Since we adopted this approach it has made my life easier by putting the onus for change back where it belongs and getting me out of the policeman role."

The underlying shift in basic beliefs is from exacting punishment—"get their names and write them up"—to encouraging self-discipline and making employees responsible for maintaining reasonable standards of conduct. This is a crucial difference and cannot be underestimated. This shift represents a fundamental change in the assumptions and beliefs that are the under-pinnings for a system of discipline and cannot be taken lightly or covered quickly or superficially in one management meeting. If managers simply use new language as they continue to behave in the same old parent–child man-ner, employees do not feel supported in recommitting to anything but a job search. Employees are smart enough to recognize the change de jour or "flavor of the month" bandwagon and simply assume that the managers have been to another workshop and are now using different words to "bring them back in line." Harvey (1986, p. 3) is adamant about this awareness as he writes, "the impact of the change on the organization will be no more than that of putting a Mercedes emblem on the hood of a rusty Pinto. What is required is a total organizational commitment to an entirely different approach to the issue of managing people, performance and professionalism."

Treating employees as responsible adults (i.e., expecting responsible behavior) may well require intentional work with managers about how to give feedback and what to do when the conversation does not go well and employees decline to take ownership of their behavior. When employees take on a victim role and blame everyone else or when they give lip service to expected behavior change, managers need coaching on how to respond in ways that are adult-like rather than acting like a critical parent, which comes naturally with frustration.

The manager must continue to uphold appropriate standards. There are always some employees who do not want to accept ownership of their behavior, but the vast majority of employees appreciate being treated as adults and being supported in efforts to change. These people recommit to the organizational standards when the situation is dealt with in a fair and professional manner. By pointing out the gap between expected behavior and actual behavior and offering to support the employee in closing that gap as they move forward together, the manager can shift focus to the future and supports commitment to that future rather than punishing for past behavior. This emphasis on moving forward rather than rehashing old patterns tends to promote a mutual respect and partnership between employees and man-agers. Obviously, this is a welcome change for managers who become more likely to confront gaps in behavior when the process they use feels more professional and affirming rather than punitive.

When managers feel more comfortable confronting marginal behavior and pointing out the gap between what is observed and what is expected, they are more likely to deal with these issues as they occur and not put them off. The majority of employees who are meeting or exceeding standards are reassured in knowing that when colleagues are not measuring up, the problematic behaviors will be addressed. When behavior does not measure up to agreed-upon standards, most employees prefer that the situation be dealt with early on rather than waiting until some event necessitates a meeting of those involved.

Experience with this approach in business for the past thirty years has also demonstrated positive outcomes with respect to labor relations. Because positive discipline relies on the employee committing to behavioral expectations and developing his or her own action plan, there is less likelihood of wrongful termination suits. Labor unions report fewer grievances since the emphasis is on problem solving and supporting the employees' efforts to change rather than "making the punishment fit the crime" (Harvey 1986).

It goes without saying that if this approach is preferred in unionized environments, if managers are more likely to deal with a performance issue instead of putting it off, and if employees are following their own identified plan for moving forward, then managers have more time to recognize and support those who are doing a good job of meeting expectations. Finally, it becomes possible to move away from having problem employees who consume so much of the managers' time and emotional energy. Most important, again, employees take ownership for their own behavior and feel more committed to an organization in which they are treated as adults and are supported in their efforts to improve (Murray 2003).

Increasing numbers of health care organizations have undertaken the philosophical shift to positive or nonpunitive discipline. Their experience has provided further evidence of the many benefits of this approach. The numbers of grievances and suspensions have been reduced, and managers have more time for recognizing high-performing employees and promoting healthy interpersonal relationships, which result in a sense of partnership among employees and managers.

For example, an employee relations manager in a tertiary care center told a story about a long-term employee whose behavior had deteriorated to the point that it was no longer meeting the organization's customer service standards. To address the customer service problem, the employee's manager initiated the positive discipline process. When the employee returned to work after a one-day leave during which she completed a self-assessment and performance improvement plan, the employee called the employee relations manager to let him know where she was in the process and that she was optimistic about her ability to get back on track. She explained that the day away had given her some time for personal reflection about how much she really wanted to keep her job. She told him, "You know, I think it is really good of my supervisor to give me this time to sort things out. . . . She could have just fired me, but instead she is working with me on this, and that makes me want to hold up my part of the deal."

Similarly, a director of nursing operations in Idaho was so impressed with the positive changes he has seen in the two years since the implementation of a positive discipline approach that he wrote about the experience salvaging good employees. In his article, "Positive Discipline Reaps Retention," he explains that "prior to implementing this approach there were 30 suspensions or disciplinary actions in process. That number dropped to 12 in the first year of implementation and was again cut in half in the next quarter" (Murray 2003, p. 20). He also reports that the implementation of this approach has been transformational for the organization because communications among employees and managers are now on a more mature level, and employees are behaving in a more empowered manner as they take responsibility for their own behavior. Managers in the organization have found this system to be much easier to use than past disciplinary programs, and much of the animosity that existed between operational managers and human resources staff has dissipated because the process is so clear and workable. Managers using this approach follow an agreed-upon policy that has also been communicated to employees and includes the following directions for managers (Murray 2003):

- Informally communicate to employees that their role and expertise is highly valued.
- Build the confidence level of employees by reminding them that they have the ability to change.
- Provide direction and guidelines by communicating expectations for change and continued success.
- Draft a standard-of-expectations memo when formal communications are needed.
- Determine whether the employee will accept responsibility for his or her actions or continue to deny ownership.
- Continue with positive reinforcement for behavior change, and if the behavior does not change, provide the employee with a day off with pay as a time for reflection.

It should be noted that the policies on positive discipline typically stipulate that the one-day self-assessment/decision-making leaves are offered only once per employee. The employee typically returns from this day of leave having reflected on his or her willingness and responsibility to change. During the day off the employee develops a plan for sustaining the needed changes. This plan is reviewed with the manager and signed by both the employee and the manager (Murray 2003).

The employee relations manager in a large tertiary medical center reports that four years after implementing positive discipline, a steady improvement in the Gallup Employee Engagement survey has been seen as the relationship between managers and employees has become less adversarial and more like a true partnership (Wedman 2008). One of the items from this survey, "My supervisor cares about me as a person," has shown consistent improvement over time.

This manager tells the story of a twenty-year employee who has been known for relationship issues and poor interactions with co-workers throughout her tenure in the organization. This employee would never take ownership of her performance issues and over the years it was assumed that "this is just how she is." A new manager decided to deal with the performance issues and over several months used coaching and counseling techniques that eventually resulted in the employee acknowledging that she had some issues to deal with. The manager expressed faith in the employee's ability to make the needed changes and offered her a self-assessment/decision-making leave for one day with the request that she return with a written letter of commitment to her job and to the organization detailing how she planned to change her behaviors.

At first the employee was taken aback by this measure and called the employee relations manager to complain. He assured her that this action proved that the manager had faith in the employee's ability to make the needed changes and that she should view this as an opportunity to keep her job. The meeting the day after the leave day went well. The employee relations manager reported that he watched the employee coming in from the parking lot a week later with flowers for her boss. Using the nonpunitive approach for disciplinary issues conveys to employees that the words on an organizational mission statement regarding a "respectful work environment" are more than just words.

Another major medical center implemented a system for positive discipline in the nonunion parts of the organization and found that, in addition to the benefits mentioned earlier, immature and acting-out behavior diminished when managers addressed employees' unacceptable behavior or performance issues in an adult manner. The director of employee and labor relations for the system commented on how impressed she had been with the quality of the performance improvement plans that employees developed. In reflecting on their progress after one year using this system for discipline, she stated, "It has become clear to me that when we treat our employees as adults and support their efforts to change, then they respond as adults and often exceed our expectations" (Searcy 2003).

The insight into culture change reflected in this comment points to a key aspect of how discipline is handled in health care organizations. The approach used with employees when the need for discipline arises says a great deal to them about the fundamental values of the organization. Authoritarian and punitive responses from managers negate whatever sentiments may be posted in the lobby about how the organization values each of its employees. "It is through the discipline system that the organization's culture is revealed most directly to the individual" (Harvey 1986, p. 5).

Slowly but surely, health care organizations are revisiting some of their basic beliefs and assumptions. According to Harvey (1986, p. 5), the success of so many organizations that have implemented positive discipline systems is encouraging:

> They recognize that whatever the "real world" may be, it was created by management behaviors and beliefs, and therefore can be changed through different behaviors and beliefs. They realize that commitment cannot be mandated—it must be built. By eliminating punishment, by recognizing

good performance, by creating effective administrative systems that emphasize individual responsibility and decision making, commitment to high performance and achieving organizational goals is for them a workplace reality.

Asking for Assistance from the Human Resources Department

Addressing performance problems is difficult no matter what system is used. Perhaps the difficulty arises from the fact that so much is at stake that people tend to look for inflexible policies to guide the process. But the most effective actions often require the application of judgment and the consideration of each case's unique circumstances at various points along the way. In the initial stages of the process, the questions that need to be asked are:

- Is the problem rooted in a system-based cause? (This is the same question posed by most nonpunitive risk management policies in an attempt to promote a safe environment.)
- Is the problem a fit issue that can be better addressed in partnership with the employee?
- Has everything been done to support the employee's ability to succeed?

At the point of taking action, it is important to ask:

- Is this a behavioral problem or a competency/skill problem?
- How serious is the problem?

Finally, the outcome of the process needs to be assessed:

- Has the performance improved to an acceptable level? If not, is a job transfer, demotion, or separation appropriate?
- Has the case been sufficiently documented in the event of litigation?

Each of these decision points is tough to face alone, and the process usually can be effectively addressed when the manager works in partnership with the human resources department. The support that human resources professionals can provide spans a number of areas, the most important of which are the development and application of clear policies and guidelines, consultation and support, and education and training.

Clear Policies and Guidelines

Clear policies and guidelines help ensure the staff's awareness of the organization's policies as well as the consistency of policy application across the organization. New employee orientation programs usually include a review of the organization's human resources policies. Orientation gives employees who are new to the organization an opportunity to ask questions and gain an understanding of the organization's expectations of employees, given that human resources policies vary depending on each organization's values and services.

Consultation and Support

By design, human resources staff bring an objective perspective to the processes of performance improvement and discipline and can readily assist the manager in determining appropriate actions. Human resources professionals deal with cases across the organization on a daily basis, so they are able to guide managers in a way that ensures consistency but accommodates any circumstances unique to individual cases. They are the repository of information on past precedents, another important checkpoint. Finally, they are professionally trained in how to conduct these sometimes difficult conversations and can serve as much-needed support for managers faced with employee performance issues.

Education and Training

It is critical that managers receive training so that they can thoroughly understand their organization's human resources policies and definitions of specific performance problems. Human resources professionals can also help managers build their counseling skills and apply performance management tools effectively. Although these steps cannot eliminate every problem associated with confronting a performance issue, they can certainly help managers stay on track and avoid predictable pitfalls.

Taking action to address performance problems is an important leadership function, and one that is best approached with adequate knowledge, skill, and support. Adequate preparation helps overcome a person's natural tendency to avoid unpleasant situations. Working in partnership with human resources during the early stages of the performance improvement process also helps managers avoid the missteps that can make the process longer or more difficult than it needs to be.

Extreme Performance Challenges

In the final section of this chapter, several difficult challenges are addressed. These include managing negativity in the workplace and dealing with especially difficult employee behaviors.

Managing Negativity in the Workplace

In some workplaces, the culture is characterized by negativity. Complaints predominate, uncooperative behavior is the norm, and coming to work just seems to become more burdensome every day. This kind of climate is demoralizing and depressing for all who work in it. Sometimes this negativity has been a long-term characteristic that simply worsens over time, especially if left unchecked for years, while in other instances it may be a more recent development, perhaps in response to a specific situation such as employee layoffs or severe financial difficulties.

Most people become frustrated with constant negativity and complaining. And worse, the impact on productivity is significant. As noted in chapter 4, a strong business case is to be made for creating a workplace in which people are happy, and the reverse can be extrapolated from the research.

When people are unhappy, creativity is lower, satisfaction is less common, absenteeism is higher, attention spans are shorter, problem-solving abilities are decreased, and cooperation is nil.

This entire book is about creating a positive work environment. While specific suggestions are made in chapter 4 for finding happiness in the workplace, not all workers achieve this state. This section briefly summarizes steps that can be taken to deal with a negative work environment. It begins with a short review of workplace incivility.

Workplace Incivility

In some organizations and departments, the negativity has reached a level so serious that it is referred to as workplace incivility. Workplace incivility is commonplace in too many departments and organizations and is of great concern because of its tremendous cost and its very real potential to escalate into workplace violence. It creates a toxic, destructive work environment that harms all who work there or pass through. "The financial cost of workplace violence is 4.2 billion dollars a year. . . . Workplace incivility is distinct from workplace violence, both verbal and physical, in that it has an ambiguous intent to harm. In other words, as long as the intent of the act is unclear, then it is incivility" (Hutton 2006, p. 22). This behavior is usually in violation of workplace norms for healthy relationships and mutual respect. When the intent to harm is clear, the incivility has escalated into workplace violence. Violence can be physical or verbal.

Hutton (2006) says that in addition to physical violence, there are low levels of violence such as mobbing, bullying, and ostracizing. Workplace incivility is considered low-level deviant behavior and can include leaving the copier jammed or out of paper for the next person, eating someone's lunch that was stored in the department refrigerator, using someone's supplies without permission, withholding information, and excluding people from department-based activities. Gossip about co-workers or others can also be considered incivility. Clear intent to harm may not be present, but passing along negative information indirectly harms the person about whom the gossip is spread.

The issue of verbal abuse has received a lot of attention in recent years. Three sources in particular cause concern in health care organizations. The first type of verbal abuse comes from a manager or supervisor. This type is closely related to a second form that emanates from physicians. In both of these situations, a hierarchical element is in play that can lead to abuse. What may seem like a harmless remark to the speaker may be perceived by the recipient as more significant than intended. The third type of verbal abuse is especially disturbing: the incivility and negativity expressed between peers or co-workers. This is referred to as horizontal violence.

From the Manager/Supervisor

Not only is there significant financial impact when the workplace is negative but there are other impacts as well. Research has found that managers who are rude, grumpy, or discourteous to employees have wide-reaching impact in the workplace. It can be truly miserable reporting to a supervisor with these characteristics. Even employees who only hear about the situation secondhand are affected. "The mere thought of being on the receiving end of verbal abuse hurts people's ability to perform complex tasks requiring creativity, flexibility, and memory recall" (*Harvard Business Review* 2008, p. 21). The studies indicate that after exposure to rudeness, people think hard about the situation, and whether they are just ruminating or trying to formulate a response, these thought processes take cognitive resources away from the other tasks at hand. Research conducted by Hutton and Gates (2008) found that workplace incivility from supervisors and patients was linked to lower levels of employee productivity. Even if the incivility is toward others, it leaves a person wondering when it could be directed toward him or her.

From Physicians

Another common source of verbal abuse comes from physicians in health care workplaces. In a poll of nurses, physicians, and health care executives, 96 percent of nurse respondents said they have witnessed or experienced disruptive behavior by a physician (Lazoritz and Carlson 2008). In 2003, a study including nurses, pharmacists, and other hospital workers reported that nine of ten respondents experienced subtle to overt intimidation by a physician. They listed "condescending language, tone of voice, lack of patience, and refusal to answer questions or return phone calls as major issues causing stress and conflict in the workplace" (Gegaris 2007, p. 44). Additionally, 61 percent of the nurses and pharmacists were dissatisfied with the organization's ability to deal effectively with these physicians. They often refuse or are unable to see the effects of this behavior.

When the interchange is between a physician and another professional, the patient may be the unwitting loser. A positive correlation exists between healthy working relationships and patient safety outcomes (Johnson, Martin, and Markle-Elder 2007). Unfortunately, research has also found that physicians are less likely to believe that these incidents influence employee morale and turnover rates or create a potentially unsafe patient environment.

The Joint Commission has recently released standards on behavioral expectations for hospital employees as well as physicians. The new standards require the hospital to establish a code of conduct that clearly defines both desirable and disruptive behavior as well as a process for dealing with deviant behavior. It requires physicians to deal with disruptive behavior by other physicians. The American Medical Association defines disruptive behavior as "personal conduct, whether verbal or physical, that affects or potentially may affect patient care negatively" (Lazoritz and Carlson 2008, p. 20).

These behaviors can be classified into four categories:

1. **Intimidation and violence:** yelling, throwing objects, exhibiting threatening behavior, pushing or hitting others, finger pointing, displaying outbursts of anger, or invading another's space
2. **Inappropriate language or comments:** making demeaning comments (such as referring to the staff as stupid); voicing racial, ethnic, or socio-

economic slurs; uttering profanities or obscenities; making sarcastic, cynical, or cutting remarks; criticizing staff in front of others; making comments that undermine a patient's trust in another physician or nurse, other staff members, or the facility; or using other disrespectful language

3. **Sexual harassment:** making inappropriate advances, jokes about sex, or comments with sexual innuendo

4. **Inappropriate responses to patient needs or staff requests:** failing to respond to repeated calls, replying late to pages, giving inflexible responses when asked for help, leaving retaliatory notes in the patient's record, hanging up the telephone on people, disregarding established policies, or blaming others for adverse outcomes

Every organization must establish a code and a process for dealing with disruptive physician behavior. (Multiple examples of medical staff codes of conduct and behavioral policies are available at http://lazoritz.com/sample behaviorpolicies.html.) These mechanisms clearly spell out the kinds of behaviors considered disruptive, the steps to take in dealing with them, and the consequences of noncompliance. Using these established guidelines can educate both staff and physicians about appropriate behavior.

From Peers

Most horizontal violence, acts of aggression perpetrated by one colleague toward another, is verbal or emotional abuse. It can also include physical abuse, and each form can be subtle or overt (Longo and Sherman 2007). Repeated acts of horizontal violence against a co-worker are referred to as bullying and are addressed more thoroughly later in this chapter. Longo and Sherman (2007) identify common examples of horizontal violence, including nonverbal behaviors such as the raising of eyebrows or making faces in response to comments by the victim; verbal remarks that could be characterized as snide, or abrupt responses to questions raised by the victim; activities that undermine the victim's ability to perform professionally, including refusing to give assistance; acts of sabotage that deliberately set victims up for negative situations; formation of cliques that exclude certain employees; scapegoating an individual; failure to talk directly with a co-worker to resolve conflict, and instead complaining about it to others; failure to respect the privacy of others; and sharing information given in confidence.

Pervasive incivility can create a negative work environment that hampers the work group's ability to achieve excellence. It can also cause harm, sometimes irreparable, to people. The manager's role in creating a positive workplace may include dealing with widespread negativity.

Six-Step Process for Addressing Negativity

Six specific steps can be taken by a manager to address negativity in the workplace:

1. Undergo self-examination of one's own behavior and then make necessary adjustments.

2. Establish clear expectations for behavioral norms.
3. Address deviations in acceptable behavior in others.
4. Set a zero tolerance policy for negative and destructive behaviors.
5. Give each other direct and honest feedback.
6. Use deliberate approaches for helping people substitute the positive for the negative.

Step 1: Examine One's Own Behavior

A manager attempting to deal with a negative workplace begins by asking, Am I part of the problem? The research on emotional intelligence has revealed that the emotions and behaviors of the leader have a significant impact on those of the people with whom the leader works. And in any workplace, people are usually closely involved, at least geographically, with the people around them. Increasingly complex, difficult organizational challenges help create a work environment in which emotions are running high and difficulties require a lot of energy to surmount. The leader (and anyone) can perform a quick self-assessment by answering the following questions:

- How do I respond to problems and issues?
- Do I still have faith and optimism that most problems can be worked out?
- Do I have the ability to rise above the difficulties of the day and hold fast to a new vision for the future? Or am I so tired and bogged down with the everyday details of my work that I am as demoralized and downtrodden as anyone in the department?
- How do I respond to the good news that people bring? Do I reinforce it, or am I cynical and pessimistic?

A quick self-assessment by a manager can reveal opportunities for immediate change and improvement. Of course, if the individual is a paragon of positivity, there may be no room for improvement and work on step 2 can begin.

Steps 2 and 3: Establish Clear Expectations and Address Deviations

Steps 2 and 3 are inextricably linked. Establishing clear expectations was discussed briefly in chapter 6. This intervention works most effectively when done with the active involvement of employees. The basic approach is to facilitate a discussion with staff members about what the mutual expectations should be in order to create a more positive working environment. In some instances, however, a great deal of negativity exists in the department, and significant resistance is encountered from people as this development of expectations is facilitated. The group may come together, but members may sit back, not contribute and refuse to participate. In this situation, the manager can say something like this:

> Okay, I've asked for your help in establishing our expectations of each other. You don't seem to be willing or interested in doing so. That means you are granting me the authority to set these for us. The trade-off here is

that when I develop these expectations, you will be responsible for living up to them. They will become our "contract" for working with each other and I will let you know if and when I see deviations from the expectations. So, let's be clear here. You are telling me you want *me* to do this?

There should be no hesitation if the manager has to resort to this tactic. Resistant or obstructionist behavior on the part of employees ought not keep the leader or group from establishing expectations for a more positive workplace. Some members of the work group will be secretly glad this issue is being tackled because they may be facing tremendous pressure from their peers to be negative.

This is an instance, however, of where working closely with a colleague from human resources as well as the next level of management is important. They can review the expectations to determine whether they believe they are realistic and clear. It will also be helpful to have their support, as employees are held accountable for meeting these new expectations.

As employees' deviations from the newly established norms are addressed, working closely with specialists in human resources helps the manager go as far as needed in order to deal with any deviant behavior. If particularly toxic employees are influencing the rest of the staff, simply dealing with one or two firmly sends the message to others that destructive or inappropriate behavior will not be tolerated.

Once the expectations are established, an important next step is to share them with employees. The manager can begin by saying something like:

It feels like we have gotten very negative here in our department. This makes it harder for all of us to come to work, and I believe it is beginning to affect the quality of service we are providing. This is a good time to start fresh with clear expectations. Let's look at what I have developed. I would be happy to hear your feedback and additional suggestions.

Pointing out to people that this is a new start puts everyone on an equal footing. Furthermore, it does not hurt to let bygones be bygones.

Developing concrete expectations for a positive workplace is not easy. There is a perception that it is too difficult to be concrete and specific enough around attitude issues, and, as a result, these problems are often ignored and not addressed. The leader has a right to maintain certain expectations for the people with whom he or she works. For example, it is possible and even desirable to say that the organization needs employees who:

- Speak positively of others
- Encourage others around them
- Have a can-do attitude
- Find the positive about an idea or situation before complaining about the negative
- Treat each other courteously and kindly
- Work interdependently with others
- Have a positive and upbeat approach to tasks and circumstances

Step 4: Set a Zero Tolerance Policy for Negative Behavior

A zero tolerance policy for negative and destructive behaviors must be in place, even if these behaviors are in the realm of workplace incivility and harm may not have been intended. The problem with these behaviors is that they can, and often do, escalate into workplace violence, either verbal or physical. Perhaps a co-worker, out of frustration and fatigue, makes a sarcastic or cutting remark to another, who takes it personally and responds in kind. This type of interchange, fueled by the pressures and stresses of the harried workplace environment, can quickly escalate into a shouting match. This in turn can lead to mobbing behavior, where one party entices and encourages other co-workers to retaliate. Before long, the workplace is hostile and distressing to all who are there.

A zero tolerance policy means no gossip, bullying behavior, mobbing, demeaning of other people, disrespectful comments, spiteful and retaliative behaviors, or blocking behaviors will be tolerated. Policies such as this can be established within any work group, but it is much more powerful if this is a systemwide policy. If housewide, the human resource department needs to take a leading role and commitment must be obtained from senior leadership that these behaviors will be addressed, whether they are exhibited by the CEO, a physician, a supervisor, or a co-worker. In one organization, a female nurse who worked in a physician office was sexually accosted by a surgeon who was an employee of the local hospital. Charges were brought by the employee, and during the investigation the surgeon's wife came into human resources to plead for her husband. She said he was under extreme pressure because he was studying for his certification board exam and asked if he could be given "some slack," as he needed an outlet for his stress during this time. Furthermore, she requested that the female employee be transferred to another department. The surgeon's employment was severed by the hospital.

Behavior that is deviant to the norms of the group must be addressed immediately and action taken. Absolute consistency must be exercised in application of this practice, or its intent will not be met, and worse, the credibility of organizational leaders will be seriously jeopardized. Research has found that employees hold the manager culpable for incivility due to lack of disciplinary action (Hutton 2006).

Step 5: Give Direct and Honest Feedback

The process of giving feedback was explored more fully earlier in the chapter. This step can be difficult if it is taken in a hostile and negative workplace. However, both managers and employees must be committed to delivering feedback, or individuals will not understand how they have deviated from the expectations. Admittedly, this process takes a significant amount of energy in the beginning when people test even the best of intentions and strongest fortitude. It is human nature to challenge limits that have been placed on behavior. The individual who feels constrained wants to see whether the manager plans to live up to his or her statements and expectations. In addition, everyone involved needs to be willing to develop the skill to hear feedback on behavior without becoming defensive or angry.

Step 6: Help People Substitute the Positive for the Negative

Chapter 4 explains specific interventions from the field of positive psychology that can help increase happiness levels in individuals and in the workplace. These include approaches such as writing gratitude letters, performing the Three Good Things activity, letting go of grudges, and performing acts of intentional kindness. All of these exercises can substantially improve the atmosphere at work. Other techniques presented in this book are also useful. For example, using appreciative inquiry as an approach to issues is more positive than focusing on problems.

Additional Interventions

In addition to the approaches discussed in earlier chapters, leaders can use a variety of other interventions to help substitute a positive approach for the negativity that surfaces within their organizations. The following three additional approaches are helpful for addressing common issues.

Balancing Exercise

During times of great change, occasions often arise when staff members can only grumble and see the negative side of the situation. This is pretty normal in any work group. The balancing exercise can be performed quickly during a department meeting or as an individual intervention. It is simple and consists of making a list on a piece of paper. On one side are listed the things that may be gained as a consequence of the change, and on the other side are listed the things that are likely to be lost because of the change. The individual thinks of as many ideas as possible. Then, working with a partner, the list is reviewed, and the partner adds two to three new items to each column.

People who focus predominantly on the losses change brings have a harder time dealing with change. Those who can see only the positive also have difficulty coping with change because they fail to anticipate their losses and often experience them as unpleasant surprises. This simple activity helps a person or work group achieve a balanced perspective and find a much healthier approach to change. Even in the most devastating change, positives outcomes may result.

Reframing

Reframing is another powerful technique for focusing on the positive. Reframing means simply changing the frame in which an event is perceived in order to change the meaning of the event. When the meaning changes, so do responses and behaviors to the event. This approach was developed years ago in Bandler and Grinder's (1982) work on neurolinguistic programming. It is best illustrated by an ancient Chinese Taoist story about a farmer in a poor country village:

> [The farmer] was considered very well-to-do, because he owned a horse, which he used for plowing and transportation. One day his horse ran away. All his neighbors exclaimed how terrible this was, but the farmer simply said, "Maybe."

A few days later the horse returned and brought two wild horses with it. The neighbors all rejoiced at his good fortune, but the farmer just said, "Maybe."

The next day the farmer's son tried to ride one of the wild horses; the horse threw him and broke his leg. The neighbors all offered their sympathy for his misfortune, but the farmer again said, "Maybe."

The next week conscription officers came to the village to take young men for the army. They rejected the farmer's son because of his broken leg. When the neighbors told him how lucky he was, the farmer replied, "Maybe."

This approach can be used in the workplace to change the context of the complaint or issue toward which people feel negatively. For example, one emergency department charge nurse used the reframing technique when employees were complaining that they had held a patient in the department for almost three hours and an inpatient bed still was not available. The charge nurse said, "Look at it this way, we're now three hours closer to getting that patient upstairs." They laughed and grumbled good-naturedly, but it did give them a different way of looking at the situation. Using reframing is a way to identify the positive aspects of an issue. In this way, a difficult customer service situation gives a person the opportunity to hone skills in conflict resolution and perhaps to make a needed improvement in the system. A difficult day in the department reveals more information about the skill levels and working relationships of employees. Reframing is not just putting a superficially positive spin on things; it is truly finding what is positive about the situation.

Reframing is a key aspect of resiliency—the ability to bounce back after difficult events happen. For example, having an attack of acute appendicitis that requires surgery and postpones a long-anticipated vacation can lead to disappointment initially, but relief later when one realizes it would have been much worse to have become ill while on vacation. Another example are the people described earlier in this chapter who were laid off and availed themselves of placement services and found themselves in better jobs that they enjoyed more. Reframing recognizes that although a person would not be happy about being laid off, new opportunities might arise that they would never have considered before. People who cope well with adversity usually use reframing as a technique.

Forward-Focused Meetings

Forward-focused meetings are meetings during which the manager or leader deliberately ensures that the process does not deteriorate into a gripe session. When a meeting starts to deteriorate, the leader can take one of several different steps. The first is to remind people of the parameters of the discussion. For instance, if the discussion has gotten off track and has become a primarily negative discussion of an unrelated issue, reminding the group that it has only a certain amount of time left in the meeting can bring it back onto the subject it needs to deal with. Another way to deflect the negativity is to ask, "Is this something we have any control or influence over?" In other words, if the group has little authority to influence the issue, talking about it is just a waste of time. Bringing the focus back to what is working and why it is working is another way to convert negative to positive energy in a group.

Converting a negative departmental climate to one that is positive is time consuming and challenging. However, a chronically negative workplace is a tough place in which to exist. Even small improvements can make a big difference to the people there. When the organization's climate is pervasively negative, the challenge is even greater.

Dealing with Extreme Behavior

One of the most difficult challenges faced by managers, leaders, and employees alike is coping with the extreme behavior of others. Toxic, caustic, and destructive behavior in the workplace leads to the development of a toxic workplace. "The operational definition of a toxic workplace: it's a place where people come to work so they can make enough money so they can leave" (Webber 1998, p. 156). When destructive, negative behavior is tolerated, no one feels safe.

Sometimes extreme behavior is caused by a personality disorder or a more serious mental health problem. A detailed discussion of the impact of severe mental illness and substance abuse on health care workers and organizations is beyond the scope of this book. In no way is this brief discussion intended to provide a manager with enough information to diagnose or treat a psychiatric disorder. However, presented here is a brief discussion on dealing with employees who have mental health issues and personality disorders resulting in two kinds of extreme behavior that lead to a negative workplace: disruptive personalities and bullying.

Mental Health Issues and Personality Disorders in the Workplace

Extremes in behavior are often the result of mental illness, and like the general population, employees in health care organizations are vulnerable to psychiatric disorders such as clinical depression, personality disorders, and substance abuse. Although managers usually are not expected to handle these issues directly, mental illness among employees and managers can have a drastic effect on individual job performance as well as a negative impact on co-workers and patients. In its most extreme forms, mental illness, especially substance abuse disorders, among health care providers can actually place patients and co-workers at serious risk for physical harm.

Most managers in health care organizations are not equipped to recognize specific psychiatric problems manifested among their colleagues and employees. However, personality disorders, depressive disorders, and anxiety disorders, as well as substance abuse disorders, are as common among health care providers as among the general population. Managers are not expected to be mental health experts, but they should be able to recognize the warning signs of the most common psychiatric disorders as well as the symptoms of alcohol- or drug-related impairment so that they can refer troubled individuals to a source of professional mental health services as soon as possible. It may be useful to ask the director of the organization's employee assistance program to provide an in-service for the management team on the subject of recognizing and managing employees with these health problems.

Some mental health problems are the result of acute illness (for example, a treatable episode of clinical depression); some are chronic but treatable (such as posttraumatic stress disorder), while others (particularly personality disorders) are relatively permanent features of behavior. Working with or managing employees with psychiatric disorders can be a challenge, as can managing employees whose behavior is affected by substance abuse or addiction and other forms of impairment.

The first step in dealing with a troubled employee should always be to refer him or her to the organization's employee assistance program. Managers should also document their efforts to intervene with troubled employees and discuss any related problems with the employee relations manager in human resources as early as possible. It is important that managers maintain complete records of the conversations and coaching and counseling efforts they provide for use in any possible litigation in the future (Cavaiola and Lavender 2000).

It is also essential for the manager to maintain the confidentiality of employees with mental health problems. Employees with mental health problems deserve the same level of respect as employees with medical problems. Tossing around diagnostic labels when referring to employees is inappropriate.

Without realizing it, everyone encounters people with personality disorders every day. In fact, most individuals with personality disorders do not even realize that they have a problem. To them, and often to their families, friends, and co-workers, their behavior seems perfectly normal, if not sometimes a little difficult. Still, some of the most common personality disorders can result in a significant amount of disruptive behavior inside and outside the workplace. They can also be at the root of individual performance problems, and when that is the case, significant change becomes much more unlikely.

Most people in the work world have had a co-worker who was extremely difficult to deal with. Managers often say, "We have this one employee who just keeps things stirred up, and I'm at my wits end as far as how I can deal with her!" This exasperation should be a clue for managers that they may well be dealing with an issue that is more significant than the usual interpersonal differences encountered every day in health care's stressful work environments. It is relatively easy for managers to address everyday interpersonal problems by providing feedback or coaching, and most employees eventually recognize their part in a conflict and are able to change their behavior and maintain those changes over time.

When the call for change goes unheeded, however, or when employees refuse to recognize how their own behavior contributes to a problem, the possibility exists that the employees involved may be suffering from a common mental health problem called a personality disorder. Dr. Vicki Lachman

(2001), a well-known nurse consultant who also has a private practice in psychotherapy, defines personality disorders as:

> Enduring patterns of perception or behavior that are inflexible and mal-adaptive and cause significant stress. Personality-disordered individuals often see themselves as victimized by the "system" and have little insight into how they contribute to their own problems or how to change. The individuals' personality problems often appear to be acceptable and natural for them. . . . They typically are not compliant with agreed upon standards, goals or counseling agreements and may discount their need to change by claiming they have "always been this way." They manage their anxiety by acting out rather than [by] talking out their issues.

The American Psychiatric Association's Diagnostic and Statistical Manual estimates that about 10 percent of the general population in the United States meet the diagnostic criteria for having a personality disorder. In addition, an individual can be diagnosed as having more than one personality disorder at the same time. Another complicating factor is that people with personality disorders are prone to developing additional mental health problems, especially clinical depression and substance abuse disorders.

Some individuals with personality disorders display behavioral patterns that are relatively mild and manageable (for example, perfectionistic or overly dramatic behaviors), while other individuals with more severe personality disorders may behave in more maladaptive ways that have a damaging impact on interpersonal behavior and vocational functioning. For example, individuals with borderline personality disorder can be very volatile, and they often engage in intense and stormy interpersonal conflicts that disrupt an entire department.

In their classic book on this issue, *Toxic Coworkers: How to Deal with Dysfunctional People on the Job*, Cavaiola and Lavender (2000, p. 6) make note of the fact that all too often, "personality disorders go unrecognized and yet they create a substantial amount of stress in the workplace." They offer a list of the personality disorders that are most commonly found among employees in the workplace (Cavaiola and Lavender 2000, pp. 4–5):

- Paranoid personality disorder, which is characterized by highly suspicious and distrustful behavior
- Schizoid personality disorder, which is characterized by behavior indicating no desire for affiliation or friendship
- Antisocial personality disorder, which is characterized by an apparent disregard for social morals and the rights of others
- Narcissistic personality disorder, which is characterized by self-centered and grandiose behavior that indicates a lack of empathy for others
- Histrionic personality disorder, which is characterized by dramatic, overly emotional behavior
- Borderline personality disorder, which is characterized by moody, intense, and angry behavior and stormy interpersonal relationships

- Obsessive-compulsive personality disorder, which is characterized by extremely perfectionistic and inflexible behavior and overconcern for details

In the health care workplace, as in any other work setting, many of the personality traits mentioned in this list are present. At one time or another, a person can find himself or herself feeling a little suspicious or moody. The difference between a personality trait and a personality disorder is the maladaptive and inflexible nature of personality disorders, which can adversely affect occupational functioning and interpersonal relationships. Without medication and psychotherapy to help them control their emotions and gain insight into their behavior and perceptions, people with personality disorders are usually unable to change their inappropriate behavior. It is obvious that employees with personality disorders have the potential to disrupt teams and undermine employee morale.

In her coaching seminars for nurse managers, Lachman (2001) identified narcissistic personality disorder and borderline personality disorder as the personality disorders that have the most impact on a typical work environment. The narcissistic personality characteristically manifests as grandiose, flamboyant behavior. Narcissistic individuals are also hypersensitive to criticism. At the same time, they lack empathy for others, although they are sometimes able to take advantage of the feelings or needs of others for their own personal gain. They require excessive admiration and often have fantasies of brilliance (Lachman 2001). They are very manipulative in getting their own needs met, and for these reasons they create problems for work groups. The common phrase "it's all about me" might well be the motto of individuals with a narcissistic personality disorder.

For the manager or leader dealing with someone with a narcissistic personality disorder, it is important for the manager to respond in the following ways:

- Be aware of ways you can be manipulated. When the employee gives you effusive praise or extensive accolades, you should be prepared for the demands for special treatment that may soon follow.
- When employees complain about the ways in which the individual with a narcissistic personality has taken advantage of them, be prepared to coach the staff on ways they can negotiate for better outcomes next time.
- Be honest in giving feedback to this individual, but begin with the things they are doing well before coaching them on the areas in which they need to make changes (Lachman 2001).
- Help the person to set realistic goals and to have a more realistic understanding of his or her skills and abilities. Coach the individual in specific ways to be a team player (Cavaiola and Lavender 2000).
- Provide positive feedback and recognition when there is evidence that the person is empathetic to others or is making an effort to work as a member of a team.

- Build bridges with a narcissistic individual rather than engaging in confrontation.
- Stick to your agenda, not the individual's. You may want to correct his or her errors in logic, but it is best not to (Cavaiola and Lavender 2000).

Equally challenging are people with a borderline personality disorder. Just as a "the world revolves around me" attitude is often a sign of narcissistic personality disorder, people with borderline personality disorder can often be recognized by the intensity and changeability of their moods and the comments people make about them ("she runs hot and cold and you never know what to expect" or "we are all walking on eggshells wondering what will trigger his outbursts this time"). A person with a borderline personality has no real sense of self-identity, and so even slight changes in the environment can trigger an overreaction. Their impulsive behavior and intense anger are particularly problematic in a work setting (Lachman 2001). Co-workers quickly learn that they may be viewed as friends one day and enemies the next. Needless to say, this state makes team building and establishing healthy working relationships difficult. The turmoil created by the overreactions or intensity of people with borderline personality disorder often makes the workplace feel like a soap opera. Perhaps the movie *Fatal Attraction* provides the most memorable example of the havoc that can be created by an individual with borderline personality disorder. In a work setting, such employees can often be recognized as the ones who "keep things stirred up" and "act out" rather than processing an issue and choosing a more mature response (Lachman 2001).

A manager who steps in to manage an employee with this disorder should consider the following pointers:

- Help the employee see the gray in an issue rather than the black-and-white thinking that often leads to an intense emotional response.
- Set limits, but expect the limits to be tested repeatedly. The broken-record assertion technique may be helpful.
- Seldom, if ever, make special arrangements for the employee; this will likely lead to additional requests for special treatment.
- Deal promptly with strong, emotional responses and role-play what the employee should do the next time a similar situation comes up.
- Notice nonverbal behavior (for example, rolling of the eyes, turning away) and ask about the employee's feelings so that he or she is less likely to have an explosive emotional reaction (Chambers 1998, p. 138).
- Let the employee know about an upcoming change ahead of time so he or she is not caught off guard (Lachman 2001).
- Expect some moodiness, but avoid overreacting to the employee's mood state (a simple "I hear you" is usually sufficient).
- When possible, limit the employee's contact with others (the less stimulation in the environment, the better).

- Provide positive feedback when good decision making or effective coping is observed (Cavaiola and Lavender 2000).
- Help the employee transfer effective behavior to new situations, but do not be surprised when the employee is unable to apply the same skills in a similar situation.

Bullying Behavior in the Workplace

One of the most challenging situations in the arena of workplace interpersonal relationships involves the presence of individuals who use bullying behavior to get what they want. "Bullying is not something confined to schoolchildren. It is a widespread form of abuse to be found in all forms of employment, cultures, and religious congregations" (Arbuckle 2000, p. 25). Obviously, bullying is extremely costly in both human and financial terms. "In the United States, businesses are losing an annual five to six billion dollars in decreased productivity alone, due to real or perceived abuse of employees" (Arbuckle 2000, p. 25).

Arbuckle (2000, p. 25) defines bullying as "persistent, unwelcome action or verbal, psychological, or physical aggression that is knowingly or unknowingly directed by an individual or group against people who normally are not in a position to defend themselves. It is irrational behavior, evoking strong emotions in both the bully and victim." Bullies try to force other people to do what they want them to do and are willing to try any kind of intimidation to achieve their goal. One form of bullying, horizontal violence, has recently received increasing attention in health care workplaces. It represents damaging behaviors that occur between two employees. It must be noted, however, that bullying behavior is not limited to employee–employee relationships. Managers and supervisors also use bullying behavior and intimidation tactics to coerce others in ways that are self-serving rather than beneficial to the organization as a whole and the people within it.

Abrasive and abusive behaviors used by managers and supervisors include both engaging in the toxic behavior themselves and ignoring the behavior in others. In one hospital, a director of perioperative services was being bullied by physicians who did not want to make changes that needed to be made. Several physicians threatened the manager and her family with bodily harm during a meeting attended by the organization's chief executive officer, who did nothing to stop the attacks. In a self-protective effort, the director began parking in a variety of different places from day to day because of threats to her person and property. The manager was actually pushed down a stairwell in the hospital, and still no action was ever taken against the bullies. Most of us find it hard to believe that this kind of behavior can occur, but naïveté is no excuse for refusing to see or deal with bullying behavior.

Bullying behaviors on the part of managers include (Ryan and Oestreich 1991, p. 74):

- Chilling silence
- Glaring eye contact

- Abruptness, shortness
- Snubbing or ignoring people
- Insults and put-downs
- Blaming, discrediting, or discounting others
- Aggressive, controlling mannerisms
- Threats about the job
- Yelling and shouting
- Angry outbursts or losses of emotional control
- Physical threats
- Sexual harassment

Bullying behavior among employees can range from mild forms such as making sarcastic comments, refusing to help others, or not including individuals in normal kinds of department activities to more serious and dangerous behaviors such as threats and actual physical assaults. Farrell (1997) offers a "professional terrorism" list that sorts the various kinds of bullying behaviors on the basis of whether they are active or passive, verbal or physical, and direct or indirect. Figure 10-5 includes some of Farrell's examples as well as others reported in the literature.

Thomas (2004) has done extensive research on how nurses handle their anger and reports that one of the most disturbing aspects revealed is the vehemence of nurses' anger directed at each other. The anger described in the research interviews is not a healthy kind of anger that can occur in

Figure 10-5.   Examples of Bullying Behavior

	Direct	Indirect
Active	**Verbal** Expressing disdain Making snide remarks Constant criticism Screaming at each other Racial slurs **Physical** Assault Property damage Sexual harassment	**Verbal** Talking behind your back Sabotaging behaviors Reporting false information Malicious gossip Persistent nitpicking **Physical** Inciting others to act; riling them up
Passive	**Verbal** Cattiness Chilly silence **Physical** Refusing to help Refusing to speak to a colleague Turning away Humiliating behaviors	**Verbal** Withholding information from a colleague **Physical** Refusing to move out of the way Ignoring a colleague Blocking opportunities

any workplace, but destructive anger. Thomas writes about the faultfinding, bickering, backbiting, needling, snapping, and cutting remarks that are common in the work environment. Furthermore, she reports that nurses "were constantly writing each other up," which included nasty notes on locker-room doors as well as reporting each other to supervisors. "Today, hostile messages from coworkers can be transmitted even faster in workplaces with networked computers—in those snippy e-mails with a little zinger at the end" (Thomas 2004, p. 116).

Sometimes the bullying results in performance that can actually threaten patient care. In one department in a large tertiary care center in the Midwest, one employee in the department was a vicious bully who embarrassed and humiliated other employees and then employed the threat of physical harm to keep her victims from complaining to management. When the behaviors came to the attention of the assistant manager, he addressed the issue and involved the department manager. As a result, the individual's employment was terminated. However, this woman had quite a following in the department, and the assistant manager soon found himself the target of retaliation in the form of employees calling in sick on his shift and refusing to come in and work when they were needed. The situation actually became quite dangerous for patients before it was addressed. In the end, the assistant manager transferred to another department just to alleviate the situation.

There is no doubt that bullying and other disrespectful behaviors can result in negative outcomes in the workplace. In one study of rudeness, insensitivity, and disrespect in the workplace, the investigator found that most people who were the targets of bullying behavior at work retaliated against their employers rather than the bully. Twenty-eight percent lost work time to avoid the bully, 22 percent decreased their efforts at work, 10 percent decreased the amount of time they spent at work, and 12 percent changed jobs to avoid the bully (Lee 1999). Jeffrey Pfeffer (1999), the Thomas D. Dee Professor of Organizational Behavior at the Stanford Graduate School of Business, insists that organizational loyalty is not dead; instead, toxic companies are driving people away. He says that "there isn't a scarcity of talent—but there is a growing unwillingness to work for toxic organizations" (quoted in Webber 1998, p. 154).

So how can the manager deal with this dysfunctional and destructive behavior? The first step is to be aware of the possibility of bullying and to recognize it for what it is. Dealing with the behavior directly prevents it from escalating out of control. Here are some specific suggestions for dealing with a bully or bullying behavior in the workplace:

- Develop a zero tolerance policy for bullying behavior. Be very clear that it will not be tolerated, regardless of where it is found. Work with the human resources department to develop appropriate policies and protocols.

- Keep accurate information about the times and places the bullying behavior occurs. Documentation is critical. Work with human resources specialists to ensure that documentation is complete and adequate.
- People who successfully use bullying behavior love to dominate. The person who is the victim of abuse should not meet with the bully alone. Support must be available from the manager or a peer. As a manager, do not expect employees to handle these behaviors alone. Often, managerial authority is necessary to deal with this dysfunctional behavior. As a manager, this is not a time to tell employees to "just work it out." That approach amounts to the manager throwing his or her support on the side of the bully.
- Logical and rational arguments usually do not work with bullies. When such people are confronted with factual information or when their deviant behavior is addressed, they often become more enraged and vindictive. The person addressing the behavior should not expect a reasonable response. Calmness must prevail; the manager losing his or her temper only escalates the emotion in the situation.
- A true bully wants the victim to feel guilty, humiliated, and powerless. Victims of the bully are encouraged to respond with nonviolence but to avoid appearing humiliated. In other words, they should not remain passive but instead should find some nonviolent way to reassert their dignity, perhaps by taking actions or responding in a way that embarrasses the bully (Arbuckle 2000).
- Deal with the unacceptable behavior, and do not blame the victim. The victim must feel safe and be assured that someone understands what is happening to him or her. "To overlook what is happening is to collude in the intimidation" (Arbuckle 2000, p. 32). And while whistle-blowing increases a person's chance of becoming the target of the bully, it is the only ethical course of action under the circumstances.
- Recognize that in some instances the victim of a bully may need the support of a counselor to deal with the aftermath of emotion. In one study, the researcher discovered that health care workers who experienced bullying behavior often showed symptoms of posttraumatic stress syndrome (Doherty 2002). A referral to the organization's employee assistance program or to another source of professional help may be appropriate.
- Develop an action plan to enlist the help of other employees and managers. If possible, get agreement and commitment from others to help make the work environment a safe and positive place.
- Teach employees how to respond to horizontal violence. Research has found that when employees are taught to depersonalize the behaviors or remarks and practice cognitive responses to the offensive behavior, they are able to confront the destructive behavior directly (Griffin 2004).

Summary

Influencing the performance of others is an important aspect of creating a positive work environment. For leaders and managers, this means working in partnership with employees on performance improvement and skill development. Important aspects include being actively engaged in coaching and giving helpful feedback even when it is difficult. In some instances, sculpting the job to better take advantage of an employee's signature strengths may be the intervention required. In cases where performance or behaviors are not acceptable, the manager needs to apply appropriate processes that are implemented fairly and in full partnership with the employee. Finally, dealing effectively with toxic behavior prevents deterioration of morale.

Influencing and managing performance and problem behavior are probably among the toughest challenges faced by organizational leaders. Yet these are directly linked to quality of work life for people in the organization and must be undertaken without fail. The payoff is worth the effort in the end. Finding allies and support in human resources is a strategy that helps lighten the burden and ensures that support is available for both managers and employees in the system.

Conversation Points

Organizational Perspective

1. How effectively does the organization's current formal performance appraisal system work? Is it motivating to employees? Are employees treated as partners in the process, or is it a manager-driven approach?
2. How do managers feel about the performance appraisal system? Is it connected to pay increases?
3. Are organizational managers expected to be actively engaged in coaching employees? Or are work schedules so full of meetings and other commitments that proactive, consistent coaching from the manager is rarely possible?
4. Is there ongoing dialogue and feedback among people throughout the various levels of the organization? Are employees taught how to receive feedback? Is there an openness about sharing feedback even between levels in the hierarchy?
5. Is corrective discipline or positive discipline the approach used in the organization?
6. What are the underlying assumptions about employees and the employee–manager relationship that are driving the development of policies and practices in the system? Are they positive or based on negative perceptions about employees?
7. Is there a zero tolerance policy on bullying behavior in the workplace? Is it applied equitably and fairly at all levels of the organization? For example, how is physician bullying behavior dealt with? What recourse does an employee have who is being bullied by a manager?

8. Is there a policy for dealing with disruptive physician behavior? Is it used? Have physicians, managers, and employees been taught about the process?

9. Are there any pockets of negativity in departments? What level of support is available for managers and staff dealing with this problem?

Leader Perspective

1. How actively are you involved in coaching and developing your employees and colleagues? Is your coaching proactive and consistent or sporadic and related only to performance problems?

2. How comfortable are you with giving difficult feedback to others? Do you use a model for scripting difficult feedback? Have you taught the model to employees? How comfortable are you with receiving feedback from those around you? Are you able to listen without becoming resentful or defensive? What could you do to improve your skills in giving and receiving feedback?

3. What is your working relationship with the specialists in human resources? Do you engage human resources early when you suspect that you are facing a potential problem situation?

4. How thorough is your documentation of performance issues? Is it complete and appropriate or sketchy and inadequate? How might you strengthen your approach to documentation of performance issues?

5. Is chronic negativity a problem in your department? If it is, how have you tried to deal with this issue? Do you have specific techniques or approaches for keeping things focused on the positive?

6. Do you see or suspect any bullying behavior in your area? If you do, who is the bully? Does this person have a following? How have you tried to deal with this behavior? How has it worked? What resources do you have to help you? If you do not see any evidence of bullying behavior, have you ever had to deal with this issue?

7. Are there issues of physician disruptive behavior or incivility? How do you handle these? Is there support in the organization for doing so? Are employees comfortable coming forward about these issues?

8. Do you see any of the personality disorder behaviors in people with whom you work? Are the behaviors you see just personality traits, or are they more persistent? What is the effect on the work group?

Employee Perspective

1. How do you prepare for your annual performance appraisal? Do you refer to the goals established at different points throughout the year, or does the form go in your file, only to be reviewed when next year's date rolls around? Do you provide any sort of self-assessment in preparation for the appraisal?

2. Do you find the performance appraisal system helpful and motivating? How would you change it if you could?

3. Is there someone who actively serves as a coach for you in the workplace? How helpful is your coach? What kinds of things does this coach work on with you?

4. How open are you to receiving feedback? Do you actively seek out opportunities in your daily work life to ensure you are taking advantage of the feedback around you?
5. Do you feel comfortable giving your co-workers or manager feedback on behavior that you would like to see them change?
6. What is your knowledge of the corrective action or positive discipline process in your organization? Have you ever experienced it firsthand? Did you feel like you were supported in the process and encouraged to improve?
7. What is the climate like in your department? Is it predominantly positive or mostly negative? Why? What are the behaviors you see that make it so?
8. Are there any bullies in your workplace? Who are they? What bullying behavior do you see? Does management know about it? How is bullying behavior dealt with in your organization? Do you feel supported and safe in your workplace? Why?

III

Special Challenges

THE FIRST PART of this book reviews several bodies of literature and provides the foundation for understanding approaches for creating a positive health care workplace. Part II presents research on what exemplary health care managers do to create a culture of engagement and follows with five chapters on techniques and approaches that can help. Although every health care organization today faces common challenges, such as the need to manage fluctuating financial resources and constraints, a turbulent business environment, increasing demands and expectations of consumers, and dealing with the availability of rapidly changing technology, some challenges are also unique to a particular organization.

Part III explores some of these challenges. The first set of challenges relates to unique characteristics of the organization that are thought by some to make the attainment of a positive workplace more difficult. These challenges may be environmental conditions such as the size of the facility, the type of setting, or other characteristics such as the presence of union representation of employees. These are explored in chapter 11.

Chapter 12 explores two challenges that are universal and that are identified as difficulties by managers. Changing demographics have resulted in two major issues. The first is the increased complexity in the workplace because, for the first time in human history, employees from four generational cohorts are now working together. This age diversity results in a tremendous challenge for the manager as it can often lead to increased friction and conflict in the workplace. Additionally, each generation has a distinct set of characteristics, values, beliefs, and preferences. Understanding these differences and blending them in the workplace challenge even the most experienced and capable leader. Chapter 12 identifies the characteristics of each generation and explores the challenges they create for leaders in establishing a positive health care workplace.

The second, closely related issue is the challenge of managing the transition of workers out of the active workforce. With the rapidly approaching collision of demographics, the retention of the mature or older worker is a crucial issue for maintaining a viable workforce into the future. Workforce shortages strike at the heart of the organization's ability to attain its mission and strategic initiatives. As presented in chapter 1, alarm is growing about the challenge this issue will present in the future, and it affects virtually every category of worker and every professional discipline. Clear evidence in the literature indicates that a cycle of employee shortages tends to become self-perpetuating. Strategies for retaining the mature or older worker are identified and presented. Managing knowledge transfer through succession planning is related to this issue and is briefly addressed.

11

Unique Organizational Challenges to Creating a Positive Workplace

Jo Manion

*Social sector organizations increasingly look to business
for leadership models and talent, yet I suspect we will find more
true leadership in the social sectors than in the business sector. . . .
True leadership only exists if people follow when they have
the freedom not to.*

—Jim Collins

WHY DOESN'T every health care organization have a positive work environment? The obvious answer is, "Because it isn't easy to do." Less obvious answers might be, "it's not important," "it doesn't make that much difference to the bottom line," "managers are too busy just trying to keep things afloat on a day-to-day basis, there isn't time for the 'fluff,'" or "it can't be done here because _____ " (fill in the blank: there's a strong union, this is long-term care, this is home health, there are too many tenured faculty, and so on). The truth is that there are many reasons offered for not creating a positive work environment or that explain why the organization is failing on this important indicator of health and vitality. Too often these reasons begin to sound like excuses. So the question is, when does a challenge become an excuse?

Challenge versus Excuse

Bilbrey (2008b) explores this question in a provocative article in which she notes that excuses lead to complacency, and when complacency becomes widespread in an organization, it severely hinders the organization's pursuit of excellence. "One critical role of a great leader is fighting complacency by refusing to accept excuses, and instead giving life to the challenges" (Bilbrey 2008b, p. 26).

When circumstances present a challenge to the achievement of a goal, the pursuit of that goal requires more persistence and diligence than those goals that are easily attained. The danger of significant challenge is that it may cause a person's commitment to the goal or desired outcome to waver or actually be broken. As a result, the desired outcome is not attained. However, a significant challenge or difficulty can also lead to a positive effect on commitment: to make one's commitment even stronger. Adversity can cause a person to re-examine the commitment, reaffirm that commitment, invest even more in the chosen course of action, and ultimately achieve the desired outcome.

Perhaps the challenge, then, becomes an excuse when the individual or organization gives up on the commitment and uses the challenge as a reason for why it is impossible to proceed. For each of the challenges identified and addressed in this chapter, there are leaders and organizations that have created a positive workplace in spite of the presence of these difficult situations. In all cases, leaders must be honest with themselves and hold themselves accountable for their thoughts, words, and actions. Only the individual can determine whether he or she is using the challenge as an excuse.

Certainly, some situations and organizations have no intent or desire to create a positive workplace. Jettisoning a negative, toxic workplace may be a frequent topic of conversation, but more often in organizations like these this conversation is just lip service, with no significant follow through or application. Individuals within these systems have basically three options: speaking up, staying put, or getting out.

Speaking Up

The first and most assertive option is to give voice to the situation. Providing feedback about observations and the potential consequences of the current course of action is a healthy alternative to saying nothing. This alternative is not without risk. The risk can be objectively assessed, and the individual can determine how he or she will deal with potential subsequent consequences.

Speaking up and speaking out is neither as easy as it sounds nor as common as one would think. Defert and Edmondson (2007) have researched reasons why employees do or do not speak up when they have a good idea, opinion to offer, or concern to express. Their research found that self-censorship was common from all levels in the organization, from point-of-service personnel all the way to the occupants of the executive suite. About half of the people interviewed in their study felt it was not "safe" to speak up in their organization. The reason? Self-preservation. Defert and Edmondson (2007, para. 3) found that "the innate protective instinct [is] so powerful that it also inhibited speech that would have been intended to help the organization." So, even sharing positive ideas and contributions was felt to be risky. The perceived threat and risks of speaking up felt very personal and immediate to the employee, and, in the case of good ideas, the possible future benefit to the organization was uncertain at best.

The self-censorship that causes a person to not speak up may be based on a previous actual experience in which a negative consequence occurred. In one acute care facility, the chief executive officer (CEO) and the vice president of human resources held townhall meetings on a quarterly basis to share information and hear from employees. At one of these meetings, a supervisor raised a question, not in a discourteous or challenging manner, about a new policy. Within two hours, she was in her vice president's office being admonished and told that her question was inappropriate. Not only did this woman get the message that it is not safe to speak up, but her experience became widespread cultural lore in the organization and clearly conveyed the message, "keep your mouth shut."

Interestingly, the self-censorship is not always from actual experience but may result from unspoken and untested assumptions that the employee holds: "If I speak up, it could cost me my job," "If I share this idea in the meeting, my boss is going to be upset because this is his project," "If I bring up this concern at the management meeting, with others present, my boss may feel like I'm making her look bad," or "I've brought this up before and nobody has been interested in doing anything about it." This kind of thinking easily causes a person to be reticent about his or her ideas and concerns.

It is also important to consider the consequences of *not* speaking up. When an individual remains in an unhealthy, toxic, or destructive work environment, he or she pays a high cost that may not be readily apparent. By remaining in the environment or keeping silent, the person is basically condoning or allowing the dysfunction to continue. It is destructive to the human spirit to remain in such a situation. If the individual has tried everything he or she deems possible and has spoken up in a confident, assertive voice and the impact on the environment is disappointing or unacceptable, staying put and getting out are two additional options.

Staying Put

A second, less healthy choice is to make the decision to remain. Albert O. Hirschman (quoted in Beck 2004) says that if a person chooses to stay, it has to be with the willingness to support the organization. Hirschman calls it "uncomplaining loyalty." Although taking this option does not mean the person never speaks up again, it does mean that the person sees the organization with all of its faults and says, "I am staying. I know this place is not perfect, but I will not become a negative saboteur trying to destroy the system." It implies a level of loyalty that precludes the person from continually "bad mouthing" the organization and the people within it, or actively engaging in sabotaging behaviors. The concern in selecting this approach has to do with the compromise in the individual's values and the resulting personal ethical issues. For example, the person may believe that the stability and security offered by the job are more important than quality of work life. People face these decisions at various points in their careers, and each person handles them in his or her own way. However, it is important to be ruthlessly honest with oneself about the trade-offs and compromises being made. And, if one chooses to remain within this system, in return for the rewards of the job, the expectation is that there is a certain level of loyalty to the organization.

Getting Out

The third choice that is available is to exit from the organization. This action can be either a physical exit that involves separating from employment or the less healthy emotional, or psychological, termination mentioned in chapter 1. Psychological termination is not recommended for a long-term option; however, it can be very effective as a short-term strategy. Beck (2004) refers to this as the "Monte Cristo technique." The Count of Monte Cristo was imprisoned and remained sane because he was continually digging his way out of the prison, until he eventually escaped. In the workplace, this may describe the time after an employee decides to leave when he or she puts things in order to make it a positive transition. The person may stay long enough, for example, to obtain additional certification or education, graduate the last child from high school or college, take that long-awaited dream vacation, or find a new position. But in the meantime, the individual has separated emotionally from the job.

Next Steps

The techniques and strategies presented throughout this book have all been aimed at preventing options number two (uncomplaining loyalty) and three (exit) from occurring. However, in some instances these responses are certainly justified. The recommended next step is that the individual focuses on what he or she can do within his or her sphere of influence and responsibility. Much can be changed and influenced if the person stays within his or her loci of control. As personal effectiveness increases with success, the person's influence within the system also expands. Fully one-third of the managers who participated in the research reported in chapter 5 were working in organizations that were quite difficult. These managers said their larger organizational culture was dysfunctional and basically nonsupportive of their efforts in trying to create a positive workplace. The managers were clearly able to prevail within their own work area and create a positive environment. However, it was at great personal cost to the individual, and whether or not this effort could be sustained over time remains to be seen. There are times when everything has been tried that the individual is willing to try and the situation does not improve. In these cases it may be time for the person to seek out a system or an environment that is already positive or at least amenable to change.

The Challenges

For each of the challenges discussed below, there is a solution. However, the solutions are custom-made for each organization by each organization (or the strong leadership and employees within). It is probably fair to point out that what may be seen as a challenge in one organization may not be perceived in the same manner in another. There is no silver bullet that works for each challenge each time. For every situation that has been identified as a difficult challenge, there are examples of people making it work. Different challenges are faced by individuals in every possible situation in health care. However, the basic principles in the first part of this book apply to all of the challenging situations mentioned here.

When health care managers, educators, and executives were interviewed for this chapter, virtually every one of them indicated that he or she clearly believed that the principles for creating a positive workplace are universal and can work in any setting or any circumstance. It takes good people with solid, highly effective leadership skills applying the same basic principles regardless of the situation. The challenges of four specific settings are considered here: a large and small environment, a union environment, a long-term care environment, and an academic setting. Before considering these settings, a significant challenge is discussed that is universal: leadership in a social-sector organization.

The Challenges of Social-Sector Leadership

Jim Collins (2005) describes a significant difference between leadership in a business setting and that in a service-sector setting. In a business setting, the top executives have what is referred to as executive power. In other words, once they make a decision, it is expected to be carried out (some leaders may be more participative than others). In the service sector, it is understood that even executives do not have the full power of decision making. They face what Collins refers to as a "complex and diffuse power map. When you add in tenured faculty, civil service, volunteers, police unions, or any number of other internal factors, most nonbusiness leaders simply do not have the concentrated decision power of a business CEO" (Collins 2005, p. 10).

These factors led Collins (2005, p. 11) to hypothesize that there are two types of leadership skills: executive and legislative.

> In executive leadership, the individual leader has enough concentrated power to simply make the right decisions. In legislative leadership, on the other hand, no individual leader—not even the nominal chief executive—has enough structural power to make the most important decisions by himself or herself. Legislative leadership relies more upon persuasion, political currency, and shared interests to create the conditions for the right decisions to happen.

These differences mean that leadership in health care organizations is far more complex and challenging than in a comparable organization in the business sector. The effective leader in health care must have a compelling combination of personal humility and professional will that creates credibility and influence. Otherwise, those being led are not going to imbue the leader with the power to lead. The leader's role in social-sector organizations is not to make the decisions but to ensure that good decisions are made.

The Challenges of Size and Location

In some cases the setting or other environmental characteristics of the organization or facility may create a challenge.

The size and location of the facility can affect the positivity of the work environment. A more isolated rural setting has distinct advantages and disadvantages over an urban or suburban setting. There are advantages to being a smaller facility where everyone knows one another, relationships are more long term, and the sheer logistics are not as complex. The difficulty in a smaller organization may be in creating true culture change where people have worked for a long time and have entrenched beliefs on the direction of the organization. If working relationships are not healthy, it may be harder to address them when negative co-workers also happen to be neighbors or fellow members of the local church or the parent-teacher association.

A larger organization may have more resources that can be tapped for expert help and assistance, such as organizational development specialists. It also has more locations and jobs within which to move people who may be underperforming or in need of a greater challenge. Due to the larger community of people in an organization of this size, geographical differences can also influence the ease with which a positive workplace is created. However, it is quite likely that the differences are just that, uniqueness that has some impact on strategies and outcomes but does not determine whether the goal itself can be achieved.

The Challenges of Union Presence

Many health care managers and executives may believe employee representation by professional labor unions presents a unique challenge for the organization. Furthermore, some managers believe the presence of unions automatically creates an adversarial climate that is contradictory to a positive workplace. However, this assumption is false, as there are many organizations with excellent work environments whose employees, or a portion of them, are represented by labor unions. In fact, in approximately 10 percent of all health care organizations that have received Magnet designation, the nurses are represented by professional labor unions (Moran 2008). Many factors and strategies help determine the quality of the management–union relationship that are worth considering.

The Nature of the Relationship between Management and Union

If an adversarial relationship exists between management and the union, it will be very difficult to create a positive environment. This kind of relationship is characterized by supervisors, managers, and executives who feel contempt for the union and believe the union is unrealistic and greedy in its demands and has selfish ulterior motives for representing employees (to fill union coffers). And if union staffers believe that the organization's management is selfishly exploiting employees, does not care about service excellence, and treats people unfairly or abusively, it sets up a cycle of negativity that can be difficult to interrupt. The length of time the union has been in place can affect these impressions and feelings.

Length of the Relationship

If the organization has just undergone a successful organizing effort by a union, there may be intense negative feelings in management that must be resolved before a healthy relationship can be established. These campaigns often resort to strategies that increasingly polarize employees and management against each other in order to gain votes or to defeat the union. Typically, organization managers and executives are presented in the worst possible ways and promises are made that employees want to believe will be met. The same process occurs in the U.S. political arena, especially during presidential campaign years. Parties too often foment doubt and mistrust of the opposing candidate to convince voters to vote for their position or candidate. The small issues are magnified and the larger, more important issues ignored. Votes are frequently cast based on emotion rather than critical thinking and analysis of the issues. Unfortunately, the more polarization created, the more difficult it is for people from the two sides to come together after the vote and work together in good faith to achieve desired goals.

Most managers would consider a successful union organizing effort as a severe blow to their pride and an indication that they had failed as leaders. For employees to feel like they need a third party to speak for and represent them often implies the ultimate failure from a leadership perspective. The outcome of the vote can also trigger very human reactions that range from grief and loss to embarrassment and humiliation. These reactions can result in managers simply resigning themselves to the new reality in a passive way, leading to psychological termination and distancing. Other managers and leaders may become aggressive and ultimately vindictive. In one organization, managers openly were pleased about the inability of the union to effectively negotiate a contract for its nurses for as long as sixteen months after the successful vote. They were delighted in what they saw as ineffectiveness that would reinforce the "sheer stupidity" of the employees' decision. And it was apparent that many managers held the not-so-secret belief that this might cause the employees to vote the union out.

If the union loses the vote to represent employees, feelings on the part of the organizers also run the gamut. However, because the union is not physically present, some of the emotions may not be visible to organizational leadership. If the unionizing effort was successful, starting the relationship on a positive note is important. If the union begins its relationship with management with overtones of arrogance or gloating, or a "gotcha now" mentality, it bodes ill for the quality of the future relationship.

So, if the presence of the union is new or recently expanded, one can expect to see higher intensity of emotions. External support for those involved may be necessary to help begin to heal the rawness of feelings and get the relationship started in the right direction. Organizations with an internal labor relations department have an advantage because these staff specialists can help managers understand the new relationship and see it in a business light rather than as a personal issue. At the heart of the challenge is the recognition and acceptance by managers that the union exists in the organization because employees wanted it there for one reason or another, and as leaders, a primary responsibility is to support what employees need or feel they need in order to do a good job. If managers continue with the attitude toward the union that "we hate you and wish you weren't here," the work will be much more difficult (Watson 2008). The leader who holds the belief that there is merit in the existence of the union and that he or she wants to work well with the union because it represent employees will find it much easier to form a healthy working relationship with this new entity. The underlying philosophy is that "employees matter a great deal in this organization, and union representation is what matters to the employees." So, in this respect, the union will be supported.

If the union or unions have a long-term history in the organization, the challenges are slightly different. In some instances, the relationship may feel like an arranged marriage. In other words, the relationship was already established by others who may feel more strongly about it than does the current manager, but now it is up to him or her to make it work. There may have been no sense of connection to or interest between the parties initially, but the hope is that a good relationship can be developed. In other instances, the relationship can take on the characteristics of a long-term marriage. The parties begin to take things for granted and perhaps slip into a bit of complacency. The challenge is to not take each other for granted and to keep the relationship on a steady, productive path.

The Importance of Partnership

Organizations that work productively with the unions that represent their employees often find that the healthiest relationship is one that is a true partnership. The fact that the original partnership between employer and employee has just expanded to a threesome is one of the biggest challenges represented by this circumstance. One executive said, "It's like inviting a third party to a marriage" (Balik 2008). This expansion of parties often means that roles and expectations need to be renegotiated. Furthermore, the complexity of the relationship and everything associated with it has amplified.

In chapter 6, partnership relationships were briefly examined. Healthy partnerships are not easy to establish, but the potential outcomes make the effort worthwhile. Several elements of a healthy partnership are worth addressing here in relation to the management–union partnership. The word itself comes from the Latin *partaker*, meaning "to share." The first essential element of a healthy partnership is willingness and intent to work together interdependently as well as the capability to do so. It is very difficult to engage in this relationship with a partner who has no intention of working together at this high level of relationship maturity. Any healthy relationship features complementary skills, and these can often at least initially form the basis of the partnership. In other words, each partner contributes something to the relationship. This unique contribution is recognized, valued, and respected. In the case of the union–management partnership, the union may be bringing to the table the unique ability to speak for employees, to give voice to the needs and desires of the union members in a way the employees felt unable to do on their own. Management may bring the opportunities represented by providing employment in the organization and the authority and resources to create a positive work environment.

Equitable rewards are also a key component of a healthy partnership relationship. All parties to the partnership must benefit, or it will not be productive. Moreover, each must contribute something substantial to the partnership, or there will always be a perceived unequal balance of power and the parties will vie for stature. The equitability issue may explain why the attitude of executives who see the union as something that helps their employees will be more likely to engage in a full partnership, and vice versa.

Finally, all of the elements of a healthy partnership must be present. These include trust, mutual respect, support, and open communication. They are built in much the same way as in any relationship. Clarity of mission and purpose must be established. When both management and the unions have the same outcomes in mind, for example, the establishment of the best possible workplace for employees so that the overall mission of the organization is met, this alignment can begin to establish trust. One human resources executive said that when a manager clearly has the best interests of employees at heart, a bond of trust develops between union and organization leadership.

Establishing and agreeing upon working expectations of each other is another key way to build trust. This approach includes defining *trust*, *support*, *respect*, and *communication*. For example, if a manager overhears an employee talking negatively about the union, the manager may be tempted to fan those flames of frustration, especially if there are still strong feelings following a campaign. This can also be an opportunity for the manager to support the employee and the union partner in a positive way. The manager might begin by coaching the employee in using strategies to bring his or her issues forward to a union steward. Managers who are advocates for their employees act with consistency and pay attention to what is fair and reasonable. Just because a union is involved does not mean that the manager loses his or her feelings of advocacy for the employees. These actions and attitudes of members of management usually form good relationships with both employees and the involved unions.

Being partners does not always translate into agreement about approaches or strategies. But organizations that take a very practical approach to working with unions tend to be more successful at creating successful partnerships. Many examples of this approach can be seen around the United States. Kaiser-Permanente in California has extensive experience in establishing a formal partnership model for management and labor. Mount Sinai in New York City has established labor–management partnerships whose focus is creating a more positive workplace. All partners come together based on the realization that their futures are one and the same, tightly linked together. The single consideration for their decision making is what will make patient care better. This alignment of focus and mission provides the impetus for endless possibilities. And other organizations, although their contract may not be labeled a labor–management partnership, are indeed working in just this way.

Clarity of Responsibilities

The relationship between the organization and the unions is a business one and must be understood from this light. In the same way, the relationship between employees and their union is also a business relationship. Each party has certain responsibilities to uphold. The union has legal responsibilities and obligations as well as legal rights. Some are negotiated in the contract with the organization, while others are determined by the National Labor Relations Board. Every manager in the organization needs to understand the contract (including the terms and conditions of employment) to reduce conflicts and misunderstandings. In one large system, for example, the contract precluded management from determining and distributing bonuses and financial incentives to employees without formal involvement of the union. Managers were recommending and wanting to give exceptional employees bonuses and did not realize they did not have the legal right to do so.

Filing a grievance is an appropriate approach for a union member to make his or her voice heard. And the union has a legal responsibility to represent its members, whether it believes there is merit to the claim or not. Even in organizations where managers have never been counseled about or criticized for having employees file grievances, often the mind-set on the part of the manager is that the occurrence of a grievance means "I have failed in some way." There is a fear that others may see them as ineffective or poor managers, or that these events will find their way into the manager's annual performance review. This unspoken fear can potentially lead to damaging results if it influences a manager's handling of performance or behavioral issues. A manager may unwittingly abdicate his or her legitimate authority for dealing with issues because he or she is afraid of grievances and lawsuits. Managers must understand that it is the union's responsibility to represent its members and that it is each member's responsibility to follow the proper protocol. Filing a grievance is not necessarily meant to be a personal attack on a manager.

Understanding the relationship between all three parties as a business one accomplishes two goals. First, it helps the manager remove himself or herself personally from the situation. Seeing the opposition as the existence of a difference of opinion and as a business issue can help the manager or executive retain appropriate boundaries. When leaders react personally to issues, they are more likely to lose their objectivity. They are also more likely to respond in a competitive vein, which only further polarizes the issue (Sheehan 2008). Second, when this relationship is clearly recognized and accepted as a business relationship, it necessarily requires that managers have current, concrete knowledge about that relationship and its business aspects.

Increased Complexity

Most organizational leaders agree that the increased layer of complexity that union representation brings to employee relationships makes it more of a challenge to lead and manage within the organization. The circumstance of dealing with a union demands exquisite leadership skills in order to be successful. However, on the positive side, it can also hone a person's development of leadership skills to an even higher level. Due to the availability of the process of official filing grievances, managerial missteps are highly visible. This visibility requires leaders to continually be at the top of their game. One executive said that when dealing with unions, "Good leadership and good management is more important than ever" (Balik 2008).

In one organization, a new manager initiated the disciplinary process for a long-tenured nurse who had had performance and behavioral problems for years that had never been addressed. These issues were affecting others in the workplace. Even though the manager wanted to do something about the issues, there was a significant lack of documentation. The union business agent (union employee) representing the employee in question pulled the hospital human resources specialist supporting the manager and hospital aside and told her, "I wouldn't want this nurse taking care of my family member either . . . and we don't really want to be defending bad nurses, but when you don't do your job documenting poor performance and then try to fire them, we're obligated to file a grievance. Just do your job." What many managers do not realize is that the union has a legal obligation to represent the member, and failing to do so can violate its contract with its members.

It is helpful to approach problems such as the above with the belief and attitude that management and union goals are the same: to provide for the best possible workplace for employees. Union staffers do not want to be in a position of defending employees that are dragging the workplace down. Several executives mentioned instances where the union staffer was of tremendous assistance in dealing with difficult employee behavior. In some cases the union staff member pulled the employee out of the room and basically delivered the message, "If what they are saying is true, you had better clean up your act or you will lose your job." And in the reverse case, the presence of a powerful third party advocating for an employee may ensure that the person is treated fairly and with appropriate due process.

Hidden Agendas

Some managers and executives have a hidden agenda: If we can make the employees happier, they'll vote to decertify the union. The primary motivation of major cultural changes or organizational initiatives must be because there is inherent value in the initiative, not for a potential secondary gain. The latter would fall under the category of doing the right thing for the wrong reason. Furthermore, if it is known that managers and executives have expressed a clear intent to "bust the union," then the adversarial climate is only increased.

Union employees can have hidden agendas as well. In one organization, over time, one union staffer created significant disruption in the workplace, often displaying the very behaviors that were contradictory to established expectations for a respectful workplace. This individual seemed to take great delight in badgering and being mean-spirited to managers. In one instance, the human resources specialist and a director had just finished a meeting with the union staffer and one of the managers. At the end of the meeting, the manager said, "That was the worst meeting I have ever been in." The other two organizational representatives were somewhat taken aback and realized that they had become so habituated to this union staffer's bad behavior that they had been accepting behaviors that should have been addressed. Although it is hard to know what this union employee's true agenda was, it clearly was not in fostering a healthy relationship that benefited employees and the organization.

This realization spurred action against this individual. Parameters were reconfirmed, and when the individual behaved outside the acceptable standards, she was called on her inappropriate behavior. Instead of allowing her tirade against a manager, for example, she was stopped, reminded that disrespectful language was not tolerated or management would leave the meeting. This scenario happened so frequently that work was not being accomplished. After repeated instances, legal action was taken against the union employee, and she was removed from her role in the facility.

Importance of Human Resources Support

In organizations with unions, the role of human resources becomes even more crucial. Its members must be the experts in employee and labor relations, using effective strategies, providing guidance for managers, and understanding the legal aspects of all proceedings. Human resources must be clear about management's role as well. Some organizations can develop a long history of not wanting to upset the union and a tendency to keep the union happy at all costs. This rarely is an effective strategy for creating a vital and vibrant organization capable of surmounting today's challenges. The balancing act is how to not paralyze managers while also not ignoring the rights and obligations of the unions.

Personnel processes may actually be more transparent in a union environment because the structure and process is so clearly defined, often in a legal contract. This reality forces management to be more diligent in its process. Additionally, more grievances may come forward because employees feel like they have third-party support in doing so.

Too often the basic relationship between operational managers and human resources staff needs work. As mentioned earlier in this book, some managers tend to believe that they could not possibly document thoroughly enough to convince their human resources counterpart that necessary action against an employee, such as termination, needs to be taken. The human resources specialist is there to help and support the manager treat the employee in a fair manner and also to coach and counsel the manager so that he or she, as well as the organization, is protected. The human resources specialist can be an objective set of eyes in evaluating the strength of the data upon which the manager is basing his or her decision.

One human resources executive described an example where the manager was determined to terminate an employee for a particular behavior that was inappropriate and embarrassing to the manager. When the documentation was reviewed, it was clear that it was not adequate. There may well have been justification for the recommendation, but the data available for review created only a flimsy case. The human resources executive counseled the manager by saying, "If you terminate this individual, given the documentation here, the employee will grieve it, it will go to arbitration and you will lose. That is so much worse than the position you are in right now. Let's work on this so that when you do terminate this person's employment, you have your ducks in a row and your decision will be supported." Basically, the specialist was saying, "This is my recommendation based on my experience. If you think you are embarrassed now, how will you feel when you are forced to accept this employee back because your recommendation is overturned?" Giving the manager clear direction and support in taking appropriate steps is the role of human resources. It is not their role to make the final decision.

Communication Is Critical

Effective methods of communication are essential in any organization and in every leadership role. However, communication may not be as transparent in early stages of the relationship with a union nor in an adversarial long-term relationship. Open communication is a major way to build trust, especially in the beginning of the relationship between the union and the organization. Clarity around shared purpose and goals and establishing alignment in values and beliefs can help set the stage for a productive future relationship. The communication must continually occur with and between all members of the partnership.

One executive, whose organization faced a collective bargaining organizing effort that was later withdrawn by the union involved, said that the experience resulted in tremendous positive benefits. It was an eye-opening process for the entire leadership team. Although senior leadership believed they were receptive and listened well to employees' concerns, it became clear that there are different levels of listening. There is the "Hi, how are things going?" level of interchange, and then there is the "What are you having problems with? Is there any equipment that isn't working right? What took you too long today? What do we have you doing that makes it hard for you to do your best?" level of interchange that uses and relies on deeply probing questions to get to the real issues. And, of course, this team found that the more superficial level of listening is not enough. Listening with the intention of following through and getting results is core leadership work (Natale 2008).

Communication must be iterative, well planned, and effectively orchestrated. Passive communication through e-mail and the posting of notices is simply not enough. One executive talked about the work his team was doing in partnering with the marketing department to find new ways of formatting and displaying information, based on the recognition that everyone is inundated daily with more information than they can possibly manage. The new approach involved identifying the few items that are crucial for the recipient to internalize and leaving information in the message that gave the recipient the next place to go for more detailed information (Natale 2008).

This executive also suggested establishing objective criteria for determining when communication was effective. For example, if, when asked what their performance improvement measures are, 75 percent of all point-of-service staff can answer the question correctly it is likely the communication plan has been effective.

An effective approach for increasing the level of understanding between union and management is for either of the parties involved to put themselves in the other person's position to try and determine what is important to that individual or group. For example, several administrators found that they were far more effective in working with union staffers when they consciously put themselves in the position of the staffer to try and see the situation from his or her point of view. This shift of perspective opens up possibilities that otherwise might not be considered. It helps increase understanding and the likelihood that a new solution will be found.

Again, being in partnership does not mean that agreement will always be reached on all sides. What is important is expressing opinions, respecting the ideas of others, and being willing to persist until mutually agreeable solutions and approaches are found.

Things Take Longer

A challenge of the complexity of union–management relationships is one that often happens when multiple partners are involved. To put it simply, things may take longer to get accomplished. When more people need to be involved in communication and decision making, the process can be extended. However, this process is not much different from the models of shared decision making implemented in organizations. Nor is it different from what managers experience who involve employees in determining solutions to problems.

When the right people are at the table making the decisions, the decisions are usually better and a higher level of commitment to the solution is achieved. If decisions are made by managers and executives—those further removed from where the actual work is being accomplished—the first thing the manager must do is explain the decision to others in a way that gains their commitment. This step is usually much easier if those with a heavy investment in the outcome are included in the decision-making process.

Keep It Positive

The unique challenges in organizations where the partnership includes management, employees, and union can also provide solidarity and strength if creating a positive work environment is a vision shared by all partners. However, it is interesting to note that all of the executives and leaders interviewed agreed that if employees in the organization are highly engaged, the workplace is positive, and no collective bargaining units are in place, it is very difficult for a union to organize.

The Challenge of Long-Term Care Facilities

A long-term care (LTC) facility provides complete services for supporting the resident and his or her quality of life. It is important to remember in discussions of LTC facilities that care is being provided to individuals with diverse and complex care needs. The recent change in care needs, such as acute long-term care, and the reimbursement for care has helped to alter the LTC environment, as has the fact that the length of stay in LTC facilities is now shorter than in years past. Some LTC facilities may include a combination of care for individuals with chronic ventilator use; special programs for individuals with dementia; and care for residents requiring intravenous therapy, blood products, or rehabilitation before returning home following a hospital stay. Other types of facilities are too difficult and complex to describe because regulations and definitions can vary for facilities such as assisted living, adult homes, and independent living.

In long-term care, more emphasis is placed on the environment from the resident's perspective. A key difference between an acute care facility and a long-term care living facility is length of stay. In an acute care setting, the patient is clearly expected to make adjustments, and although a tremendous amount of work is being led by organizations such as NRC Picker to create a patient-centered environment, the unspoken assumption is that the patient is in "our" facility now. In fact, the explicit justification for admission of a person to an acute care facility is that he or she needs complex nursing services and the diagnostic and testing capabilities of the organization.

In long-term care, the facilities are considered *living facilities* and they are the home of the residents. Employees are there to support and provide services that the resident is unable to provide for himself or herself. In the best of these facilities, employees recognize that they are in the resident's home. Even the physical plant in some of these landmark facilities is homelike with atriums, courtyards, areas designated as neighborhoods, and shorter corridors. Traditional approaches in other support staff areas are slowly converting to more homelike practices. For example, offering buffets that residents can choose to access during the times most convenient for them is replacing the idea of a dining room where everyone eats the same thing at the same time.

Creating a positive work environment has become a major focus in recent years in LTC facilities. The work environment affects the quality of the resident-centered care as well as employee vacancy and turnover rates. "Vacancies and turnover in long term care compromise quality and increase costs. Studies indicate that the supply of well trained nursing staff is a key factor in the quality of care in long term care" (American Health Care Association and National Center for Assisted Living 2007, p. 1). This study reports that the current annual turnover rate for registered nurses (RNs) is 49 percent and 71 percent for certified nurses' aides (CNAs). This rate results in an annual cost of more than $4 billion a year for nursing facilities. This extraordinarily high cost of turnover is a long-accepted historical fact for long-term care, even as this level of turnover affects resident outcomes.

Most managers and executives believe that the principles for creating a positive workplace are the same in any setting. Good leadership, along with the right strategies, builds the positive environments present throughout the chapters of this book. However, the unique environment of the LTC facility presents challenges to creating a positive work environment that are not present in the acute care facility.

Education Level of Employees

Unlike an acute care facility where a higher percentage of highly educated and credentialed employees works, in LTC the majority of point-of-service workers do not have the benefit of high levels of advanced education. In many facilities, the more highly educated professionals are not always physically present. For instance, in the dietary department, a registered dietitian may only make periodic visits to the facility to oversee the development of menus and delivery of nutrition services. The director of nursing may be an RN, but most supervision of the point-of-service workers, the nursing assistants, is provided by licensed practical nurses (LPNs). (This lack of highly credentialed employees does not always hold true, for example, in facilities dealing with the care of ventilator-dependent patients.) Additionally, even the more highly credentialed employees have had little to any formal education related to geriatric care. Geriatrics has only recently been added to the curriculum of academic programs.

This challenge can be overcome by education. Educational programs for the staff in LTC facilities are critical. The implementation of an educational program demonstrates great respect for the contribution and role of the point-of-service worker. Facilities often send the primary staff (CNAs) to outside educational programs as well as offer in-services on a routine basis. Nursing homes that offer CNAs training programs have fewer ambulatory care-sensitive conditions that are likely to result in hospitalization (Intrator, Zinn, and Mor 2004). In one facility, the nursing assistants had the option of being designated as rehabilitation nursing assistants. They were provided with the opportunity to receive additional training in techniques such as Tai Chi and therapeutic massage. With these expanded educational opportunities, they became an ever greater resource in their facilities.

Additionally, those who are interested in furthering their education should be encouraged to take advantage of any tuition reimbursement program that may be offered at the facility or through the organization at large. Helping employees get more education helps the facility as a whole, even while the employees are still in school. The employee-students use their new knowledge and their work experience to inform both their day-to-day work and their class work. They become both better caregivers and better students.

Involvement in Decision Making

For nurses and therapists, working in long-term care often offers an opportunity for autonomy in their practice that does not always exist in other clinical settings. Almost all of the residents' needs fall within the scope of nursing practice. However, in LTC, most of the direct care is delivered by CNAs. Often an assumption is made that individuals without advanced formal education are not interested in or capable of being involved in decision making. This is a misconception that needs to be challenged. One facility experienced an 80 percent turnover rate for CNAs. A retention committee was launched comprising the nursing director, a couple of LPNs, and both experienced and new CNAs. The committee implemented a variety of initiatives including a well-designed orientation program that used assigned volunteer preceptors, or tutors, for new hires. The committee also made a commitment that employees in orientation would not be pulled and used to staff when a vacancy occurred. Within a year, the turnover rate had dropped to 20 percent, well below industry standards.

In another facility, the CNAs are involved in developing the care plan for residents based on their day-to-day working relationship with the residents. They are also included in the daily report that occurs between employee shift changes. Bringing the caregivers into care conferences and talking with them about the residents' needs has demonstrated respect for the employees' contributions and has improved care (DeRosa 2008).

Involving employees in decisions about their work is important for creating a positive workplace. In one facility, at a recent staff meeting, it was brought to the director's attention that a resident with Alzheimer's disease needed one-on-one staffing. This situation was creating a tremendous strain on the staff. The director talked with the affected staff members about the situation, shared several possible ideas, and asked them to think about it for a few days. Several days later the employees had developed a rotation of two-hour slots to help spell the primary CNA and help the department get through this difficult period of time with one of its residents. They also made changes in the overall care plan so that the one-on-one staffing requirement did not go on indefinitely.

Creating a Homelike Atmosphere

Perhaps one of the greatest challenges facing LTC facilities is that the atmosphere itself can often seem miserable. If the environment is depressing or demoralizing, leadership will be hard-pressed to get workers to stay for long. As discussed in chapter 5, a pleasant environment is part of what makes a workplace positive. So the facility and its characteristics are important in long-term care. When the physical plant resembles the more antiseptic, sterile environment of an acute care hospital, it is difficult for both staff and residents to feel like they are in a domestic environment.

Creating a homey atmosphere means doing away with features like long hallways, standard institutional decorating schemes, and the occurrence of overhead pages, if feasible. The ability to access the outdoors is also an important factor, as is the presence of plants and animals. The rhythms of home life are also considered. Special events throughout the year are occasions for celebration. If residents are unable to go home for their holidays, the staff can make certain that the celebrations occur in the facility. Staff can decorate and invite members of the community to come for the celebration.

If the facility is simply a department in a larger organization, the challenge to create an environment that is inviting and homelike for the residents can be great. However, some facilities have met this challenge through relatively simple programs. Resources may not be available to redesign the department environment physically, but employees can redesign the environmental atmosphere into a cheerful and positive place. And the more positive the place, the better chance that the workers will stay. The work itself of making the workplace into a home for the residents might inspire the workers to stay.

Changing the Culture

Successful LTC facilities are working to overcome the history of long-term care. A stigma is often attached to long-term care, not just from employees but also from residents. There can be the belief, on the part of everyone involved, that the individual has entered the facility and will remain there until death. Transforming the attitude of all involved to see the facility as a long-term living facility is a crucial culture change that must be made. The resident is not coming into long-term care to die, but instead to live. It is a challenged faced by every LTC facility trying to foster a positive environment for residents and employees. If the residents are not miserable, it is less likely that the caregivers will be.

Not so many years ago, the approach of the employees of these facilities was to do everything for the resident. The individual's strengths were not identified and consciously reinforced. Inadvertently, this approach created unnecessary dependence on the part of the resident. Today the movement is toward resident-centered care and the philosophy is for the staff to be a support for what the resident needs. Finding out the individual's normal preferences and habits is crucial for building a schedule and activities around his or her interests.

The primary value is quality of life. This means encouraging residents to be active, move about the building, and become involved in the events around them. Perhaps the normal metrics used for evaluating quality of care need to be reassessed. For example, in one facility, because of the emphasis on encouraging residents to be active, the fall rate is higher. Due to the concern for quality of life, the facility's philosophy is to not physically restrain the residents. If a resident cannot be up on his or her own or is confused or delirious, it may mean that a staff member must be present at all times. When decisions are made about a resident's requests, this philosophy is taken into account. For example, the facility tries to stress the resident's independence. If a resident wants to use the commode chair, it is more important for him or her to do so than to always try and control the process for the sake of cleanliness. If a resident is having skin issues but wants to go to the mall and participate in the other activities, the rule is, "life trumps." In other words, the quality of life as perceived by the resident is the most important consideration. This is a major cultural shift that also benefits the employees. The work environment is a more positive place when the residents are happy and feel freer to live their lives closer to the way they did in the past. And it is easier for staff members to keep their own spirits high and engaged in their work.

However, caregivers might feel overwhelmed by letting those in their care live in such a variety of ways. Teamwork is the key, and breaking down the silo mentality of employees is critical for creating an approach that best benefits the residents. In the past, for example, recreation staff members were the ones who initiated activities for residents. Recently a concept called Simple Pleasures has been developed. It is based on the concept that every employee should do something that the residents might find enjoyable. For example, one resident needed nail care, and the person working with her decided to do a nail spa day. She gathered all the residents who might enjoy the pleasure of having their nails done and created a spa-like atmosphere. The employee did not worry about which resident was assigned to whom. Through the Simple Pleasures concept she knew that what she was doing would, on some small scale, positively affect the lives of many residents as well as her co-workers. Many of these small-scale actions end up in the long run helping to overcome the challenges of enacting cultural change at an LTC facility. These actions help make the place less one where residents are to die and more one where they are at home to live.

Interpersonal Relationships

As discussed throughout the first portion of this book, positive relationships with others is a key factor in determining whether an individual perceives his or her workplace to be positive or not. A huge advantage in long-term care facilities is the length and depth of the interpersonal relationships that form between caregivers and residents. Unlike many clinical settings in which the employees' relationship with the clients consists of brief encounters, long-term care affords the opportunity for staff to develop long-term relationships with residents and their families and the ability to witness the outcome of their interventions. Staff members are often assigned in as consistent a manner as possible, and they work with the same residents over long periods of time. In one facility, some CNAs had been caring for the same residents for as long as ten years. This situation creates a deep bond between employee and resident and is a positive aspect of LTC. However, it also makes it more crucial that the relationship is based on healthy principles and that there is a fit between the personalities of the resident and employee. In instances where problems begin to develop—both personality conflicts and overly personal relationships can occur—active coaching and support are needed. Employees can be reassigned, but in many cases they do not want to "give someone up."

One disadvantage of these long-term relationships is seen when a resident or a family member dies. In many cases family members become very close to the employees. One manager noted that it is extremely difficult to lose a resident, because in many cases it can also include the loss of a family member. This sentiment can be especially true when workers are there when family members come in and visit. Bonds with the resident's family can become very strong. Support in the form of grief counseling and special services can be helpful.

Fighting the Mundane

Long-term care offers the employee more diversity in his or her work life. "Residents and their families come from a wide range of cultural and religious backgrounds that significantly impact care and that must be considered in providing services that enhance a high quality of life" (Eliopoulos 2007, p. II-1). In addition, the clinical complexities of the residents' situations require workers to be knowledgeable in a wide range of clinical specialties. Conversely, several employees confess that it is a constant battle to fight the boredom of the everyday. Long-term care facilities are very busy places, but the pace is different from acute care facilities. The work is about supporting the daily living of these elders, and it can become mundane after a period of time. Continually finding ways to create fun, excitement, and passion is important in these organizations. Generating excitement is beneficial to both residents and employees.

One facility celebrated Nursing Home Week in high style with its residents (Kerfian 2008). The week's activities were focused around the theme "Love is ageless." The first day began with a mayoral proclamation and a special breakfast. That evening, the local Veterans of Foreign Wars post sponsored a dinner dance for residents and employees. The second day was designated "'50s Day" and the facility was decorated with pictures of motorcycles and old cars. The dining room was converted to a drive-in theatre where movies were shown and root beer floats were served. Employees wore saddle shoes, poodle skirts, and rolled-up jeans. A jukebox played music from the era throughout the day and employees, residents, and visitors all danced. On Wednesday, keeping with the week's theme, eight couples renewed their wedding vows. The dining room was transformed into a showplace by a local wedding decorator. Employees dressed as befitted the wedding ceremony, families of the couples were present, and a reception was held afterward. Thursday was "Intergenerational Day," with a carnival theme, a petting zoo, and visits from children from the local schools. The final day was "Casino Day." The week was filled with events to remember for residents, families, and staff.

Special events like the one mentioned above help break the monotony of the LTC facility. But it is vital for management to reinforce the importance of this work and its contribution to the community. Recognizing the residents as people with a full and vital past helps breaks through the mundane tasks of the everyday. One long-term care nurse summarized this sentiment beautifully: "When you look at this old woman's hands, you see the wrinkles, arthritic knuckles and age spots. I look at this woman's hands and I see a mother's young hands holding her first child, hands teaching her granddaughter how to tie her shoes, hands comforting her children and husband. I see all she is and has been."

Fewer Resources

In LTC, resources tend to be more limited than in acute care, and managers and employees must work within the resources they have. Many workers in the LTC field feel like second-class citizens in the broader picture of health care. This feeling creates a critical challenge for managers and executives to communicate the uniqueness and importance of their mission. The many interventions and suggestions throughout earlier chapters are ideas for ways to tackle this issue, such as understanding the intrinsic motivators from chapter 2. The challenges of the LTC facility can be considered unique opportunities for the staff members to create a positive environment and, quite simply, a better world for people who are not only their residents but also their personal charges.

The Challenges of Academic Settings

Academic settings are distinctly different in many ways from service-only settings. One aspect that the two settings share in common is workforce shortages. In academic institutions a shortage in nursing faculty is escalating. Other health science programs are more likely experiencing competition for a faculty position, that is, more people are applying for positions than positions are available. With these growing nursing faculty shortages, a cycle is created that affects the workforce for all health care organizations. For example, it limits the number of nursing students the academic program is able to admit. This situation highlights a unique difference between service and academia: Workforce shortages affect these settings in different ways based on how the flow of customers (patients and students) is controlled.

Acute care hospitals rarely close their doors to patients. People continue to become ill and need treatment or hospitalization regardless of whether anyone is available to take care of them. There is no turning them away. In many cases they are admitted to the hospital whether there are resources to provide for their care or not. Some organizations have developed a diversion policy in the emergency department when inpatient rooms are filled to capacity. However, when all hospitals in a community are at capacity with patients, somehow, patients are still accepted.

Just as the patient is the direct customer of the hospital, the student is the direct customer of the academic program. Academic settings do turn away potential students based on their resources, such as faculty availability and adequacy of clinical sites. They limit student admissions and create waiting lists of potential students when they do not have the resources to provide services. Faculty may be asked to increase their workload, but they receive workload credit for this increase, with a commensurate increase in financial compensation. And the work is not beyond the point of capability, unlike frequent instances in acute care hospitals. Lab work and diagnostic tests are ordered for the acutely ill patient whether or not enough staff are working in the lab or imaging department. Inpatient units are filled to capacity regardless of the number of nursing staff available. This does not mean to imply that there is no concern for this practice, and, of course, at some facilities, worker availability determines whether patients are accepted or turned away. However, this policy seems to be the exception rather than the rule on the acute care side.

The shortage of nurse faculty does not affect individual faculty members in the same manner as it affects staff or a manager in an acute care facility. There are limits to numbers of students in a course, as there are limits to the number of students a faculty member may take for clinical supervision. And although the faculty may be asked to increase their workload, it is most often the faculty member's individual choice whether or not to do so. There is no mandatory overtime or working double shifts to cover for staffing vacancies. Those with administrative responsibilities are not automatically pulled back into the classroom or given increased teaching assignments. Faculty members are able, and in fact expected, to continue their research and scholarly activities. On the other hand, the manager in an acute care hospital whose department is experiencing a worker shortage often is expected to step in and do the clinical or technical work of the department until the situation calms down again. Management and administrative work is often deferred, either to be taken home and done in the manager's leisure time or simply not completed.

A temporal aspect is at play here as well. For a faculty member, to take an increased workload is a much longer time commitment, usually for the course of a semester or term. On the other hand, a manager in a hospital may experience this acceleration of workload for a shorter period of time, perhaps for a shift or a week. Organizations where this increased demand for covering worker shortages is unremitting for managers find they have severe long-term difficulties. At some point it becomes impossible to dig out of the backlog and to regain the enthusiasm and commitment of their severely depleted managers.

The challenges for both the academic setting and the service setting are many but varied. The academic setting has more problems creating a positive workplace besides a lack of staff. A handful of the rest of these challenges are explored here.

Financial Compensation

Faculty pay is often cited as an underlying, if not a major, reason for the shortage of nursing faculty. Ample evidence exists to show that academic settings do not provide a baseline compensation package for their faculty that compares with what the individual would be paid in a service setting. It is financially more lucrative to be in a practice/service setting regardless of one's profession.

Although significant dissatisfaction with financial compensation is evident, this issue may actually be a result of a sense of equity more than compensation. Faculty members are often some of the most highly educated members of their field. It has to be demoralizing for them to have worked for and achieved the highest levels of academic preparation and to have decades of experience and know that new practitioners in the service arena have salary packages that match or exceed theirs. The resulting sense of inequity may foment dissatisfaction. Of course, there are trade-offs, and often these are not fully considered nor appreciated. For example, the salary may be for a nine-month contract. Many academic settings not only allow but encourage faculty to remain active in their clinical or professional practice to at least some degree. This activity can take the form of a part-time or occasional work, consulting, publishing, or speaking engagements. The additional financial compensation supplements what many consider a relatively meager salary. Moreover, there are other perks and benefits that might not seem apparent. For example, one faculty member noted that if one has a bad semester, it will pass and before long a new group of students will arrive with whom one can start over, unlike the service arena, where there is rarely a new beginning.

Obviously, those who choose to become educators and work in an academic setting find satisfaction there. Reported levels of nursing faculty satisfaction are quite high. Added to this finding is the fact that once the faculty member makes it through the first two to three years, he or she tends to stay. When academic faculties are examined and compared with a management team in an acute care setting, length of employment for individuals is likely to be longer in academic settings. It reportedly is also easier for individuals nearing the end of their career to transition into a stage of lesser work requirements. For example, administrative faculty can more readily ease back into partial teaching or research assignments. It is more difficult for a manager or hospital executive to move back into his or her original clinical or professional role. Recent changes in the educational process also facilitate this transition. In many academic settings, more and more courses are offered online. A faculty member may teach the course and provide advisement to students totally through electronic means online. The faculty member can be traveling in Italy and adequately manage his or her teaching assignment. The new technology allows a freedom of movement and availability unlike anything widely seen in the service setting.

In regard to compensation, one factor related to the academic benefit packages may indirectly affect the shortage of faculty. Faculty tend to have longer lengths of employment, and many work in state government systems. Due to this, the retirement benefit may be more robust than in other health care organizations. One factor that contributes significantly to a person's decision to retire is whether he or she can manage it financially. Thus, if the educator reaches a point in his or her career where he or she is able to retire and the workplace is not positive, he or she is more likely to choose to leave either physically or psychologically.

The Tenure and Promotion System

Another unique challenge to the academic setting is the issue of hierarchy. Hierarchy in an academic setting has nothing to do with the legitimate authority level based on a supervisory, management, or executive position. Academic hierarchy is based on tenure and the achievement of specific academic status. It can create a sense of elitism based on ranking. One faculty member is regarded as better than another because he or she has a particular credential or academic achievement. As discussed in chapter 6, unconditional and mutual respect is an essential component of healthy working relationships. The system of tenure provides a visible, sanctioned ranking more likely to result in conditional respect in the workplace. Unconditional respect does not mean that one does not extend respect for another person's achievements, it means that respect is not withheld because an individual does not have the same achievements. Yet tenure is often the basis of committee assignments and involvement in decision making. Some university settings have powerful committees on which only tenured faculty are allowed to serve. For example, in one academic setting, when a new doctoral program was being developed, only faculty members with a particular degree were allowed to be involved in the decision making about the new curriculum. The result of this kind of common practice is that decision making tends to not be inclusive but exclusive and can easily lead to an insular thinking pattern resulting in less effective and creative solutions and strategies.

Tenure has another potential negative outcome: difficulty removing a problematic individual. The original purpose of a tenure system in academia was to provide protection for a faculty member within a highly political system. Once a faculty member achieved tenure, it ensured that he or she was afforded academic freedom and could hold and express divergent opinions from administration without fear of losing the position. The positive aspect of this concept is that faculty members are certain of the stability of their jobs and they value the academic freedom they enjoy. However, if these tenured individuals exhibit toxic, negative behavior, not much can be done to remove them from the environment. The toxic behavior of one individual, as addressed in chapter 10, can infect the rest of the workplace community, which in this case consists of the faculty and the students they teach. It takes extreme or gross negligence or misbehavior to remove a tenured professor. This can make it very difficult to hold people accountable for their behavior and its impact within the work group. As long as this individual meets the minimum requirements for research, scholarship, and service, he or she has a job.

Tenure's most deadly aspect is that it is an entitlement system. In other words, once the status of tenure is gained, there is less incentive for the individual to continue to strive and achieve at the high level it took to attain the status initially. It is easy for the individual to come to believe that he or she is "owed" and deserves the benefits of the position regardless of whether he or she has done anything recently to earn them. Tenure may have been granted for achievements from decades earlier, and yet protection continues. One faculty member with 40 years of experience in service and academia said that in her experience, after achieving tenure, approximately 75 percent of her colleagues begin to coast. In other words, they consider that meeting the minimum requirements is enough. Regardless of the percentage, it is clear from Bardwick's (1991) work on entitlement that when people feel extremely safe in their jobs, it often leads to lower productivity. After all, the job is guaranteed and no one can do anything about lackluster performance. This attitude is ultimately destructive to the human spirit and its drive to continually improve, be responsible, and excel. And it can create unintended negative consequences for the organizations that use the system.

Academic settings use objective systems of promotion based on individual performance measures. Faculty members face the challenge of meeting concrete, objective requirements for research, scholarship, and service. If these requirements have not been met, promotion does not occur. Several factors create special challenges for creating a positive work environment. First, the demands placed by these requirements are quite high. Doing original research requires a massive amount of time as does writing for publication. Balancing these demands is a juggling act that is comparable to what is experienced by managers in the service side of health care. However, the objectivity of the promotion system means that a clear emphasis is placed on what moves one forward and what does not. Staying current in the practice arena can be very difficult, even if the faculty member does clinical supervision.

Faculty members are not rewarded in any substantial manner (other than personal satisfaction) for additional activities such as mentoring a new faculty member or participating in a faculty shared governance council. These aspects of the role require significant effort and yet are not counted toward workload or merit requirements. And both of these activities— mentoring new members and participation in shared decision making—are clearly associated with a more positive work environment. Thus, the very structure in the system makes it less likely that faculty will participate readily in activities that might improve the situation because they require a great deal of effort that goes unrecognized in the promotion system.

Isolationism

Teaching is basically an individual activity. Although some academic settings use team teaching, it usually occurs on only a limited basis within the setting. And even though a course may be taught by a team, it often is not the same kind of team as discussed in chapter 7. Each member has a unique assignment and component of the workload for which he or she is responsible. Educators do not often teach together in the same place at the same time. Many faculty members talk about the interaction with their students, but little interaction takes place with other faculty colleagues. In some cases it is possible to go for weeks without really interacting with another colleague.

Recent changes in how teaching occurs only accentuate this aspect of the role. With more and more education being presented virtually through the Internet, instances occur where the faculty may seldom or never meet the student face-to-face. Although electronic classes offers students maximum flexibility in the logistics of how they complete course work, they provide little human contact. For faculty whose primary human connection with other people was through their students, this format can create a significant sense of aloneness and isolation. For the individual who went into education to work with students, having only electronic discourse and contact with them may provide limited satisfaction.

Meeting the challenge of staying current in the practice area is also a challenge posed by the isolationism of academia. It is difficult to stay current on practice issues, technology being used, and current trends in the service arena when most of the academic's work is individual work.

Preparation for the Role

Another challenge of the academic setting is the preparation of the new faculty member for his or her role in the new setting. There are two aspects to this challenge. The first relates to preparation for the individual faculty— the point-of-service worker in academia. Most individuals who become faculty members come from a service setting. It is hoped that interest in or passion for teaching others draws them into the academic arena. And although these individuals tend to be highly credentialed, their expertise is in practice, not necessarily in teaching others. Few have actual academic preparation for their educational role. They may have attained the highest level of academic credential for their field, but along the way they may have had no coursework related to educational principles or how to facilitate the learning process. An individual might have a PhD in biophysics and decide to join the faculty, but if no one has taught him or her how to teach, the endeavor may not be a success. Unfortunately, this lack can perpetuate ineffective teaching methodologies. A new faculty member without training in the art of teaching may simply teach the way he or she was taught. If his or her teacher also did not know how to teach, a perpetual cycle of misunderstanding about how to teach is propagated.

Administrative faculty members often experience the same issue. Although they come from leadership and management positions in the service sector, the very skills needed for an individual to be successful in these roles are often only secondarily considered during the interview and selection process. The successful applicant for a deanship, for example, must have a proven track record of academic and scholarly achievement, such as an extensive list of publications and an impressive research agenda. Although these are certainly remarkable achievements, they do not necessarily result in an individual with successful leadership qualities and capabilities. In the hiring process, the greater emphasis seems to be on individual achievement. This philosophy may be antithetical to the very nature of an outstanding leader.

Collins (2005) concluded from his research of organizations (both business and social sector) that successfully made the transition from being merely good to becoming great that a different level of leadership was apparent in these organizations. Those organizations that became great (on very objective measures) were those with what he refers to as "Level 5" leadership. These leaders are "ambitious first and foremost for the cause, the movement, the mission, the work—not themselves—and they have the will to do whatever it takes (*whatever* it takes) to make good on that ambition" (Collins 2005, p. 11). The people being led must believe that the leader is motivated first and always for the greater good, the greatness of the work, not for himself or herself. The contradiction here is that the accomplishments required to be considered a successful executive in academia may be of a more individual nature and not the other-directedness of high-level leadership.

Leadership Skills Required

The challenges of the unprepared leader can be met only with the knowledge of what a prepared leader can do to successfully guide an academic program. The effective leader must be extremely skilled at leading by consensus. As discussed earlier, Jim Collins characterized effective leaders in the social sector as being skilled at legislative rather than executive leadership. Acute care hospitals, long-term care living facilities, home health agencies, and freestanding medical facilities all exist within the social sector of our society, and as such, they are different from the business sector as described by Collins. However, a strong business aspect still exists within these organizations that allows for some level of executive leadership compared with legislative leadership. In academic settings, administrators must have strong legislative leadership skills if they are going to be effective. They must be able to tap into and use the power of inclusion, language, shared interests, and coalitions. Effective leaders in an academic setting are only successful if they are able to lead by consensus. It simply is not effective to tell a tenured faculty member what he or she will do.

Effective administrative faculty members are also responsible for another aspect of the job that is different from the service arena—fund-raising. The amount of money obtained through grants is important. A culture in which fund-raising is an expectation leads to elitism, which can be very dissatisfying. Large sums of money are often donated to schools of medicine rather than to the other schools within the health sciences (physical therapy, social work, occupational therapy, nursing, and so on).

The On-Boarding Process

A unique challenge to academic settings is bringing new faculty members into the system. This process is somewhat different from that of a new hire in a service setting. Academic settings are just beginning to develop formal systems of mentoring or assigning preceptors to the new person. As in service, the first several years are the most vulnerable for the new person. What makes the situation unique in academia is that the new faculty member likely has moved from a position where he or she felt knowledgeable, respected, and successful. The initial expectations of the new faculty member may be based on inaccurate assumptions and impressions about teaching that have little basis in reality. When the new person discovers that it is harder than expected, he or she can become frustrated. It is extremely labor intensive to develop coursework, and there are few supports in the system to offer help. Add to this the discovery that although the individual was very effective in the previous role, there may be a lot to learn in the arena of how to teach others. All of these factors occur in the presence of clear, continual, and perhaps not-so-positive feedback from students, who have their own high expectations. In the absence of a colleague-mentor or a system support, this pervasive sense of failure may cause the person to give up teaching prematurely.

Although it is almost necessary to the new faculty member, other faculty may not voluntarily step in and provide the support needed simply because of the significant time commitment it can require. And, as pointed out earlier, although mentoring is unarguably a crucial activity, no workload nor merit consideration is given for it when evaluation time rolls around. On many faculties there can be a sense of competitiveness that affects the willingness of one member to help another because the new person may eventually outperform the mentor.

Process of Creating Change

A key positive benefit that exists in an academic setting is the freedom a faculty member has in pursuing individual interests. If an idea or activity intrigues the person, it is possible to focus a great deal of time on this interest. It may become the focus of the person's research or publishing pursuits. Individual faculty members have the freedom to choose their interests; they are not assigned as they would be in many other workplaces. Not a lot of time is spent working on projects that someone else has designed.

Paradoxically, however, creating broad system change in an academic setting occurs only at glacial speed. As Donna E. Shalala, former secretary of Health and Human Services, said when asked about whether it was easier to get things done at the University of Miami or in the government, "moving faculty toward change is like moving a cemetery." For example, an individual faculty member may feel strongly about teaching a particular concept to students and adds it to the course syllabus. But this act does not change the overall curriculum of the program. The possibility of an individual faculty member significantly influencing a curriculum revision is unlikely at best. One faculty member said, "It takes an act of Congress to change the curriculum. We just don't have the energy to fill out all of the forms required." The process of changing curriculum is burdensome, to say the least.

Decision making may not be speedy in the service arena, but it is slower in the academic setting. Issues are considered, debated, and examined, and then the process starts over again. New ideas can be shot down by a small minority. People in these systems become worn down by the effort it takes to get a good idea heard, which induces people to leave the academic setting either physically, by resigning, or psychologically, by giving up.

Summary

Successful leaders recognize and meet the unique challenges they experience in trying to create a positive work environment, no matter the type of environment in which they lead. They use the challenges to inspire and call others to action rather than allow the challenge to be used as an excuse. Virtually any characteristic or situation can be either employed as an excuse or seen as a challenge regardless of size or location of the facility, type of facility, or the presence of difficult union–management relationships. The types of challenges can reach the limits of the imagination, including financial downturns, natural disasters, or unfortunate media events, to name a few. These challenges call forth the best effort on the part of capable leaders.

Conversation Points

Organizational Perspective

1. What are the unique challenges of this organization?
2. What is the level of success in creating positive work environments? Has this been taken on as an organizational challenge?
3. Are there currently any temporary situations that are especially challenging (for example, new senior leadership, a financial downturn, or recent negative media event)? How are they affecting the workplace?

Leader Perspective

1. What are the unique challenges that make it difficult for you to create a positive work environment?
2. Do these challenges ever become an excuse for not doing more?

Employee Perspective

1. What are some of the unique characteristics of your department that make it hard to create a positive workplace?
2. Are there any temporary situations that are affecting the level of positivity in your workplace?

12

Age Diversity in the Workforce

Jo Manion

*There is a problem in the workplace—a problem derived not from
downsizing, rightsizing, change, technology, foreign competition,
pointy-haired bosses, bad breath, cubicle envy, or greed.
It is a problem of values, ambitions, views, mind-sets,
demographics, and generations in conflict.*

—Ron Zemke, Claire Raines, and Bob Filipczak

THERE ARE two main challenges related to the demographics of the workplace. The first has to do with the age diversity brought by a multigenerational workforce, and the second is related to retaining the older worker who is nearing retirement. Eventually, all employees do retire. However, retaining these workers for a longer period of time and having someone in place to succeed the individual in the position can make a positive impact on an organization.

In many health systems—and, for that matter, entire countries—the workforce is the most age diverse in history. For the first time, as many as four generations of employees are working together. This diversity can be overwhelming for managers trying to understand the implications for their practice. Much has been written concerning the different experiences and values of members of the different generations, as well as their needs and behaviors in the workplace. However, the practical implications of managing and balancing the impact of these differences are less clear. Although a number of authors suggest implications for managerial approaches, little research actually tests these suggestions and recommendations.

Managing the Multigenerational Workforce

The complexity created by a multigenerational workforce is often cited by managers as one of the toughest challenges they have to creating a healthy, productive, positive practice environment. For this reason, managers need skills in dealing with the diversity represented by a multigenerational workforce. While diversity in the workplace can lead to increased creativity

This chapter is adapted with permission from the policy paper *Managing the Multi-Generational Nursing Workforce*, 2008, for the International Centre for Human Resources in Nursing (ICHRN) and the International Council for Nurses (ICN).

and a greater richness of values and skills, it can also lead to value clashes, disrespect of differing viewpoints, and increased conflict (Swearingen and Liberman 2004; Kupperschmidt 2006). Today's health care organization, struggling with matching resources to needs, cannot afford the high cost of generational enmity.

Defining the Generations

Generational groups are often referred to as cohorts, the members of which are linked to each other through shared life experiences during their formative years. As each cohort ages, it is influenced by what sociologists call generational markers. As products of their environment, members of the cohort are influenced by events that have an impact on all members of the generational grouping (Zemke, Raines, and Filipczak 2000). They share birth years and history, and they develop a collective personality as a result of these generational events. It is believed that each generation possesses unique characteristics and cultural dissimilarities from that of preceding and subsequent generations. An acute awareness of these differences began surfacing in the early 1990s as distinct variations became apparent between workers of the different generations.

Although the mean age of the global population is declining, with 50 percent of the world's current population younger than 20 years of age, the trend has not yet reached developed countries (Alexander 2006). Upcoming population shifts in developed countries result in increased concern with the needs and desires of middle-age and older citizens (Dychtwald and Flower 1990). A combined senior boom and a declining birth rate in many developed countries has resulted in an increase in population of persons over 65 years of age. In the higher-income countries, the ratio of active workers to retired persons is declining.

After World War II, births rose dramatically in many parts of the world. In some countries this birth spurt lasted only a few years. However, in the United States, Canada, Australia, and New Zealand, the so-called baby boom lasted for nearly two decades. Called Baby Boomers, this generation of individuals was born between 1946 and 1964. This large population cohort has dramatically increased awareness of generational differences, both as their experiences entering the workforce differed from their parents and as the succeeding generations' experiences entering the workforce differed from theirs. Other factors have also precipitated increased awareness of generational differences. For example, in Italy, the time set by law for retirement previously was 39 years in the workforce. When this time was increased, the number of older workers (nurses in the case studied) wanting to remain employed also increased (Palese, Pantali, and Saiani 2006), and thus generational differences became increasingly apparent.

The four defined generations in today's workforce include:

- Veterans (born between 1922 and 1945)
- Baby Boomers (born between 1946 and 1964)

- Generation Xers (born between 1965 and 1979)
- Millennials (born between 1980 and 2000)

The years encompassing these generations vary somewhat by author, based on each researcher's experiences with how the members of the cohorts think and act. There are no hard stops that indicate when one generation ends and another begins. These time frames are only guidelines. People born during these years share a common history as a result of the events that occurred during their formative years as well as the conditions of the workplace when they entered it.

The danger of stereotyping or labeling can occur when characteristics of a particular group are identified and presented as absolute fact. Such identification certainly does not mean that these characteristics or attributes are shared by every individual born between the years being discussed. Although generational differences account for diversity in the workplace, so do many other factors, such as cultural heritage, personality traits, and individualized experiences. However, understanding generational information can help explain the sometimes baffling and confusing differences in an individual's unspoken assumptions about how the world operates. It can serve as a beginning point in determining what people believe and hold important. Insight into the values of the different generations helps increase understanding of how these values influence organizational values and the interface between work and family. The following is a summary of the most common differentiating factors of the various generations reported in the literature. More thorough descriptions of these generational cohorts are offered by Duchscher and Cowin (2004).

The Veterans (1922–1945): "The Loyal Generation"

The Veterans grew up in hard times, including the Great Depression in the United States and World War II. They rose to the challenge of rebuilding nations and economies and creating a new foundation for generations to come. Most came of age during the transition from a primarily agrarian way of life to a manufacturing mind-set (Zemke, Raines, and Filipczak 2000). Living through economic and political uncertainty groomed them to be hardworking, financially conservative, and cautious (Sherman 2006).

Veterans like consistency and uniformity, and they are impressed by size, flash, spectacle. They tend to be conformers and value organizational loyalty. Longevity and tenure are, for them, appropriate bases for progression and promotion in their career. They are disciplined and believe in propriety and logic. Members of this generation value the lessons of history and tend to look back and reflect on precedents set that might be helpful and applicable in the present. Their most enduring workplace legacy is the hierarchy and the old command-and-control management style (Zemke, Raines, and Filipczak 2000). They do not take their job for granted and are used to working hard to get things accomplished.

The Baby Boomers (1946–1964): "The Loved Generation"

The Baby Boomers grew up in optimistic, positive times. In many of the developed countries, this was a time of expansion. Most people of this cohort were raised in child-centered nuclear families and grew into ego-centric adults who have continued to rewrite the rules rather than follow the traditional path (Zemke, Raines, and Filipczak 2000). Boomers learned about collaboration and teamwork as they were growing up and brought those sensibilities into the workplace. They pursued their own personal gratification relentlessly and without regard to the cost on relationships and others. Baby Boomers are still optimistic and believe in the infinite possibilities in the world today.

As the Baby Boomers turn fifty, work is slowly slipping down on their list of priorities. As a result, the workplace is becoming more informal and more humane (Zemke, Raines, and Filipczak 2000). The Baby Boomers have redefined and popularized every phase of life as they have passed through it. They form the largest cohort of health care workers, and the oldest segment of this group is within a few years of reaching retirement age. One survey found that "more than two-thirds plan to work after retiring. Most plan to work part time, and a few will even pursue a new career full time" (Zemke, Raines, and Filipczak 2000, p. 89).

Generation X (1965–1979): "The Lost Generation"

This unique generation is a group that went basically unnoticed until the late 1990s. As a generation it is defined more by what it is not, than what it is. Maligned and misunderstood, much of what has been written about this generation is through the eyes of Baby Boomers who simply see them in contrast to themselves rather than as a unique generation. They are often described as "Baby Boomers' children who inherited Boomers' social debris: divorce and dual-career parents resulting in Latch Key Kid experiences" (Kupperschmidt 2006, p. 3). They grew up independent and self-reliant. They saw their parents sacrifice time with them to further their careers, only to be later downsized or restructured out of their positions.

Zemke, Raines, and Filipczak (2000) believe that a person's first job experience significantly affects their values and expectations of the workplace. For example, many Generation Xers' (or GenXers) first work experiences occurred during a time of national recession and massive reorganization and restructuring efforts in health care. The lessons they learned are that there is no such thing as job security, hierarchical reverence is worthless, and "paying your dues" is just a worn-out cliché from the previous generation. Instead, increasing your own marketability through additional job skills and development is the path to success. One way they achieve this level of marketability and develop skills and personal attributes is by changing jobs frequently. Santos and Cox (2000) report that the GenXers in their study clearly indicated they anticipated moving out of their organization and even the profession during the course of their work life. "They indicated this arrogance was not arrogance at all but the need to be self-reliant as they have had to be throughout their lifetime" (Santos and Cox 2000, p. 12).

The Generation X cohort is smaller than that of the Baby Boomers. Add the fact that fewer GenXers chose health care careers in the 1990s, and it becomes clear that a demographic collision is waiting to happen as the Baby Boomers are beginning to transition from the active workforce. The good news is that more GenXers are choosing health care as a second or even third career (Kupperschmidt 2006; Sherman 2006).

The Millennials (1980–2000): "The Linked Generation"

The Millennials, or Generation Y as they are sometimes referred to, are the second largest cohort in the general population (Raines 2002). Raised by nurturing parents, they have lived structured and incredibly busy lives filled with activities and scheduled events that rival the most workaholic Baby Boomer. They value their families highly and remain close within them. During their childhood they saw violence, terrorism, and drugs become realities of life. They are the first truly global generation and have incorporated multiculturalism as a way of life. They are the most connected generation in history. Advanced computer technology and instant, constant communication through cellular phones and text messaging are a way of life for them.

In the qualitative study conducted of Italian chief nurses (charge nurses), Palese, Pantali, and Saiani (2006, p. 179) report that "'fragility' is a characteristic found in all of those belonging to Generation Y, having grown up in a family environment in an overprotective society which tended not to give them responsibility." This is also the generation that grew up with the "everyone gets a blue ribbon" and "everyone gets selected to the team" mentality. Some managers are finding that in working with members of this generation, they also must contend with the employee's parents, who are so overly involved in their child's life that they become part of the workplace relationship as well, communicating with the manager about issues, giving approval for schedules, and even attending performance appraisals sessions.

Conventional wisdom suggests that there are differences in characteristics of generational cohorts—ask any parent. Although little empirical research has been done to substantiate this claim, many authors offer observations on the core values of each generational cohort as well as project their assets and liabilities on the job. These factors are summarized in table 12-1. This table is a brief overview of the differences between the generations for purposes of understanding the challenges faced by health care managers.

Managerial Issues Related to the Multigenerational Workforce

The incredible amount of diversity in today's workplace places demands on current managers unlike any previously experienced. Diversity is not limited to generational differences; however, the presence of diversity in other areas simply increases the importance of leadership skills for effectively dealing with diversity. The current generational diversity is also unique in a rather striking way: The generations in today's workforce are more likely to be

Table 12-1.   Generational Differences

	Veterans	Baby Boomers	GenXers	Millennials
Core Values	• Dedication/ sacrifice • Hard work • Conformity • Law and order • Respect for authority • Patience • Delayed reward • Duty before pleasure • Follow the rules • Honor	• Optimism • Team orientation • Personal gratification • Health and wellness • Personal growth • Work • Youth • Involvement • Like to belong	• Diversity • Thinking globally • Balance private and work life • Technoliterate • Fun • Informality • Self-reliance • Pragmatism • Apolitical • Prefer no ties • Start at the top	• Optimism • Civic duty • Confidence • Achievement • Sociability • Morality • Street smarts • Diversity • Idealistic • Prefer no ties
Assets on the Job	• Stable • Detail oriented • Thorough • Loyal • Hardworking	• Service orientation • Driven • Willing to go the extra mile • Good at relationships • Want to please • Good team players • Focused on the job	• Adaptable • Technoliterate • Independent • Unintimidated by authority • Creative • Focused on career • Want variety	• Collective action • Optimism • Tenacity • Heroic spirit • Multitasking capabilities • Technological savvy • Ambitious
Liabilities on the Job	• Inept with ambiguity and change • Reluctant to buck the system • Uncomfortable with conflict • Reticent when they disagree	• Not naturally budget minded • Uncomfortable with conflict • Reluctant to go against peers • Overly sensitive to feedback • Judgmental of those who see things differently • Self-centered • Sacrifice for the job • Little faith in authority	• Impatient • Poor people skills • Inexperienced • Cynical, skeptical • Will not sacrifice for the job • Lack of respect for authority	• Need for supervision and structure • Inexperience, especially handling difficult people issues

mixed at all levels of the organization. In the past, older workers were often at the more senior levels of management, with younger workers on the front line. However, generational status is no longer tightly linked to job status. Even relatively young Millennials can be found at senior levels in some organizations. Whereas in the past the question from Baby Boomer managers was, "How do I manage these young GenXers?" the question today is just as often from the Generation X manager who asks, "How do I manage these Baby Boomers?"

The uniqueness of this situation is seen in another way as well. As the age of new health care professional graduates continues to rise, generation-specific understanding becomes important for faculty and academic settings. Students in the health sciences are no longer most frequently a 21- or 22-year-old young man or woman. Increasing numbers of second- and even third-career workers are choosing health care.

As with the issues identified in chapter 11, although creating a positive workplace may be more challenging in an age-diverse environment than in a workplace without this diversity, the presence of a multigenerational workforce does not make it impossible to achieve. Strategies for managing a multigenerational workforce include the following:

1. Create a workplace culture and environment that engages all workers.
2. Remain adaptive to current circumstances and respond with flexibility in approaches and practices.
3. Deal with the culture clash and conflict that can occur between members of the different generations.
4. Recognize and use generation-specific interventions and approaches.

Strategy 1: Create a Workplace Culture that Engages All Workers

This book has already made the case that the highly effective health care manager is one who recognizes the importance of creating a workplace that supports a positive, healthy practice environment (Stuenkel and Cohen 2005). While clearly potential differences exist between members of the various generational cohorts, focusing solely on these differences can create a sense of hopelessness or unfounded pessimism. It is helpful to remember that although members of each generation may be different in many ways, they are also alike in many ways. And, ultimately, focusing on the universality of human experience may serve as a more productive beginning point for the leader focused on retention. In fact, some research suggests that the differences in the values of the four generations, at least in the nursing workforce, are not as divergent as sometimes reported. McNeese-Smith and Crook (2003, p. 266) report that "Generation X had higher values for both variety and economic returns. However, no other significant differences were identified."

Chapter 2 presented findings from the psychological, sociological, and organizational development research on human motivators and why people work. Understanding the five basic intrinsic human motivators serves as a starting point for creating a positive environment. These intrinsic motivators have been presented in-depth earlier in the book; they are healthy working relationships, the belief that one's work is meaningful, competence, autonomy or decision-making ability, and seeing progress as a result of one's efforts.

However, a few cautions and clarifications about using these intrinsic motivators are in order. First, not all of the intrinsic motivators are equally important to everyone. Members of generational cohorts may vary in the following three distinct ways. First, what is most important to them as a cohort may be different. For example, Baby Boomers are said to value relationships and attach a great deal of importance to the meaningfulness of their work. Generally, GenXers value their competence and self-efficacy as well as having jobs that stress independence, autonomy, and choice. Again, however, this does not mean that there cannot be overlap in individuals in these various generational cohorts.

A second way the members of the different generations may be distinct in their valuing of the intrinsic motivators is in how they define the meaningfulness of their work. The Millennials have a strong sense of civic duty and are likely to define meaningful work as work that contributes to societal good, while GenXers may define meaningful work as work that advances their career or helps them develop a broader range of skills in order to become personally more marketable. Members of the Veteran generation may define meaningful work as that which provides safety and security for their family and community.

And yet a third way the generations may be distinct is in what they are likely to do if the workplace does not provide for their most important values or needs. For example, Baby Boomers may be more inclined to stay with an organization because they value security and longevity. GenXers are more likely to leave and go on to another job. One GenX manager demonstrated this when she told her colleagues, "When I stop learning anything new in this job, I'm out of here." This sentiment not only relates to the universal human motivator of competence but also illustrates a generational difference in how she will handle her disappointment when her job fails to provide what is important to her.

Strategy 2: Remain Adaptive to Current Circumstances and Respond with Flexibility

It has long been recognized and accepted that a hallmark of leadership effectiveness is the ability of the leader to assess what is needed in a given situation or interaction and to respond flexibly, choosing a response that matches the situation. In the 1960s, the model of situational leadership was developed and is still of practical value in today's work world. To be effective, the leader accurately diagnoses the situation and uses an appropriate style to supplement what the follower lacks. This effort requires flexibility on the part of the leader. In the same way, the high level of diversity in the workplace means that an effective leader must adapt his or her style and employ a flexible style and approaches that meet the needs of the follower. Managers who put their employees first are more likely to find that employees put the patients or customers first. Flexibility and versatility require both keen judgment and the ability to move between various styles and approaches.

This challenge is daunting, to say the least. It is based on understanding that one approach does not fit every person or every situation. One key principle, however, can make meeting the challenge easier. Instead of assuming all employees fit the defined characteristics of a particular generational cohort, ask employees directly what is important to them or how they want to be treated. Nothing can substitute for knowing employees well and matching the workplace culture with what they believe is important.

One potential difference between the members of the various generations is in what they expect from their manager. Wieck, Prydun, and Walsh (2003) studied nursing members of the "entrenched generations" and the "emerging generations" to determine what they want from their leaders. Interestingly, out of fifty-six characteristics, seven appeared on the characteristics list of both groups. No statistical differences were found in how the characteristics were ranked between the older and younger generations. Honesty was high on the list for both groups. Eight of the ten characteristics identified by the younger nurses could be categorized as "nurturing." "These traits—motivational, receptive, positive, good communicator, team player, good people skills, approachable and supportive— all depict an environment in which younger nurses feel nurtured and supported" (Wieck, Prydun, and Walsh 2003, p. 287). In further research, as yet unpublished, Wieck reports that the generations seem to have similar desires for their managers. The characteristics depict a flexible, nurturing manager.

Strategy 3: Deal with the Conflict that Can Occur between Generations

Conflicts occur more readily when people hold different values, especially in the high-stress environments that characterize health care organizations. Many authors are reporting a particularly negative subculture within health care that includes high levels of horizontal violence and dysfunctional interpersonal behaviors (Santos and Cox 2000; Swearingen and Liberman 2004; Kupperschmidt 2006; WHO 2006). Nursing comprises about 60 percent of the health care workforce, and any characteristic of this group will ultimately affect the organization. This type of negative culture can lead to toxic behaviors such as discounting each other, making rude or cruel comments about people who are different, withholding important information, and other forms of disrespect. Kupperschmidt (2006) contends that mutual respect is a key factor in reducing intergenerational conflict in the workplace. An effective manager is aware of what is going on in the work area and addresses negative behaviors immediately.

Examples of important managerial interventions for dealing with conflict resulting from the clash of these different cultures include the following:

- Establish clear expectations for behaviors based on the elements of healthy relationships.
- Lead the work group in establishing its behavioral expectations of each other, developing a code of conduct or an operating agreement that clearly spells out what behaviors are desired and what are not acceptable.
- Set a no tolerance policy for gossip, behavior that demeans others, toxic aggression, chronic negativity, bullying, mean-spiritedness, or disrespect.
- Ensure that employees have skills in healthy conflict resolution and giving each other feedback, both positive and constructive.
- Engage employees in value-clarification exercises that focus on the different values each holds.
- Continually re-emphasize the common mission or purpose that binds people together.
- Emphasize the similarities between people rather than the differences.

In their study of chief nurses in Italy, Palese, Pantali, and Saiani (2006) report that there did not seem to be any real conflict between the generational groups. Instead, they found that the coexistence of a number of different generations in the workplace led to the formation of small groups of individuals who are similar in attitude and behaviors but at odds with groups made up of staff from different generations. They report that these small groups did not seem to compete among themselves, but instead had different objectives. And when employees separate into generational groups, "the staff lose the opportunity of a reciprocal exchange of information which would benefit both the staff and the patients" (Palese, Pantali, and Saiani 2006, p. 181).

Strategy 4: Recognize and Use Generation-Specific Interventions and Approaches

The final challenge facing the leader is to become knowledgeable about generational differences and skilled in using generation-specific interventions and approaches. Although it is dangerous to assume that the characteristics discussed above apply equally to all individuals within a cohort, it can be just as dangerous to assume everyone from all cohorts is alike and needs to be treated exactly the same. An understanding of generational differences can be a beginning point in making sense of behaviors and beliefs. Many authors (e.g., Kupperschmidt 2006; Lancaster and Stillman 2002; Sherman 2006; Wieck 2000, 2003; Zemke 2002) offer specific guidelines for recruiting, orienting, training, motivating, and coaching individuals from different generations. These are summarized in table 12-2. Although they may be helpful, it is important to remember that no or only limited empirical research has tested these managerial interventions.

Table 12-2. Managerial Ramifications of Generational Differences

	Veterans	Baby Boomers	GenXers	Millennials
Recruiting	• Know they like part-time work and projects • Stress their valuable experience • Be courteous and respectful (say please, thank you, etc.) • Communicate messages that speak to traditional work values	• Acknowledge experience • Set a challenge • Stress a humane environment • Give them credit and respect for their achievements • Show them how they can be a star	• Emphasize balance • Stress merit • Discuss changes expected • Create a fun, intimate environment • Emphasize technology • Emphasize independence • Implement flexibility in scheduling	• Sell organization solidly • Show opportunity • Emphasize organization's importance • Sell them on the job • Tell how organization meets its civic duties • Customize job opportunities • Be flexible
Orienting	• Take the time to explain • Share the organization's story • Bring them into the goals of the group, and explain how they will contribute	• Emphasize goals and challenges • Show them the opportunity	• Show technology, allow for exploring • Show who's who list, who knows what • Repeat the work-life balance message • De-emphasize the politics	• Be clear on expectations • Show opportunities • Emphasize equality • Sheltered, will need lots of support
Training	• Need technology training, but don't underestimate • Take time, use an older trainer • Use large text in printed materials	• Share strategy, budgeting, etc. • Use their book knowledge • Give developmental assignments • Use books, tapes, and videos	• Give multiple opportunities • Stress self-development • Understand they are self-directed learners • Be more task and not process oriented • Know they dislike groups and meetings • Be brief • Stress project opportunities	• Provide how-to training • Assign mentors • Use lots of details • Understand they like collaborative action, group work, and high levels of involvement • Use interactive approach • Didactic lectures are boring to them

(Continued on next page)

Table 12-2. (Continued)

	Veterans	Baby Boomers	GenXers	Millennials
Motivating	• Use the personal touch, notes, and calls • Provide traditional perks • Use them as mentors • Reward is a job well done	• Personal relationships are important • Public recognition • Work perks • Name recognition (get them quoted) • Reward hours and efforts • Talk about legacy • Know they like involvement and participation	• Provide opportunities to develop skills • Provide opportunities for promotion • Assign multiple tasks and projects • Give feedback but do not micromanage • Allow laxness • Give freedom as a reward	• Provide competitive pay and benefits • Provide good environment • Show opportunities for advancement • Provide career planning and counseling • Know they are socially conscious • Understand they like feeling they do a job well • Their reward is meaningful work
Coaching	• Be tactful • Be private • Build rapport • Be respectful • Ask permission to coach • "No news is good news"	• Be tactful • Create harmony, warmth, agreement • Use questions, not statements • Treat as equals • Ask questions to get to the issues • Give yearly feedback with documentation	• Be direct and honest • Value equity and fairness • More relaxed and informal • Feedback needs to be continual and focused on "How am I doing?"	• Like public recognition • Develop trust • Be honest and direct • Listen • Show confidence • Treat like an adult • They expect feedback with the push of a button • Need detail and structure

While all employees must be held to the same work expectations and organizational policies and procedures (Hart 2006), managerial approaches can take generational differences into account. For example, according to Lancaster and Stillman (2002), the way members of the different generations perceive authority can be somewhat disconcerting unless understood. Veterans tend to believe in and follow the chain of command, while Baby Boomers expect a change of command; they want to rewrite the rules. GenXers believe in self-command, and Millennials collaborate rather than believe in command.

Rewards are important to individualize as well. Veterans value a job well done, while Baby Boomers like titles and recognition. GenXers want the reward of freedom to do things their own way, and Millennials seek a sense of meaningfulness of the work. Hart (2006) reports that Baby Boomers are more influenced by money and the younger generations by time off. Finding ways to meet the needs of the different generations is the challenge for today's organizations.

How they view job changes can also explain the difficulty in retaining younger generations. While Veterans see changing jobs as a stigma, Baby Boomers find that changing jobs causes them to lag behind others in their career progression. GenXers see it as a necessity, while Millennials consider a job change almost as routine. Baby Boomers are focused on the job, while members of the younger generation are focused on a career. Palese, Pantali, and Saiani (2006) found that a sense of belonging was important to older nurses, while younger nurses wanted few ties in the workplace so they would be free to be nomadic.

A Cautionary Note

It is widely believed and accepted that the values, ambitions, views, beliefs, and behaviors vary according to generational cohorts—simply listen to any group of health care managers in the cafeteria. Certainly reports of these differences are surfacing globally, especially from developed nations, and the extent to which they hold true in developing countries remains to be seen. Swearingen and Liberman (2004, p. 55) believe that "similarities of experience within and differentiation of experiences between age group cohorts are observable in every culture. Similar functioning is imposed by society on those sharing an age cohort at a particular time. The same is true of any major event in personal history, which is identified by age."

A cautionary note must be re-emphasized. Much has been made of the differences between members of the various cohorts. However, the truth is that many factors influence what is important to people in their work. Generational differences certainly account for and explain part of the situation. The members of different generations have had different lived experiences, and these influence the way they view their work and their behaviors in relation to their careers. However, there are likely other significant factors that are less frequently discussed. One striking factor is simply that people need and value different things at different ages throughout their lives.

It makes sense that younger workers entering their field are likely to be focused on gaining mastery and building their level of competence. When these younger workers begin raising a family, their needs and desires about workplace benefits, working schedules, and opportunities are affected by this major life change. Workers nearing the end of their career are more interested in their legacy and planning for transition to a reduced work life or retirement. Social issues also affect what is important to people in the various generations and in different countries. For example, the frequency of grandparents raising grandchildren is increasing, which affects retirement age as well as needs for better work-home life balance.

And a final reminder: Pronouncements of certain values or attributes never apply consistently to all members of the age cohort, no matter how well researched these characteristics might be. Individual personalities and experiences affect behaviors and values as well. And although some of these generalizations may be helpful, ultimately they must be validated with the individual or work group to determine their applicability.

As mentioned earlier, when members of different generations focus on and emphasize how they are different from one another, they can raise barriers and create increased conflict between themselves and others. An alternative strategy is to recognize the possibility of differences, yet understand that there are many universal elements of the human experience. When a manager recognizes and builds on similarities, he or she may ultimately be more successful in bringing people together. Thus, a key managerial strategy is to build on how employees are alike while respecting how each is different.

Managing Workplace Exits through Retirement

The United States has the largest professional health care workforce of any country in the world. While physicians and nurses have been studied most extensively, all health care disciplines and categories of workers—as well as other fields—are experiencing the same phenomena at a rapid rate: the aging of the active workforce. This situation results in the following considerations. The first is, what can be done to delay an older worker's exit in order to retain the experience and productivity of the individual for as long as possible? The second consideration is, how does one manage the knowledge transfer so that when a seasoned, highly experienced individual does leave, invaluable information and resources are not lost to the organization? This issue is of such importance that an alliance of more than twenty organizations, called the Alliance for an Experienced Workforce, is working to cultivate best practices on matters such as employee benefits, workplace design, and recruitment strategies (Thrall 2006).

From a review of the literature it is clear that employers, as well as governments, that are concerned about the vitality and size of their future workforce consider the retention of the older worker as a strategic initiative that has the potential of helping them achieve their goals. This is an issue that extends well beyond health care. The testimony before governmental bodies, appointment of special committees, and commissioned research have all focused on what might be done to successfully retain the older person in the workforce (Armstrong-Stassen 2004; Commonwealth of Australia 2003; Hatcher et al. 2006; Walker 2007).

In testimony before the U.S. Senate Special Committee on Aging, Walker (2007, p. 4) sums up the issue based on U.S. population statistics: "The aging of the baby boom generation, increased life expectancy, and fertility rates at about the replacement level are expected to significantly increase the elderly dependency ratio—the estimated number of people aged 65 and over in relation to the number of people aged 15–64." This ratio was one person over 65 per every eight people age 15–64 in 1950. The ratio is projected to increase to one person aged 65 and over for every three people age 15–64 by 2050. This trend results in an enormous impact on the U.S. federal government programs of Social Security and Medicare. There will be fewer younger workers to support those drawing benefits.

Other indirect ramifications are in store for any national economy. Two of the most significant include fewer available workers to produce the goods and services that drive the economy and less taxable income resulting in lower government revenue. With increasing life expectancy, people who retire at earlier ages will spend more years in retirement and draw on these pension benefits for a longer period of time. Extending the length of time older people remain active in the workforce not only provides necessary labor for a country but also delays their drawing on retirement funds. As older people remain in the workforce, their income also remains taxable, thereby continuing to bolster federal revenues.

The U.S. Bureau of Labor Statistics released nursing workforce projections for 2004–2014, which included an increase in the 55–64 age cohort of more than seven million. The number of workers 65 and older is expected to increase nearly seven times as fast as the total labor force. Hart (2007), reporting on nursing demographic changes, suggests that workers postponing retirement account for this upswing in the older categories. The most recent national registered nurse (RN) survey conducted by the Health Resources and Services Administration estimates the average age of the registered nurse as 46.8, which is more than a year older than the estimated average of 45.2 from the 2000 survey. A statistic of concern reported by Buerhaus (2002 p. 4) is that "Between 1983 and 1998, the number of RNs in the workforce younger than 30 years fell 41%." In 2002, more than 60 percent of the nursing workforce was older than 40 years of age.

Similar statistics are reported from other countries as well. Spinks and Moore (2007) report that across the Western world the average age of the working population, not just in health care, is increasing. In 2010, older workers (age 55–64) will outnumber younger workers (age 20–29) for the first time. Canada leads the industrialized world in the speed at which the over 45-year-old labor force is increasing. By using simulation models for workforce planning, O'Brien-Pallas and colleagues (2005, p. 18) report that "results indicate that if nurses retire by age 65, 13% of Canadian nurses will be lost to retirement or death by the year 2006. However, if nurses retire by age 55, Canada will lose almost 28% of the workforce by early 2006."

Similar reports have emerged from Australia. More than 61 percent of nurses are 40 years of age or older (O'Brien-Pallas, Duffield, and Alksnis 2004 p. 298). As these nurses near retirement age, staffing difficulties in health care organizations are predicted to be exacerbated. The Royal College of Nursing, Australia (2004, p. 4) reports, "The proportion of workers aged over 45 increased by 17% between 1987 and 2001 and the under 35 decreased from 54% to 30% in the same time period." The report goes on to note that an aging nursing workforce is not simply an Australian problem. "Figures for England show that in 1996, 40% of National Health Service (NHS) nurses, midwives and health visitors were under 35. By 1999 the proportion under 35 had dropped to 33% (and, in Scotland it was 21% in 1998). At the same time the proportion over 45, that is, within ten years of retirement, has increased from 27 to 29%." In the United Kingdom all nurses and midwives who intend to practice must be registered, and in the space of just nine years a significant age shift was seen. "The proportion in the youngest age groups halved, whilst those in the older age groups have correspondingly increased" (Buchan 1999, p. 819). These nurses have retirement rights enabling them to retire with full benefits at age 55.

In countries where life span is increasing, the demands for health care services expand. Because of the size of the generational cohorts, as aging Baby Boomer health care workers approach and reach retirement, inadequate numbers of younger workers are available to replace them. And at a time when demand for health care services will reach an all-time high, it is no wonder that this rapidly approaching collision of demographics has led to the need for careful management of this transition of workers from the active workforce.

In *Wisdom at Work: The Importance of the Older and Experienced Nurse in the Workplace* (Hatcher et al. 2006), it is reported that of American nurses age 40 and over, more than 82 percent plan to retire in the next twenty years. "One in five nurses in the UK is aged 50 years or older" (Buchan 1999, p. 818). Projections in other developed countries mirror this finding. It is little wonder that workforce experts believe a viable strategy for easing this daunting potential nursing shortage is to retain these nurses in the workforce for as long as possible. Canadian forecasters used simulation models to project the probable result. O'Brien-Pallas and colleagues (2005) conclude that almost half of the projected losses from nurses retiring could be avoided if the health care system retained 100 percent of nurses age 50–54, 75 percent of those age 55–59, and 50 percent of those age 60–64. Although other disciplines have not been studied as extensively as nursing, the same basic principles are likely in operation.

Factors Influencing Older Workers' Employment Decisions

A key issue rarely addressed is how amenable older workers would be to employer strategies and public policies designed to encourage them to remain on the job. In a Canadian study, Morissette, Schellenberg, and Silver (2004) asked retired respondents what factors might have influenced them to continue working. The participants included 1.8 million persons who retired between 1992 and 2002. Overall, 60 percent of recent retirees indicated a willingness to continue working if certain incentives had existed. These incentives included a reduction of work schedule without pension being affected, more vacation leave, salary increases, and availability of suitable caregiving arrangements (which included flexibility in scheduling, respite care, and access to caregivers so that the employee could continue to care for an elderly parent or loved one). One-third of the recent retirees left the workplace because of health reasons. Another third would not have continued working for any of the reasons offered. The researchers concluded that the remaining third of healthy retirees would have been willing to remain in the workforce (at least partially), and this category of employees offers employers the best prospect for increasing the overall supply of labor.

In reviewing these results, it must be noted that the retirees in this study are most likely members of the Veteran generational cohort. It has been suggested (Lancaster and Stillman 2002) that retirement is perceived differently by members of the different generations. Veterans tend to view retirement as reward while members of the Baby Boom generation see it as a time to retool and try other things. This perspective may explain the finding in the Canadian study that "compared to their counterparts aged 60–64, retirees aged 50–59 were more likely to report that they would have continued working" (Morissette, Schellenberg, and Silver 2004, p. 3). If the Baby Boom generation, which is fast approaching retirement age, sees retirement as a time to retool, they may actually be more amenable to incentives that keep them in the workforce.

Watson, Manthorpe, and Andrews (2003a, 2003b) conducted a study that investigated issues related to options, decisions, and outcomes for nurses over age 50 in terms of remaining in, retiring from, or returning to work in the National Health Services in the United Kingdom. The following needs were identified:

- Flexibility—in the form of part-time work, job sharing, flextime, or school term-time schedules for older nurses with care responsibilities for children
- Fitness—working in areas with reduced stress and workload as well as changes of work practices and better use of equipment to reduce physical strain
- Reduced stress—due to factors such as staff shortages, excess paperwork, and insufficient time to complete tasks properly
- Pay—higher compensation to encourage nurses to remain working
- Morale among nurses—related to nurses feeling valued for their contributions, involved decisions about their work, and respecting the older worker

Watson and his colleagues (2003a, 2003b) conducted interviews of older nurses who were remaining in the workplace or had retired from or returned to an employment setting. These are the significant findings:

- Although many older workers mentioned flexibility in conjunction with a supportive environment as influencing their own decisions about employment, examples of flexible working alternatives were not evident in the workplace.
- "There was a widespread feeling among the nurses interviewed, whether remaining or retired, that stress and the associated burnout were major influences on decision making with regard to employment over the age of 50" (Watson, Manthorpe, and Andrews 2003b, p. 38).
- A major influence on older nurses' employment decisions was money. Many of the nurses were the sole earner in their family or were working to supplement the family income.
- Pension considerations often dictated whether it was appropriate for the worker to retire at a particular time or whether it was worth it to work for a few more years to increase the pension. The need for changes in the National Health Services superannuation scheme could result in less penalty for older nurses accepting part-time work or reducing their hours and responsibilities in other ways.
- Almost all of the nurses in the study reported that little or no information was offered to them about their options. Just at a time when the employee needed sound advice before making a decision, they were left on their own to find relevant information.

Armstrong-Stassen (2004) conducted research in Ontario, Canada, to evaluate human resource management practices that are important in the decision of health care workers (in this case nurses) age 50 and older to remain in the workforce. A second objective of the research was to determine the extent to which health care facilities are engaging in these practices. The five most important human resource management practices in retaining older workers were:

1. Improving benefits
2. Showing appreciation for a job well done
3. Providing flexible work schedules
4. Recognizing the experience, knowledge, skill, and expertise of workers 50 and over
5. Ensuring that workers 50 and over are treated with respect by others in the organization

The five least important human resource management practices in retaining older health care workers were adjusting efforts to attract workers 50 and over; offering elder or parental care provisions such as unpaid leave;

offering job sharing; providing "age awareness" training programs for managers; and encouraging later, rather than early, retirement. "The retention of nurses 50 and older will be strongly influenced by human resource management practices" (Armstrong-Stassen 2004, p. 25); however, the findings of the study report several significant shortfalls in how these organizations are actually doing. These are the key findings from the respondents:

- Seventy-two percent ranked improved benefits as very important in their decision to remain in the workforce, yet only 3 percent reported that their employer was highly engaged in offering them.
- Sixty-seven percent rated recognizing the experience, knowledge, skill, and expertise of the older worker as very important to their remaining actively employed. Only 12 percent of these participants reported their hospital/agency as currently highly engaged in doing so.
- Sixty-seven percent rated flexible working options as very important, but only 14 percent reported that their hospital/agency was currently highly engaged in offering them.
- Providing educational support was rated as very important by 57 percent, and yet only 15 percent reported that their hospital/agency was currently highly involved in doing this.
- Sixty-two percent indicated that redesigning work processes to minimize the negative impact on the worker's health was very important in their decision to remain actively employed, yet only 4 percent indicated that this is occurring in their workplace. Eighty-three percent also reported that their employer was not currently engaged in reducing workload pressure and job demands of workers 50 and over.
- Sixty-three percent indicated that providing retirement with callback arrangements (re-employment of retirees on a part-time or temporary basis) is very important to their decision to remain in the workplace. Only 4 percent reported that their employer is actively involved in providing any type of phased retirement options.

These findings seem to indicate that either these organizations do not know what older workers consider important or they do not care. Few are providing the support and practices that might be instrumental in retaining the older worker in order to maintain a healthy, vibrant workforce.

A survey conducted by AARP in 2003 (reported in Feinsod and Davenport 2006, p. 20) of more than two thousand workers age 50–70 sought to determine the specific workplace attributes these workers are seeking. Among those interested in working in their retirement years, their most important aspects included:

- An environment in which their opinions are valued and in which they can gain new skills and experiences
- The ability to choose their hours, take time off to care for relatives or loved ones, and work from home

- An organization that allows people age 50 and older to remain employed for as long as they want to continue working
- The opportunity to have new experiences and learn new skills
- Access to good health benefits

In an unpublished qualitative study by Reiners (2008), it was found that those workers who had job histories of between 31 and 40 years felt that generally they were neglected by managers and supervisors. Yet they wanted to be heard, validated, and supported. The assumption on the part of the managers was that these people are seasoned, they are doing fine, they do not need the same nurturance and support the younger employees need. As a result, the older workers felt they were left on their own more often and supervisors were less likely to check in with them and offer support. Paradoxically, it seems that the very act that acknowledges the older workers value, that is, their knowledge, experience, and ability to handle things and function independently, is what led the older workers to perceive they were not valued.

Most of the research has been conducted on nursing populations, and most is focused on demographics and factors influencing the person's decision to remain in or leave the active workforce. Although an extensive number of articles suggest strategies for retaining older workers, only a limited number are based on empirical evidence. In many cases, strategies are recommended because they are thought to be helpful in retaining the older employee in the workplace.

Strategies for Retaining the Older Health Care Worker

The strategies for retaining the older health care worker most commonly suggested can be categorized into the following six areas:

1. Correcting myths and misperceptions of and about employing older workers
2. Creating a high-quality, positive work environment
3. Changing the physical environment
4. Altering the work itself (job redesign, new roles)
5. Restructuring pay and benefits
6. Instituting flexible working models

Correcting Misperceptions of and about Older Workers

Some countries offer strong incentives for persons of a certain age to retire. A culture of retirement exists that encourages workers to claim retirement benefits and stop working as early as possible. Other countries have limits to how long a worker may be actively employed and/or mandatory retirement ages that are stringently enforced. These policies create a perception in the minds of citizens that after a certain age, continued participation in the workforce is undesirable.

Another of the most common misperceptions is that older workers cost an employer more. This is based on the logic that the older worker has more tenure and is at a higher rate of compensation. It also stems from a conclusion that an older worker has more health problems than a younger worker. The U.S.-based firm Towers & Perrin studied this issue extensively for AARP and found that most of these stereotypes are not grounded in fact (Feinsod and Davenport 2006). The researchers found that motivation in workers tends to increase with age. Older workers were more engaged and thus less likely to leave, resulting in costly turnover.

The findings in other studies related to productivity and age vary. Some studies suggest that worker productivity tends to decline between the ages of 30 and 40, while other studies found no significant differences. It was found that the increased knowledge and experience of older workers can actually off-set any cognitive declines that may occur with age. This study, conducted by Feinsod and Davenport (2006), also found that the cost impact of hiring and retaining older workers is quite modest, at the most approximately 3 percent.

In studies of health care workers, on-the-job injuries are an issue. "One of the age-related employment issues of particular concern in nursing is the high incidence of back injury amongst older nurses" (Buchan 1999, p. 824). Watson, Manthorpe, and Andrews (2003a, 2003b) report that the percentage of back injuries is more than three times higher for nurses over age 55. However, overall health status may not be as significant an issue as believed. Norman (2005) found that although work setting varied with the nurse's age, there were no significant differences in self-reported health status by age. However, Norman did report that many nurses fear developing neck and back injuries from direct patient care, which may induce some nurses to leave the acute care environment. This finding is likely to apply to any health care worker who moves and lifts patients.

Additionally, many negative stereotypes about older workers are pervasive in the workplace, including the belief that these employees produce lower-quality work than their younger counterparts and do less work overall. Buchan (1999, p. 824) found that "Whilst there was general support for the desirability of employing older nurses, most managers also expressed the opinion that nursing work was 'changing' in ways which made it more challenging for older nurses." This change included more rapid patient throughput and higher patient acuity in hospitals, and higher patient dependency in community nursing. Some employers believe the older members of the workforce are more resistant to change. Organizations adhering to this conventional wisdom are missing a critical opportunity to maximize their talent base.

Under this conventional wisdom can be included the age bias as perceived by workers. Eliminating age bias is much harder than might be expected (Wolf 2001). Despite age discrimination protection, the notion persists that "older people have had their day and should make room for the next generation" (Grossman 2003, p. 1). Grossman reports the results of an AARP study that surveyed 1,500 employed workers age 45–74, which found that 67 percent said age discrimination is a fact of life in the workplace and that they have concerns about opportunities to advance. Sixty percent believed that older workers are the first to go when employers reduce their staff. Another survey he reports found that 25 percent of workers planning to retire in the next five years were leaving because they were being held back or felt marginalized because of their age.

Many older workers are reluctant to report their plans for retirement or phasing out of the workforce because of their fear of being replaced. There is a history of older workers being replaced during organizational restructurings or reductions in force. Organizations and managers must build a climate of trust where these issues can be discussed frankly. Only a partnership approach makes it possible to do adequate workforce planning. For example, if an older employee is considering altering the work arrangement to meet personal commitments such as providing care for a grandchild or simply because of desired lifestyle changes, ensuring the freedom to talk about this openly with the manager allows alternatives to sometimes be negotiated.

Suggestions for dealing with these misperceptions include the advice to:

- Confront these biases with facts.
- Seek out older workers and consider them for open positions.
- Always hire the best person for the job, regardless of age.
- Offer job retraining and educational programs to update skills or develop new skills.
- Educate managers on communication preferences and motivators for the different age groups.

Creating a High-Quality, Positive Work Environment

Clearly a crucial aspect of a positive work environment is one in which generational differences are recognized, respected, and tapped into as a source of strength. Good potential employees look for departments and organizations where everyone works well cross-generationally. To develop this kind of open, trusting culture, many employers are implementing training and educational sessions for all employees on the differences and uniqueness of the various groupings. Employers are also seeking ways to accommodate the priorities of multiple generations and are implementing work-life balance strategies that are sensitive to multiple generations.

This balance is important in retaining older employees. Once an individual is financially able to retire, if the workplace is unpleasant or a source of conflict and strife, the environment becomes a push factor, that is, an element that exerts force and pressure on the individual to leave. Thus, one key strategy for managers is to do everything possible to create a work environment where employees enjoy working together, where the connections between people are strong and healthy, and where employee needs are being met. Research conducted by McIntosh, Palumbo, and Rambar (2002) found that the most important determinant of job satisfaction among older staff members is working with helpful and friendly people.

A workplace where stress is manageable and the employee is respected, valued, and appreciated for contributions is one that is more likely to retain the older worker (Armstrong-Strassen 2004; Buchan 1999; Watson, Manthorpe, and Andrews 2003a, 2003b). "The most effective solution, experts say, is to become a good place to work" (Thrall 2005, p. 32). This sounds simplistic, but in fact it is a key responsibility of any health care manager. And the results benefit not just the older worker but workers from every age cohort.

Understanding the basic human motivators as discussed in Part I of this book and referring to the extensive literature on positive, healthy practice environments is a good place to begin building that environment.

Changing the Physical Environment

Many strategies have been suggested that take into account the older worker's physical needs. Certainly some age-related challenges can affect productivity such as a different perception of light and sound, reduced physical endurance, reduced range of motion and muscle strength, and longer reaction time. Many organizations are taking these age-related physical changes into account. In some cases, institutions have employed ergonomic experts to follow employees during their daily work to determine unnecessary stressors.

In a survey of 377 nurses, it was found that older nurses were more likely to be employed in ambulatory settings or home care (Hatcher et al. 2006). Hospital work is physically challenging, and without accommodations, many nurses leave or transfer to less demanding jobs. Some take early retirement. "Nursing is complex and taxing physical, emotional, and intellectual work. Over time this takes a toll on the nurse" (Hatcher et al. 2006, p. 22).

Many approaches have been identified in the literature, and although some pertain more to clinical point-of-service workers, many apply to anyone in the health care workplace. These include:

- New technology for lifting patients or reducing the need to lift patients (for example, stretcher beds that fold into a chair, or lift systems installed over the hospital bed).
- Implementing special lift teams.
- Bariatric patient equipment or special accommodations.
- Transport teams.
- Back care and lift safety training.
- Redesigning the work area to reduce the length of hallways and walk time with smaller more localized work stations and supply areas, and, in patient care departments, patient assignments in clusters to avoid long distances and excessive walking. Nurses often walk up to twelve miles per shift, and much of this is related to finding supplies and equipment (Hatcher et al. 2006).
- Applying principles of ergonomics to the workplace such as ergonomically appropriate chairs, supplies placed at levels where they are easy to reach, and electrical outlets placed at mid-height to prevent stooping.

- Improved lighting, larger computer screens, lowered monitor screens, larger text type, and magnifiers (reading glasses) on all crash carts, with emergency equipment, and in medication rooms.
- Relaxation rooms, employee rest areas, chairs placed strategically so people can sit, and rolling chairs in the work areas.
- Door handles that lift rather than turn and easy-to-open containers.
- Training materials that are easier to read (high contrast colors, bold typefacing, avoidance of high-gloss items and laminated pages that produce glare).
- No posting materials above eye level (due to the difficulty caused by bifocals).
- Reduction of noise levels.

Altering the Work Itself

Most of the approaches clustered under the strategy of altering the work itself involves changing the job position or classification in which the person works. Approaches ranged from reducing typical responsibilities to moving into different roles to creating new roles within the health system.

In Australia, for example, the option is offered for the employee to transition into retirement by working at a lower job classification level. While this option may not suit everyone, it is one alternative to losing individuals to retirement (Commonwealth of Australia 2003). In other countries, such alternatives may be implemented in a less formal way, for example, when managers scale down the work commitment of older workers and phase them out of certain responsibilities. This also happens in the academic setting when administrative faculty move back into teaching positions.

"From the Canadian perspective, the biggest challenge for many senior nurses is the issue of workload. Senior nurses not only need to provide direct patient care and carry a full nurse patient assignment, they also 'manage the activities' of the unit and serve as mentors or preceptors to more junior nurses or relief staff" (O'Brien-Pallas, Duffield, and Alksnis 2004, p. 301). A reduction in this workload could reduce the stress associated with balancing these three types of job demands. This approach is similar to the finding in the Robert Wood Johnson Foundation report *Wisdom at Work*, that many of the older nurses surveyed had transferred into ambulatory or home care nursing (Hatcher et al. 2006). Others may seek positions in case management, quality improvement, or other related departments and functions. Some nurses take on project work or roles that are time limited, such as coordinator for special projects.

Other systems are searching for entirely new roles that can tap into the knowledge and experience of these mature workers. Examples include putting people in positions such as chief on-boarding officer, who assists newer employees when they join the staff, or best-practice coach, who reviews the literature and research for implementation of evidence-based clinical strategies. Other examples of new roles created for senior employees are to staff community or wellness programs or to tutor high school students. Other organizations use the more seasoned employee in knowledge transfer programs, aimed at mentoring and developing newer staff to ensure the transfer of knowledge from the older, more experienced worker.

A key aspect of this strategy may involve retraining the individual for different responsibilities. In the AARP study quoted earlier, this approach is likely to be very appealing to older workers (Grossman 2003). In some instances, it is suggested that moving the older worker from his or her primary position results in the loss of tremendous clinical or technical expertise to the system. Flexible staffing patterns, compressed shifts, and improved physical work environments can all help the more mature worker handle the requirements of a traditional work setting. In terms of nursing, another option is to "shift roles so work is more appealing to older nurses, perhaps alternating patient care with other duties" (Thrall 2005, p. 34). Norman (2005) found that, in the United States, as the age of nurses increases, the percentage of nurses working in acute care declines, from 72 percent of 18–29-year-olds to only 38 percent of nurses 50 and over.

Restructuring Compensation and Benefits

Another strategy involves reviewing compensation plans and modifying traditional approaches to provide creative, appealing, and individualized benefits. However, as noted by the Royal College of Nursing, Australia (2004, p. 4), "When the average nurse retires at 55, the Government changes to superannuation will make it easier for individuals to carry on working past 55, but improvements in flexible working conditions will have to improve further." In other words, it still has to be a good place to work.

Compensation Plans

In the Australian study, some employers looked for ways to rehire their own retirees. Often this effort included modifying pension plans in ways that entice workers to remain in the active workforce. Some organizations are offering employees the option of rehiring, working, and still being able to claim their pension benefits. Other alternatives included allowing the individual to work for six months but receive pay over a year's time. The United Kingdom has a different approach. There, the worker's pension is based on the past five years of service. This discourages people from reducing to part-time work or accepting a lower-paying role in the final years of their career (Watson, Manthorpe, and Andrews 2003a, 2003b). In one area of the United Kingdom there are provisions in place to protect the nurse's earnings. "Nurses redeployed to a job with lower pay than their previous position may have their earnings protected at the level of their previous job for up to nine years, including the past five years of service on which their pension is based. In this way staff need not be scared into early retirement to protect their pension" (Watson, Manthorpe, and Andrews 2003b, p. 39).

Benefits

Benefits that were of special interest to the older worker, such as on-site or subsidized health club memberships, subsidized health care insurance coverage, and rehabilitation time are often suggested. "Considering that 38–87% of all nursing personnel have suffered a back injury severe enough to require leave from work," back-to-work programs focusing on rehabilitative needs are a sound benefit (Cyr 2005, p. 565).

Other benefits included educational opportunities that focus on the employee continuing to learn new material and skills as well as tuition reimbursement for formal academic programs. These offerings may be especially appealing to the generation of Baby Boomers. If they see their retirement as a time to retool and pursue other interests, having assistance from their current employer to do so could be very appealing. Financial literacy programs were mentioned frequently. Because people in the developed countries are living longer, they will be increasingly responsible for preparing for their own retirement.

Examples were not only confined to funded benefit programs. Other examples were more perks or rewards like reduced floating between departments and required overtime for long-tenured employees, retiree clubs, newsletters, and periodic social events. Concierge services are another group of perks that has enjoyed an upsurge of interest in recent years. Organizations are implementing these services because they can assume the responsibility for simple but time-consuming chores for employees, making their lives easier and allowing them to stay focused on their jobs. Although a few of these services have been around for years (such as on-site dry cleaning services), Lima (2007) reports on a startlingly wide and increasingly sophisticated array of other services. Examples include:

- Running errands—courier services, vehicle services, shopping, home-sitting
- Convenience services—dry cleaning, shipping and mailing, gift wrapping
- Transactional services—obtaining theater tickets, buying gifts, making reservations
- Home-based help—waiting for the arrival of a service person, handling lawn maintenance issues, watering plants, bringing in the mail, arranging for pet care
- Corporate support—conducting fund-raising campaigns, administering recognition programs
- Information research—product research, travel, contractors, recreation, sports, financial services, volunteering opportunities
- Child or elder care—researching care options, identifying programs and services
- Event planning—planning an employee recognition dinner, a business meeting, the organization's or department's summer picnic, a birthday party, a reunion, or any other event
- Travel planning—obtaining passports, arranging airfare/hotel/car rental, exchanging currency

Instituting Flexible Working Models

Throughout the literature many examples are found of the idea that "Labor force decisions of older workers are also influenced by the availability of flexible work arrangements" (Walker 2007, p. 9). Older workers find it difficult to manage twelve-hour shifts, while younger workers find clustering these longer shifts gives them a longer personal break and better work-life balance. Longer shifts are physically more demanding and can be difficult for the older worker who may be experiencing less endurance as age advances. A number of flexible work plans were identified, including the following:

- **Phased-retirement plans**—These are also called "bridge options" and usually included a transition period from full-time work into part-time work prior to full retirement.
- **Part-time work**—Not necessarily a part of a formal phased-retirement plan, it allows the worker more time for life balance. One form of this plan is a weekender option that enables the individual to work weekends only.
- **Job sharing**—This is an arrangement where two or more people share a full-time job.
- **Seasonal or temporary work**—This program allows workers to only work part of the year. Another option is the "traveler option," which offers six- to thirteen-week assignments.

  In Australia, a program called "flexible leave options," or purchased leave, can be made available to employees (Commonwealth of Australia 2003). Employees can purchase between one and four weeks of additional leave time per year. An adjustment is then made to the employee's annual salary to repay the additional leave. Another program allows employees to work half of the year and be paid over a full year.
- **Caregiving time**—This option is useful for those with eldercare responsibilities. One employer provides workers ten days off each year for elder care. In a study by Rosenfield (2007), interviews were completed with twenty-eight elder-caregiving staff members. They reported that successful management of their dual roles was based on identifying departments and shifts that fit with their responsibilities. Caregiver-friendly practices such as creative, flexible scheduling; access to social workers and financial and legal services; and increased awareness among managers about caregiver strains were recommended.
- **Project work**—This work is temporary but may be full time while the project is unfolding. Once the project is over, the job goes away.
- **Home-based work**—This allows employees to work their regular or reduced hours from another location. Medical records transcriptionists in some organizations have been working from home for years. While most health care work takes place in the presence of patients, and thereby must be on-site, some responsibilities may lend themselves to this alternative. Administrative paperwork, reviewing

research, developing programs, and other project work are just a few examples of possible projects that can be completed effectively from home. Home-based work is especially attractive to older workers who have caregiving responsibilities for an ill spouse or elderly relative where the care is ongoing but not time consuming.

In our highly connected, electronic world, opportunities will increase for long-distance assignments. This trend may also have ramifications for countries that are providing outsourcing services for other countries, for example, radiologists in India or Australia who provide interpretation of imaging results for hospitals in the United States or other countries. Another variation of this outcome is the example of hospitals using the older nurse in assignment at a central-ized monitoring station for intensive care patients. The theory is that it does not matter where the nurse is, as long as he or she is able to use a monitoring system.

- **Career breaks**—In Australia it was found that "career break schemes may enable employees to pursue interests or activities outside of the workplace, which may assist in the transition from full-time work to retirement—for example, leave to pursue volunteer activities or other special interests" (Commonwealth of Australia 2003, p. 10). These interruptions in service can also enable older workers to attend to intensive or more long-term caring responsibilities. Some organiza-tions actually encourage employees to plan a sabbatical and make it possible for the employee to be paid four years' salary over a period of five years. The fifth year is spent out of the workplace.

Customize the Approach

Due to the range of personal and organizational circumstances and prefer-ences, a one-size-fits-all approach is not likely to succeed. Approaches must be customized for the workforce for whom they are intended.

Spinks and Moore (2007) suggest that women's retirement ages are more unpredictable than are those of men because only now are large numbers of women in the paid labor force working until retirement. Because the health care workforce is largely female, this caution should be noted: "Women, more often than men, report being pulled into retirement involuntarily or prematurely as a result of spousal retirement, caregiving demands of an elderly family member, or for personal health reasons" (Spinks and Moore 2007, p. 27). Further, the researchers state that although studies have shown that people plan to work into their sixties and seventies, the reality is that very few people choose to work beyond the time at which their personal health/wealth equation permits retirement.

Cyr (2005) conducted a descriptive survey of 1,553 hospital-based nurses in central New England. Most of this sample (65 percent) anticipated retiring after 60 years of age, with 31 percent indicating they would retire at or before 60 years old. This finding differs from earlier reports that nearly half of all men and women leave the labor force by ages 60 and 62, respectively, and that nurses tend to retire earlier. Cyr ranked the factors influencing retirement decisions in terms of their frequency of mention:

1. Financial independence (75 percent)
2. Nurse's poor health (63 percent)
3. Work intensity (48 percent)
4. Spouse's poor health (39 percent)
5. Spouse's early retirement (28 percent)

The above five factors affecting the decision to retire can be influenced by the strategies discussed in this section. Nurses who said financial independence would influence their early retirement also indicated that financial incentives would encourage them to remain employed. Work intensity can be eased by managerial interventions that focus on reducing the physical demands of the workplace. Approximately half of the nurses indicated that some form of flexible work program would be desirable and would have a positive effect on the retention of older staff members.

Much more research is needed to determine the relative importance and effectiveness of these strategies. However, many of the findings and recommendations reported here are approaches that make the organization a better workplace for both younger and older workers.

Succession Planning

Eventually, despite any strategy used to postpone it, employees will retire. A closely related retirement issue is that of managing knowledge transfer, so that when seasoned employees leave the active workforce, the knowledge and expertise they represent are not lost to the system entirely. Succession planning is often the approach used for ensuring that the implicit knowledge of the experienced employee is shared with younger or more inexperienced employees.

The workforce shortages currently experienced and predicted for the future make proactive and effective knowledge transfer a key human resource initiative in today's health care organizations. With such a large faction of the workforce set to retire, not only will fewer people be doing the work but also some methodology must be in place so that the knowledge and expertise of the retiring or exiting worker are not completely lost. Cappelli (2008, p. 74) refers to this as talent management: "At heart, talent management is simply a matter of anticipating the need for human capital and then setting out a plan to meet it." In health care, this may be as basic as strong professional and management development programs, career ladders that involve increased opportunity for the employee, and a practice of promoting from within. However, succession planning is more than these initiatives. It is more than simply having an effective approach for managing replacements.

Succession Planning at the CEO Level

Few health care organizations have formal succession planning, and, if they do, it is more likely for the senior executive positions rather than for frontline workers and others throughout deeper levels in the organization. This is not just an issue facing the health care sector. A recent study reports that two-thirds of U.S. employers are doing no workforce planning of any kind (Cappelli 2008). A poorly executed chief executive officer (CEO) succession can have an absolutely devastating effect on the quality and positivity of the work environment for everyone in the organization.

Charan (2005) discusses a lack of CEO succession planning and reports that two out of every five CEOs fail in the first eighteen months. The average tenure of hospital CEOs is now around six years, and the issue is not that more are being replaced, but that they are being replaced badly. In some instances an outsider is needed to come into the organization and accomplish a particular task, such as a turnaround. However, there is a huge disadvantage of hiring from the outside when that individual brings in a handpicked management team, disrupts or dismantles a positive and healthy culture, or is a short-termer. Charan (2005) found that in North America, 55 percent of outside CEOs who departed in 2003 were forced to resign. This high rate is compared to 34 percent of insiders. Whether the CEO has been hired from within or without, a mismatch has terrible consequences for the successful moving forward of the organization.

Another consequence of failing to have a deliberate succession plan in place is the blocking of deserved promotions. One nurse executive was suddenly faced with the possibility of promotion to chief operating officer (COO), but without a prepared replacement, she did not get the promotion. This situation arises at all levels of the organization. Some businesses today have a policy that an individual must have a prepared replacement before he or she can advance.

It is particularly challenging to have a successful succession plan for the top position in the organization. One problem is that potential candidates who show great promise may not be willing to wait until the CEO's retirement or resignation rolls around. In some instances, promising executives are moved about the organization in an attempt to provide experience with a variety of functions to help prepare them for advancement. Unfortunately, the problem with this approach is twofold: First, this piecemeal education in leadership is not the same as leading the entire organization, and second, individuals often are not in a position long enough to live with any long-term consequences of their decisions. This scenario occurred in one hospital where executives were routinely shifted around. The COO, who was the heir-apparent to the CEO, was an ineffective operations manager. His lack of leadership created havoc in normally strong, well-functioning departments. When responsibilities shifted, one of his executive colleagues would be left with the assignment of fixing the mess. Upon the CEO's retirement, this individual was promoted to CEO and failed miserably within a year. The constantly changing assignments had protected him from the consequences of his ineffectiveness for years.

Succession Planning throughout the Organization

So far, succession planning has typically only been a factor at the CEO level. It is less likely to be done in lower levels of organizations. Perhaps the lessons learned at the higher levels can be used by health care organizations as they begin to implement succession planning for other key leaders throughout the organization.

There are two categories of demographic risk that organizations are facing: capacity risk and productivity risk. "When a worker retires, you lose someone to do a job and the accumulated knowledge and expertise that this person takes out the door with him. If many people are retiring and they're difficult to replace, your organization faces what we call *capacity risk*" (Strack, Baier, and Fahlander 2008, p. 120). In health care, this translates to a potentially diminished capacity of an organization to offer its services. Furthermore, "Although age and experience can make workers more effective in many positions, in certain jobs an aging workforce can create a *productivity risk*" (Strack, Baier, and Fahlander 2008, p. 121). Because many health care jobs entail physical exertion, long hours, and stressful environments, this type of risk is a concern. The issues of the aging workforce have been discussed in the previous section.

To do successful succession planning, both of these risks must be assessed for the organization. Capacity risk is assessed by projecting the future demand and anticipating worker levels required and determining how difficult it will be to hire the people to fill the vacant positions. Productivity risk is easier and more straightforward. Using the internal workforce demographics, the number of people over a certain age can be predicted along with the potential ramifications. For example, some positions may be more physically demanding, making it less likely that the individual will continue beyond a certain age. Jobs that require shift rotation are more difficult for the older worker. The strategies discussed above for retaining the older worker can be helpful for managing the productivity risk.

Buried within the capacity risk are a variety of needs for succession planning. As noted earlier, very few health care organizations do consistent, methodical succession planning, and if they do, the focus is more likely at the executive level. Middle management and staff positions are rarely considered. Yet with the workforce shortages being projected, it would seem that all positions are crucial for organizational vitality. More and more organizations are reporting great difficulty replacing managers.

The first step in addressing this issue is to understand that succession planning is a process, not an event. In other words, the process must begin years before the event occurs. Bower (2007) believes that it consists of identifying the "high-potentials" and giving them a series of increasingly complex assignments that provide the opportunity to learn skills and manage outcomes for a key piece of the organization's work. Again, this effort implies a deliberate approach rather than simply providing generalized leadership development opportunities.

Succession planning is more than replacement planning, which is basically reactive in nature. "The primary focus of succession planning is on forecasting the strategic needs of the organization. It is proactive and based on securing the human resources needed to ensure on-going solidity and affluence" (Collins and Collins 2007, p. 321). Significant problems occur when succession planning is not in place.

McConnell (2006) notes that part of the difficulty is that this process entails planning for an open position, which is a future event. He and other authors summarize the steps of a successful succession planning process as follows:

1. Select the target position(s).
2. Identify the key competencies required for one to be successful. Unique, but temporary, organizational needs should be considered here as well. For example, perhaps an individual with specific program development experience, construction management experience, or successful turnaround abilities is needed.
3. Identify internal employees who either demonstrate these competencies or are capable of developing them.
4. Determine other experiences or educational opportunities the individual may require, and plan for it to be obtained.
5. Coalesce all of this information into a professional development plan for the individual.
6. Consider a formal mentoring program to provide support for the individual.
7. Monitor the plan and periodically review the competencies to determine their currency.

Beyond the benefit of having individuals able and willing to step into a vacant role, it is also clear that investing in an employee's development and career progression is a way to cement their commitment. When organizations "help workers acquire new skills that support their professional advancement, they often win those workers' commitment—and attract loyal new employees. This gives rise to another important point: employers can promote company loyalty by helping people grow *out* of their jobs—ideally, into new ones within the company" (Johnson 2005, p. 1).

Succession planning does have its downside. Having large numbers of people who are highly qualified for positions that are not yet available can create dissatisfaction. Moreover, these people are vulnerable to recruiters from competing organizations. Studies show that people who have recently received special training or development "are the most likely to decamp, as they leave for opportunities to make better use of those new skills" (Cappelli 2008, p. 78). In some instances, outside hiring is faster and more responsive to the organization's needs. However, hiring from within is less expensive and disruptive to the system. It also demonstrates to employees that there are opportunities for advancement and that the organization is willing to make a long-term investment in its employees (Gantz 2007).

Succession planning may feel threatening to those currently occupying the planned position. One organization attempted to forecast the number of its nursing staff who would be retiring in the next five years. It intended to develop a mentoring program that would pair soon-to-retire nurses with younger nurses who could replace them. This sounds like a proactive idea that would be successful in many organizations. But with succession planning there has to be an underlying foundation of trust. In this case, it failed miserably because the nurses refused to share their retirement plans with their managers. They were afraid they would be the first to be laid off or lose their job if downsizing occurred. They felt they were considered a liability to the organization because of their tenure, higher pay, and higher rate of vacation accrual.

Effective succession planning is a way of ensuring continuity in the organization. Whether at the executive, management, or staff level, it is a responsibility of health care organizations to be stewards for the future. Gilbert (2007) clearly identifies succession planning as an ethical responsibility. This is a much healthier attitude than the executive who said, "Why should we develop our employees when our competitors are willing to do it for us?" (Cappelli 2008, p. 76).

Summary

Health care managers today are facing a significant challenge with the presence of multiple generations of employees in the active workforce. The challenges of managing a multigenerational workforce are extensive and include the need of the manager to create a positive work environment, remain flexible and adaptable, manage conflict between the generations, and understand and use knowledge of the generational differences. Not all generational characteristics and descriptors are conclusive for every member of the generation, so it remains important that managers know the people with whom they work and not generalize or stereotype based on these characteristics. Furthermore, although there are obviously generational differences, there are also many similarities between people, and it may be productive to focus on the basic human intrinsic motivators to create a workplace that is positive and appealing to employees regardless of their generational cohort.

Retaining the older worker is a key strategy for meeting current and future workforce shortages. Even delaying a worker's retirement by a few years can make a difference in avoiding critical vacancies. Using alternatives such as bridge programs, part-time options, and other flexible working arrangements can ensure that the organization retains the knowledge and expertise of these employees. Effective workforce planning that includes succession planning is a key responsibility of human resources in health care organizations and a strategy that ensures continuity into the future.

Conversation Points

Organizational Perspective

1. Is workforce planning being done in the organization? Are demographics available for all departments and categories of workers? What percentage of employees are in the different generational cohorts?
2. Has the human resources department developed a strategic initiative to create consistent succession planning throughout the organization?

3. How has succession planning been handled in the past?
4. Has education and training been offered to managers, organizational leaders, and employees about generational differences? How extensive was the programming, and is it ongoing?
5. Are generational differences considered in designing the orientation programming for new employees?
6. How does the organization support older workers? Have any adjustments been made?

Leader Perspective

1. What generational cohorts are represented in your department? Do you see characteristics of the different generations that relate to those reported in the literature?
2. Does friction occur or do clashes erupt between members of the different generational cohorts? If yes, what does the conflict seem to be related to?
3. In your experience of interviewing new prospective employees, what are the generational differences you are seeing? Are there any approaches that have been helpful?
4. What steps have you taken to develop the working relationships of staff members from the different cohorts?
5. What are the demographics of employees in your department? What is the average age? How many older employees do you have? Between 50 and 60 years of age? Over 61? What are their plans for retirement?
6. What have you done to modify the work or the environment to make it more older-worker friendly?
7. Do you have a plan for identifying and developing your successor?

Employee Perspective

1. In which generational cohort do you belong? How many from your cohort are in your department? What are the characteristics presented here that you agree with? Disagree with?
2. What is your impression of your co-workers from the other generational age cohorts? How are your values and needs different?
3. Does your manager and the organization do a good job of using generation-specific interventions in working with you?
4. How do you feel about working with co-workers who are older (defined as over 50 years of age)?
5. What could be done in your department to reduce the physical demands of the work?
6. Are you part of a formal succession plan for your career development? Would this be of interest to you? What could you do to obtain the support and resources you would need?

Going Forward

Jo Manion

If it is to be, it is up to me.
—Anonymous

APOSITIVE WORK environment is a key competitive strategy for both today's and future health care organizations. Without it, recruitment and retention of high-quality, fully engaged employees are much more difficult, if not downright impossible. And achievement of the organization's mission as well as its strategies and goals is impossible without a skilled and talented workforce. The people who comprise the workforce are the ones who attain results for the organization and its patients or clients. Even with automation poised to take over some of the more routine work in our organizations, as good as machines may become, they will never be able to care nor to innovate, both of which are necessary components of a successful health care organization. Many people in our organizations today are struggling, trying to do a good job with decreasing resources, escalating regulatory constraints, and a multitude of other intensifying pressures. In spite of difficulties, however, they are finding ways to create a positive work environment that makes theirs a better place to work.

This book explores many of the various components connected with a positive work environment. If the intrinsic motivators can be incorporated in the workplace, it is more likely that members of the workforce are motivated and enthusiastic about their work. If their working relationships with others are healthy and positive and if individuals can see how their work makes a positive difference for others and is meaningful, intrinsic motivation is more likely. If the system supports and demands personal and professional competence and offers choice and autonomy in the work, intrinsic motivation grows. And finally, hope of progress and a sense of achievement tap into people's internal sense of motivation.

The concept of organizational commitment is explored because it is desirable to employ people who not only come to work on a consistent basis but are also engaged and committed while they are there. Commitment is emotional, it engages the heart, and it provides sticking power when the going gets tough. Affective and normative commitment, considered to be the two stronger forms of organizational commitment, are explored in some detail. Specific steps for building these forms of organizational commitment are examined.

The new field of positive psychology offers much hope to increasing the understanding of what brings happiness, both at a personal and a professional level. Although the field is still in its infancy, the research findings offer guidance and evidence-based interventions for creating a better, healthier workplace. Happiness has been too narrowly defined in the past, and when it is examined in its fuller context, it offers direction for ways to increase both personal levels of happiness and happiness in co-workers. The three components of happiness include the amount of pleasure one has in life, the degree to which one is engaged in work or activities, and the depth of meaning with which one imbues work or activities. All three aspects suggest concrete, specific ways that happiness can be increased both in the personal sphere and in the public sphere of the workplace.

The second part of this book begins by reviewing a research study through which experienced, successful health care managers shared what they do to create a positive workplace. All of the study participants acknowledged that they alone could not create a positive workplace, but that they worked in partnership with their employee-colleagues to do so. Four additional key managerial strategies emerged from this research: putting the employee first, forging strong connections with people, coaching employees for their development, and focusing on results. Based on these findings, detailed strategies for achieving these goals are presented.

Focusing on relationships, at both the individual and group levels, is the theme for two chapters. Emotional intelligence, for both the manager and the team or work group, is explored. Concepts for developing teams and a sense of community in the workplace are reviewed. Another two chapters are aimed at providing strategies for getting results and understanding organizational innovation. Chapter 10 presents the issue of influencing the performance of others, detailing coaching approaches a manager can take to deal with ineffective performance or inappropriate conduct.

The final section focuses on challenges faced by organizational leaders in trying to implement these concepts. The question of "When does a challenge become an excuse?" is explored. Multiple issues are considered, including the challenge of social-sector leadership, the presence of labor unions, the difficulties found in unique settings such as long-term care and academia, and the challenges of the multigenerational and aging workforce.

Recall the question posed in the early pages of this book: "Why is a healthy, positive workplace so important? After all, when all is said and done, it's a paycheck and that's what really matters." It is important to see the truth that money is not all that matters, nor is it even the most important element in the work world. Of course, if none of the intrinsic motivators or the elements of positive organizational commitment are present, it may be only money that keeps people there. But these individuals cannot be counted on to stay, because all it takes to encourage them to leave is for another organization to match or increase the salary and benefit levels.

Most individuals spend the majority of their awake, alert time at work, employed by others. Work is capable of bringing great meaning and joy to life, if individuals would just expect it and let it. It is an avenue where people can share their strengths and talents with others. Work is an integral part of life's journey. It shapes and informs one's personal world. It is one way to leave a mark, a legacy for others. Life is simply too precious to squander in a job or an organization where one is miserable, where the negative energy drains all enthusiasm and joy and leaves only a feeling of depletion.

A positive work environment is possible. However, it will not appear, as if by magic, on its own. It is up to each individual to take action, to be part of creating a healthier environment. Those who are not actively working to make things better may be part of the problem. It is important for every employee and manager to ask, What have I done this week to make my workplace a great place to work? How many times have I laughed with colleagues or stopped to reflect on what a wonderful contribution I make? How many times this week have I encouraged someone around me or helped someone without first being asked? When was the last time I showed gratitude to others who may not hear many thank yous? Not just peers, but the chief executive officer or the department manager? Or the person who cleans the department and empties the trash, or the security guard who is in the background making certain that the environment is safe? What can I do to create the kind of workplace where I am excited about going to work? Where I find support and fellowship and the confidence of knowing I am doing good things? The power of ten small words sums it up best: "If it is to be, it is up to me."

References

AARP. 2007. Retention strategies: healthcare industry trends: recruiting and retaining older workers. [Online information; retrieved November 27, 2007.] http://www.healthcare_industry_trends_recruiting_and_retainin.html.

AbuAlRub, R.F. 2004. Job stress, job performance, and social support among hospital nurses. *Journal of Nursing Scholarship* 36(1):73–78.

Ackoff, R., Finnel, E., and Gharajedaghi, J. 1984. *A Guide to Controlling Your Corporation's Future*. New York: John Wiley & Sons.

Adams, J.L. 1986. *The Care and Feeding of Ideas: A Guide to Encouraging Creativity*. Reading, MA: Addison-Wesley.

Advisory Board Company. 2000. *Reversing the Flight of Talent: Nursing Retention in an Era of Gathering Shortage*. Washington, DC: Advisory Board Company.

Aiken, L.H. 2007. US nurse labor market dynamics are key to global nurse sufficiency. *Health Services Research* 42(3, Part II):1299–1320.

Aiken, L., Clarke, S., Sloane, D., Sochalski, J., and Silber, J. 2002. Hospital nurse staffing and patient mortality, nurse burnout, and job dissatisfaction. *Journal of the American Medical Association* 288(16):1987–93.

Alexander, J.A., Ramsay, J.A., and Thomson, S.M. 2004. Designing the health workforce for the 21st century. *Medical Journal of Australia* 180(1):7–9.

Alexander, G.R. 2006. Cultural and generational workforce diversity. In D.L. Huber, *Leadership and Nursing Care Management*, third edition, pp. 605–23. Philadelphia, PA: Saunders.

Amabile, T.M., and Kramer, S.J. 2007. Inner work life: understanding the subtext of business performance. *Harvard Business Review* 85(5):72–83.

American Health Care Association and National Center for Assisted Living. 2007. Address the shortage of nurses and critical caregivers for long term care. Washington, DC: AHCA/NCAL.

American Hospital Association (AHA). 2001. *Patients or Paperwork?* Chicago: AHA.

American Hospital Association (AHA). 2003. Staffing watch. *Hospitals & Health Networks* 7(9):22.

American Hospital Association (AHA). 2007. The 2007 state of America's hospitals—Taking the pulse. Chicago: AHA Press.

American Nurses Association. 2001. *Nursing World Health and Safety Survey*. Washington, DC: Nursing World.

Amott, T.L., and Matthaei, J.A. 1991. *Race, Gender and Work: A Multicultural Economic History of Women in the United States*. Boston: South End Press.

Anonymous. 2002. Attitudes. *Training and Development* 56(2):27.

Applebaum, H. 1992. *The Concept of Work: Ancient, Medieval, and Modern*. Albany, NY: State University of New York Press.

Aptheker, B. 1989. *Tapestries of Life: Women's Work, Women's Consciousness, and the Meaning of Daily Experience*. Amherst, MA: University of Massachusetts Press.

Arbuckle, G.A. 2000. Cultures of bullying. *Human Development* 21(1):25–33.

Armstrong-Stassen, M. 2004. *Nursing Aging Workforce Research Project: Retention Issues for Nurses 50 and Over.* [Online information; retrieved April 24, 2008.] http://web2.uwindsor.ca/faculty/busad/AgingWorkforce/Nurses/index.html.

Aronson, E. 1995. *The Social Animal,* seventh edition. New York: W.H. Freeman.

Atchison, T.A. 2003. Exposing the myths of employee satisfaction. *Healthcare Executive* (May/June):20–25.

Baggot, D.M., Hensinger, B., Parry, J., Valdes, M., and Zaim, S. 2005. The new hire/preceptor experience: cost-benefit analysis of one retention strategy. *Journal of Nursing Administration* 35(3):138–45.

Baggs, J.G., and Schmitt, M.H. 1988. Collaboration between nurses and physicians. *Image: Journal of Nursing Scholarship* 20(3):145–49.

Balik, B. 2008. Former CEO of United Hospital, St. Paul, MN. Personal communication, July 5.

Bandler, R., and Grinder, J. 1982. *Frogs into Princes: Neuro Linguistic Programming.* Moab, UT: Real People Press.

Bardwick, J.M. 1991. *Danger in the Comfort Zone.* New York: American Management Association.

Barker, J. 1990. *The Power of Vision.* Burnsville, MN: Charthouse Learning.

Barney, S.M. 2002. Radical change: one solution to the nursing shortage. *Journal of Healthcare Management* 47(4):220–24.

Barrett, F.J. 1995. Creating appreciative learning cultures. *Organizational Dynamics* 24:36–49.

Barsade, S.G., and Gibson, D.E. 1998. Group emotion: a view from top and bottom. In D. H. Gruenfeld (ed.), *Research on Managing Groups and Teams,* vol. 1, pp. 81–102. Stamford, CT: JAI Press.

Bartel, C.A., and Saavedra, R. 2000. The collective construction of work group moods. *Administrative Science Quarterly* 45:197–231.

Beck, M. 2004. Impotent rage. *O Magazine* (October):203–7.

Becker, H.S. 1960. Notes on the concept of commitment. *American Journal of Sociology* 66:32–40.

Beckhard, R., and Pritchard, W. 1992. *Changing the Essence: The Art of Creating and Leading Fundamental Change in Organizations.* San Francisco: Jossey-Bass.

Beglinger, J. 2003. The innovative organization for the 21st century. *Nurse Leader* 1(1):39–41.

Bennis, W. 1966. *Changing Organizations: Essays on the Development and Evolution of Human Organization.* New York: McGraw-Hill.

Bennis, W. (ed.). 1970. *American Bureaucracy.* Boston: Aldine.

Bennis, W. 1989. *On Becoming a Leader.* Reading, MA: Addison-Wesley.

Berry, L.L. 1992. Qualities of leadership. *Retailing Issues Letter* 4(1):1–4.

Berwick, D.M. 2003. Disseminating innovations in health care. *Journal of the American Medical Association* 289(15):1969–75.

Bilbrey, P. 2008a. A healthy dissatisfaction for the status quo. *Hospital & Health Networks Online.* [Online information; retrieved March 11, 2008.] www.hhnmag.com.

Bilbrey, P. 2008b. Challenges, not excuses. *Hospital & Health Networks* 3:26.

Blouin, A., and Brent, N. 1997. Strategic partnering: clinical and risk management concerns. *Journal of Nursing Administration* 27(6):10–13.

Bookman, A., and Morgen, S. (eds.). 1988. *Women and the Politics of Empowerment.* Philadelphia: Temple University Press.

Bossidy, L., and Charan, R. 2002. *Execution: The Discipline of Getting Things Done.* New York: Crown Business.

Bower, J.L. 2007. Solve the succession crisis by growing inside-outside leaders. *Harvard Business Review* 85(November):91–96.

Bowles, C., and Candela, L. 2005. First job experiences of recent RN graduates. *Journal of Nursing Administration* 35(3):130–37.

Bowles, M. 1991. The organization shadow. *Organization Studies* 12(3):387–404.

Bowles, M. 1997. The myth of management: direction and failure in contemporary organizations. *Human Relations* 50(7):779–803.

Brickman, P., with Wortman, C.B., and Sorrentino, R. (eds.). 1987. *Commitment, Conflict, and Caring.* Englewood Cliffs, NJ: Prentice-Hall.

Brightman, S. 2002. Former consultant with Drake Beam Morin. Personal conversation, New York, February.

Briles, J. 2008. *Zapping Conflict in the Health Care Workplace.* Aurora, CO: Mile High Press.

Briles, J. 2009. *Stabotage!™: How to Deal with the Pit Bulls, Skunks, Snakes, Scorpions, & Slugs in the Health Care Workplace.* Aurora, CO: Mile High Press.

Britton, J. 2007. Using strengths when you work. *Positive Psychology News Today.* [Online information; retrieved June 28, 2008.] http://pos-psych.com/news/kathryn-britton/20070807363.

Brown, P., Davis-Thomas, J., and Yessis, J. 2007. *Quiet Please. I'm Trying to Recover. Strategies to Reduce Noise in the Hospital Environment.* Lincoln, NE: NRC Picker.

Bryant, F.B. 2004. Capturing the joy of the moment: savoring as a process in positive psychology. Authentic Happiness coaching class, presented July 22, 2004.

Buchan, J. 1999. The 'greying' of the United Kingdom nursing workforce: implications for employment policy and practice. *Journal of Advanced Nursing* 30(4):818–26.

Buchan, J., and Calman, L. 2005. *The Global Shortage of Registered Nurses: An Overview of Issues and Actions.* Geneva, Switzerland: International Council of Nurses.

Buckingham, M., and Clifton, D. 2001. *Now, Discover Your Strengths.* New York: Free Press.

Buckingham, M., and Coffman, C. 1999. *First, Break All the Rules: What the World's Greatest Managers Do Differently.* New York: Simon & Schuster.

Buerhaus, P. 2002. Shortages of hospital registered nurses: causes and perspective on public and private sector actions. *Nursing Outlook* 50(1):4–6.

Bürkner, H. 2007. The best advice I ever got. *Harvard Business Review* 85 (December):21.

Burns, B.M. 1978. *Leadership.* New York: Harper-Collins.

Byers, J.F., and White, S.V. 2004. *Patient Safety: Principles and Practice.* New York: Springer-Verlag.

Byrne, J.A. 2003. How to lead now: getting extraordinary performance when you can't pay for it. *Fast Company* 73:62–70.

Cappelli, P. 2008. Talent management for the twenty-first century. *Harvard Business Review* 86(3):74–81.

Cathcart, D., Jeska, S., Karnas, J., Miller, S., Pechacek, J., and Rheault, L. 2004. Span of control matters. *Journal of Nursing Administration* 34(9):395–99.

Caudron, S. 1997. The search for meaning at work. *Training and Development* 51(9): 24–27.

Cavaiola, A., and Lavender, N. 2000. *Toxic Coworkers: How to Deal with Dysfunctional People on the Job.* Oakland, CA: New Harbinger.

Chaleff, I. 1996. Effective leadership. *Executive Excellence* 4:16–17.

Chaleff, I. 1997. The groupthink challenge. *Team Management Briefings*, June, p. 4.

Chambers, H.E. 1998. *The Bad Attitude Survival Guide.* Reading, MA: Addison-Wesley.

Champy, J. 2003. The hidden qualities of great leaders. *Fast Company* 76:135.

Charan, R. 2005. Ending the CEO succession crisis. *Harvard Business Review* 83(2):72–81.

Charles, R. 2000. The challenge of disseminating innovations to direct care providers in health care organizations. *Nursing Clinics of North America* 35(2):461–70.

Chawla, S., and Renesch, J. (eds.). 1995. *Learning Organizations: Developing Cultures for Tomorrow's Workplace.* Portland, OR: Productivity Press.

Cherniss, C., and Goleman, D. 2001. *The Emotionally Intelligent Workplace: How to Select for, Measure, and Improve Emotional Intelligence in Individuals, Groups, and Organizations.* San Francisco: Jossey-Bass.

Christensen, C.M., Kaufman, S.P., and Shih, W.C. 2008. Innovations killers: how financial tools destroy your capacity to do new things. *Harvard Business Review* 86(1):98–105.

Ciancutti, A., and Steding, T. 2000. *Built on Trust: Gaining Competitive Advantage in Any Organization.* Lincolnwood, IL: Contemporary Books.

Clancy, T. 2003. The art of decision-making. *Journal of Nursing Administration* 33(6):343–49.

Clancy, T., and Anteau, C. 2008. Coordination: new ways of harnessing complexity. *Journal of Nursing Administration* 38(4):158–61.

Clarke, J. 1999. *Connections: The Threads That Strengthen Families.* Center City, MN: Hazelden.

Clarke-Epstein, C. 2002. Truth in feedback. *Training and Development* 56(11):78–80.

Clegg, S.R. 1990. *Modern Organizations: Organization Studies in the Postmodern World.* London: Sage.

Cline, D., Reilly, C., and Moore, J. 2003. What's behind RN turnover? *Nursing Management* 34(10):50–53.

Coens, T., and Jenkins, M. 2000. *Abolishing Performance Appraisals: Why They Backfire and What to Do Instead.* San Francisco: Berrett-Koehler.

Cohen, M.H. 2008. Professional communication and teamwork. *Creative Nursing* 14(1):17–23.

Collins, J. 2001. *Good to Great: Why Some Companies Make the Leap . . . and Others Don't.* New York: HarperCollins.

Collins, J. 2005. *Good to Great and the Social Sectors.* Boulder, CO: Jim Collins.

Collins, J. 2008. The secret of enduring greatness. *Fortune*, May 5, 73–76.

Collins, S.K., and Collins, K.S. 2006. Valuable human capital: the aging health care worker. *The Health Care Manager* 25(3):213–20.

Collins, S.K., and Collins, K.S. 2007. Changing workforce demographics necessitates succession planning in health care. *The Health Care Manager* 26(4):318–25.

Colosi, M.L. 2007. Nurses: when supply fails demand, a patient care catastrophe looms. *Nurse Leader* 5(12):46–53.

Commonwealth of Australia. 2003. *Flexible Working Arrangements for Older Workers.* [Online information; retrieved November 27, 2007.] http://www.dcita.gov.au/cca.

Cordeniz, J.A. 2002. Recruitment, retention, and management of generation X: a focus on nursing professionals. *Journal of Healthcare Management* 47(4):237–49.

Covey, S.R. 1989. *The Seven Habits of Highly Effective People: Powerful Lessons in Personal Change*. New York: Simon & Schuster.

Covey, S.R. 1992. *Principle-Centered Leadership*. New York: Simon & Schuster.

Covey, S.R., Merrill, A.R., and Merrill, R.R. 1994. *First Things First*. New York: Simon & Schuster.

Cox, S., Manion, J., and Miller, D. 2005. *Nature's Wisdom in the Workplace: Managing Energy in Health Care Organizations*. Bloomington, MN: Synergy Press.

Coyne, K., Clifford, P., and Dye, R. 2007. Breakthrough thinking from inside the box. *Harvard Business Review* 85(December):71–78.

Creative Healthcare Management. 1994. *Leaders Empower Staff*. Minneapolis, MN: Creative Healthcare Management.

Crow, G. 2006. Diffusion of innovation: the leaders' role in creating the organizational context for evidence-based practice. *Nursing Administration Quarterly* 30(3):236–42.

Csikszentmihalyi, M. 1990. *Flow: The Psychology of Optimal Experience*. New York: Harper & Row.

Csikszentmihalyi, M. 1997. *Finding Flow: The Psychology of Engagement with Everyday Life*. New York: Basic.

Csikszentmihalyi, M. 2003. *Good Business: Leadership, Flow, and the Making of Meaning*. New York: Penguin Putnam.

Cutruzzula, J., and Cipriano, P. 2007. Over-recruiting: breaking the short staffing and turnover cycle. *Nurse Leader* 5(12):28–32.

Cyr, J.P. 2005. Retaining older hospital nurses and delaying their retirement. *Journal of Nursing Administration* 35(12):563–67.

Davidhizar, R., and Hart, A. 2006. Are you born a happy person or do you have to make it happen? *The Health Care Manager* 25(1):64–69.

Davies, G., and Chun, R. 2007. To thine own staff be agreeable. *Harvard Business Review*, June. [Online information; retrieved July 1, 2008.] www.hbr.org.

De Man, H. 1929. *Joy in Work* (E.C. Paul, trans.). London: George Allen & Unwin.

DeChick, J. 1988. Most mothers want a job, too. *USA Today*, July 19, D1.

DeCovny, S. 2007. Biotechnology: innovations by the thousands. *Harvard Business Review* 85(October):51–55.

Defert, J.R., and Edmondson, A.C. 2007. Why employees are afraid to speak. *Harvard Business Review*, 85(5). [Online information; retrieved July 16, 2008.] www.hbr.org.

Delbecq, A.L., and VandeVen, A.H. 1971. A group process model for problem identification and program planning. *Journal of Applied Behavioral Science* 7:466–94.

Denhardt, R.B. 1981. *In the Shadow of Organization*. Lawrence, KS: University Press of Kansas.

DePree, M. 1989. *Leadership Is an Art*. New York: Doubleday.

DeRosa, S. 2008. Clinical nurse specialist at Unity Health System, Rochester, NY. Personal communication, July 11.

Diener, E. 2000. Subjective well-being. *American Psychologist* 55(1):34–43.

Diener, E. 2008. *Happiness: Unlocking the Mysteries of Psychological Wealth*. Webinar presentation for International Positive Psychology Association, July 22.

Diener, E., and Diener, C. 1996. Most people are happy. *Psychological Science* 7(3):181–85.

Diener, E., Sandvik, E., and Pavot, W. 1991. Happiness is the frequency, not the intensity, of positive versus negative affect. In F. Strack, M. Argyle, and N. Schwarz (eds.), *Subjective Well-Being: An Interdisciplinary Perspective*, pp. 119–39. New York: Pergamon.

DiSciullo, M.J. 1997. *Remembering Joy in the Therapist and the Psychotherapeutic Process.* Unpublished doctoral dissertation, Pacifica Graduate Institute, Carpinteria, CA.

Dobbs, K. 1999. Winning the retention game. *Training* 36(9):50–56.

Doherty, K. 2002. Work related posttraumatic stress in nurses. Presented at the American Organization of Nurse Executives annual meeting, April 8, Orlando, FL.

Drucker, P. 1992. *Managing for the Future: The 1990s and Beyond.* New York: Penguin.

Duchscher, J.E., and Cowin, L. 2004. Multigenerational nurses in the workplace. *Journal of Nursing Administration* 34(11):493–501.

Dumaine, B. 1994. Why do we work? *Fortune* 130(13):196–204.

Durkin, S. 2006. Implementing a rapid response team. *American Journal of Nursing* 106(10):50–53.

Durning, A.T. 1993. Are we happy yet? How the pursuit of happiness is failing. *Futurist* 27(1):20–24.

Dychtwald, K., and Flower, J. 1990. *Age Wave: How the Most Important Trend of Our Time Will Change Your Future.* New York: Bantam.

Easterbrook, G. 2003. *The Progress Paradox: How Life Gets Better while People Feel Worse.* New York: Random House.

Eisler, R. 1987. *The Chalice and the Blade: Our History, Our Future.* San Francisco: HarperSanFrancisco.

Eisler, R., and Loye, D. 1998. *The Partnership Way: New Tools for Living and Learning*, second edition. Brandon, VT: Holistic Education Press.

Eliopoulos, C. 2007. *Nursing Administration Manual for Long-Term Care Facilities.* Cincinnati, OH: Health Education Press.

Ellenbecker, C.H., Porell, F.W., Samia, L., Byleckie, J.J., and Milburn, M. 2008. Predictors of home healthcare nurse retention. *Journal of Nursing Scholarship* 40(2):151–60.

Ellerbe, S., Ostermeier, L., and Shelley, S. 2006. Redesigning the recruitment function: winning at recruitment and retention of critical health care professionals. *Nurse Leader* 4(8):38–41.

Ellis, D. 2004. What if . . . the consequences of innovation. *Hospitals & Health Networks* 78(8):39–42.

Enright, R.D. 1998. *Exploring Forgiveness.* Madison: University of Wisconsin Press.

Enright, R.D. 2001. *Forgiveness Is a Choice: A Step-by-Step Process for Resolving Anger and Restoring Hope.* Washington, DC: American Psychological Association.

Erikson, K., and Vallas, S.P. (eds.). 1990. *The Nature of Work: Sociological Perspectives.* New Haven, CT: Yale University Press.

Fagiano, D. 1994. Designating a leader. *Management Review* 83(3):4.

Fairholm, G.W. 1998. *Perspectives on Leadership: From the Science of Management to Its Spiritual Heart.* Westport, CT: Quorum.

Farrell, G.A. 1997. Aggression in clinical settings: nurses' views. *Journal of Advanced Nursing* 29(3):532.

Feinsod, R.R., and Davenport, T.O. 2006. The aging workforce: challenge or opportunity? *Worldatwork* (third quarter):14–23.

Fishman, C. 1998. The war for talent. *Fast Company* 16:104–8.

Flower, J. 1990. The chasm between management and leadership. *Healthcare Forum Journal* 33(4):59–62.

Flower, J. 1999. Building the idea factory: a conversation with John Kao. *Health Forum Journal* 42(2):12–15.

Flower, J. 2002. Good to great: a conversation with Jim Collins. *Health Forum Journal* 45(5):17–20.

Fredrickson, B.L. 1998. What good are positive emotions? *Review of General Psychology* 2(3):300–319.

Fredrickson, B.L. 2001. The role of positive emotions in positive psychology. *American Psychologist* 56(3):218–26.

Fredrickson, B.L. 2003. The value of positive emotions. *American Scientist* 91(7): 330–35.

Frick, D., and Spears, L. (eds.). 1996. *On Becoming a Servant-Leader: The Private Writings of Robert K. Greenleaf.* San Francisco: Jossey-Bass.

Gantz, N.R. 2007. Succession planning: preparing the next generation of nurse leaders. *Voice of Nursing Leadership* (September):6–7.

Gegaris, C.M. 2007. Developing collaborative nurse/physician relationships. *Nurse Leader* 5(10):43–46.

Gelinas, L., and Bohlen, C. 2002. *Tomorrow's Work Force: A Strategic Approach. 2002 Research Series,* volume 1. Irving, TX: Voluntary Hospitals of America.

George, J.M. 2000. Emotions and leadership: the role of emotional intelligence. *Human Relations* 53(8):1027–55.

Gibson, C. 1991. A concept analysis of empowerment. *Journal of Advanced Nursing* 16:354–61.

Gilbert, J. 2007. *Strengthening Ethical Wisdom: Tools for Transforming Your Health Care Organization.* Chicago: AHA Press.

Gilbert, J. 2008. *Ethics and the Board: Pathways to Leadership Excellence in Healthcare.* San Diego: The Governance Institute.

Gilligan, C. 1982. *In A Different Voice: Psychological Theory and Women's Development.* Cambridge, MA: Harvard University Press.

Goleman, D. 1995. *Emotional Intelligence: Why It Can Matter More than IQ.* New York: Bantam.

Goleman, D., Boyatzis, R., and McKee, A. 2002. *Primal Leadership: Realizing the Power of Emotional Intelligence.* Boston: Harvard Business School Press.

Gottman, J.M. 2007. Making relationships work. *Harvard Business Review* 85 (December):45–50.

Gould, S.B., Weiner, K.J., and Levin, B.R. 1997. *Free Agents: People and Organizations Creating a New Working Community.* San Francisco: Jossey-Bass.

Govindarajan, V., and Trimble, C. 2005. Building breakthrough businesses within established organizations. *Harvard Business Review* 83(5):58–68.

Gowing, M.K., Kraft, J.D., and Quick, J.C. (eds.). 1998. *The New Organizational Reality: Downsizing, Restructuring and Revitalization.* Washington, DC: American Psychological Association.

Greene J. 2005. What nurses want: different generations, different expectations. *Hospitals & Health Networks* (March 14):34–42.

Gregory, D.M., Way, C.Y., LeFort, S., Barrett, B.J., and Parfrey, P.S. 2007. Predictors of registered nurses' organizational commitment and intent to stay. *Health Care Management Review* 32(2):119–27.

Greiff, B.S. 1999. *Legacy: The Giving of Life's Greatest Treasures.* New York: HarperCollins.

Griffin, M. 2004. Teaching cognitive rehearsal as a shield for lateral violence. *Journal of Continuing Education in Nursing* 35(6):257–63.

Grossman, H.Y. (ed.). 1990. *The Experience and Meaning of Work in Women's Lives.* Hillsdale, NJ: Lawrence Erlbaum Associates.

Grossman, R.J. 2003. Older workers. *HR Magazine.* [Online information; retrieved November 27, 2007.] http://www.shrm.org/hrmagazine/articles/0803/0803 covstory.asp.

Grote, D. 1995. *Discipline without Punishment: The Proven Strategy That Turns Problem Employees into Superior Performers.* New York: AMACOM.

Grote, D. 2002. *The Performance Appraisal Question and Answer Book.* New York: AMACOM.

Gryskiewicz, S.S. 1999. Positive turbulence: a climate for creativity. *Health Forum Journal* 42(2):16–19.

Hader, R. 2005. How do you measure workforce integrity? *Nursing Management* 36(9):32–37.

Hammer, M. 2005. Making operational innovation work. *Harvard Management Update* 10(4):6–7.

Hammonds, K. 2004. We, incorporated. *Fast Company* 84:67–69.

Hart, K.A. 2007. The aging workforce: implications for health care organizations. *Journal of Nursing Administration* 25(2):101–2.

Hart, S.M. 2006. Generational diversity: impact on recruitment and retention of nurses. *Journal of Nursing Administration* 36(1):10–12.

Harvard Business Review. 2008. Rudeness and its noxious effects. 86(3):21.

Harvey, E. 1986. Discipline vs punishment. *Management Review* (March) [unpaged reprint].

Hatcher, B.J., Bleich, M.R., Connolly, C., Davis, K., Hewitt, P.O., and Hill, K.S. 2006. *Wisdom at Work: The Importance of the Older and Experienced Nurse in the Workplace.* Princeton, NJ: Robert Wood Johnson Foundation.

Hattori, R.A., and Wycoff, J. 2002. Innovation DNA. *Training and Development* 56(1):24–30.

Havens, D.S., Wood, S.O., and Leeman, J. 2006. Improving nursing practice and patient care: building capacity with appreciative inquiry. *Journal of Nursing Administration* 36(10):463–70.

Heenan, D.A., and Bennis, W. 1999. *Co-Leaders: The Power of Great Partnerships.* New York: John Wiley & Sons.

Helgesen, S. 1995. *The Web of Inclusion: A New Architecture of Building Great Organizations.* New York: Currency/Doubleday.

Henry, J.D., and Henry, L.S. 2004. Caring from the inside out: strategies to enhance nurse retention and patient satisfaction. *Nurse Leader* 2(1):28–32.

Henry, L.S., and Henry, J.D. 2007. Using a strength-based approach to build caring work environments. *AAOHN Journal* 55(12):501–3.

Hesse-Biber, S., and Carter, G.L. 2000. *Working Women in America: Split Dreams.* New York: Oxford University Press.

Hirschhorn, L. 1997. *Reworking Authority: Leading and Following in the Post-Modern Organization.* Cambridge, MA: MIT Press.

Hock, D. 1999. *Birth of the Chaordic Age.* San Francisco: Berrett-Koehler.

Houck, John. 2003. Presentation at a meeting of the Maryland Hospital Association, July 29.

Hu, J., Herrick, C., and Hodgin, K. 2004. Managing the multigenerational nursing team. *The Health Care Manager* 23(4):334–40.

Hubble, M., Duncan, B., and Miller, S. 1999. *The Heart and Soul of Change.* Washington, DC: American Psychological Association.

Huff, C. 2007. How 'wowed' are your patients? *Hospitals & Health Networks* 81(11): 53–56.

Hutton, S.A. 2006. Workplace incivility: state of the science. *Journal of Nursing Administration* 36(1):22–28.

Hutton, S., and Gates, D. 2008. Workplace incivility and productivity losses among direct care staff. *AAOHN Journal* 56(4):168–75.

International Council of Nurses. 2007. *Nursing Workforce Profile 2007.* [Online information; retrieved April 20, 2008.] http://www.icn.ch/SewDatasheet07.pdf.

Intrator, O., Zinn, J., and Mor, V. 2004. Nursing home characteristics and potentially preventable hospitalizations of long-stay residents. *Journal of the American Geriatrics Society* 52(10):1730–36.

Iverson, R., and Buttigieg, D. 1999. Affective, normative and continuance commitment: some methodological considerations. *Journal of Management Studies* 36:307–33.

Iyengar, S.S., and Lepper, M.R. 1999. Rethinking the value of choice: a cultural perspective on intrinsic motivation. *Journal of Personality and Social Psychology* 76(3):349–66.

Jaramillo, B., Jenkins, C., Kermes, F., Wilson, L., Mazzocco, J., and Longo, T. 2008. Positive deviance: Innovation from the inside out. *Nurse Leader* 6(4):30–34.

Johnson, B. 1996. *Polarity Management: Identifying and Managing Unsolvable Problems.* Amherst, MA: HRD Press.

Johnson, C.L., Martin, S.L., and Markle-Elder, S. 2007. Stopping verbal abuse in the workplace. *American Journal of Nursing* 107(4):32–34.

Johnson, L.K. 2005. The new loyalty: make it work for your company. *Harvard Management Update* 10(3):1–3.

Joint Commission. 2002. *Health Care at the Crossroads: Strategies for Addressing the Evolving Nursing Crisis.* Oakbrook Terrace, IL: Joint Commission.

Jones, B.R. 2006. A smart solution to the worker shortage. *H&HN OnLine.* [Online information; retrieved February 5, 2006.] www.hhnmag.com.

Jones, C.B. 2005. Nurse turnover: why it is such a tough problem to solve? *Nurse Leader* 3(6):P43–P47.

Jones, C.B. 2008. "Revisiting nurse turnover costs: adjusting for inflation." *Journal of Nursing Administration* 18(1):11–18.

Josselson, R. 1996. *Revising Herself: The Story of Women's Identity from College to Midlife.* New York: Oxford University Press.

Kalisch, B.J. 2003. Recruiting nurses: the problem is the process. *Journal of Nursing Administration* 33(9):468–77.

Kalisch, B.J., and Begeny, S. 2005. Improving nursing teamwork. *Journal of Nursing Administration* 35(12):550–56.

Kalisch, B.J., Begeny, S., and Anderson, C. 2008. The effect of consistent nursing shifts on teamwork and continuity of care. *Journal of Nursing Administration* 38(3):132–37.

Kallenberg, A.L. 2008. The mismatched worker: when people don't fit their jobs. *Academy of Management Perspectives* 22(1):24–40.

Kangas, S., Kee, C.C., and McKee-Waddle, R. 1999. Organizational factors, nurses' job satisfaction, and patient satisfaction with nursing care. *Journal of Nursing Administration* 29(1):32–42.

Kanter, R.M. 1972. *Commitment and Community: Communes and Utopia in Socio-logical Perspective*. Cambridge, MA: Harvard University Press.

Kanter, R.M. 1997. *On the Frontiers of Management*. Middlebury, VT: Soundview Executive Book Summaries.

Kanter, R.M. 2008. Transforming giants. *Harvard Business Review* 86(1):43–52.

Kaplan-Leiserson, E. 2001. Aged to perfection. Like fine wine, workers get better with age. *Training and Development* 55(10):16–17.

Kash, B.A., Castle, N.G., and Phillips, C.D. 2007. Nursing home spending, staffing, and turnover. *The Health Care Manager* 32(3):253–62.

Katzenbach, J.R. 2003. *Why Pride Matters More than Money: The Power of the World's Greatest Motivational Force*. New York: Crown Business.

Katzenbach, J.R., and Smith, D.K. 1993. *The Wisdom of Teams: Creating the High-Performance Organization*. Boston: Harvard Business School Press.

Kaye, B., and Jordan-Evans, S. 1999. *Love 'em or Lose 'em*. San Francisco: Berrett-Koehler.

Kaye, B., and Jordan-Evans, S. 2002. Retention in tough times. *Training and Development* 56(1):32–37.

Kerfian, T. 2008. Personal communication.

King, Martin Luther, Jr. 1963. "I Have a Dream." Quoted in P. Anderson. 1990. *Great Quotes from Great Leaders*. Lombard, IL: Celebrating Excellence.

Kirby, J., and Stewart, T. 2007. The institutional yes. *Harvard Business Review* 85 (October):75–82.

Kleinman, C.S. 2004. Leadership and retention: research needed. *Journal of Nursing Administration* 34(3):111–13.

Kotikoff, L.J., and Burns, S. 2004. The perfect demographic storm: entitlements imperil America's future. *The Chronicles of Higher Education* LI no. 3, pp. B6–B10. [Cited in D. Huber.]

Kouzes, J.W., and Posner, B.Z. 1993. *The Credibility Factor*. San Francisco: Jossey-Bass.

Kouzes, J.W., and Posner, B.Z. 2003. *Encouraging the Heart: A Leader's Guide to Rewarding and Recognizing Others*. San Francisco: Jossey-Bass.

Kovner, C., Brewer, C., Fairchild, S., Poornima, S., Kim, H., and Djukic, M. 2007. Newly licensed RNs' characteristics, work attitudes, and intentions to work. *American Journal of Nursing* 107(9):58–70.

Kovner, C., Brewer, C., Wu, Y., Cheng, Y., and Suzuki, M. 2006. Factors associated with work satisfaction of registered nurses. *Journal of Nursing Scholarship* 38(1):71–79.

Krail, K.A. 2005. Retaining the retiring nurse. *Nurse Leader* 3(2):33–36.

Krentz, S.E., and Ross, J.S. 2008. Avoiding mission collision. *H&HN OnLine*. [Online information; retrieved April 30, 2008.] www.hhnmag.com.

Kupperschmidt, B.R. 2006. Addressing multigenerational conflict: mutual respect and carefronting as strategy. *Online Journal of Issues in Nursing* 11(2). [Online information; retrieved June 27, 2008.] http://www.nursingworld.org/MainMenuCategories/ANAMarketplace/ANAPeriodicals/OJIN.aspx.

Kupperschmidt, B.R. 2008. Associate professor at University of Oklahoma–Tulsa. Personal communication, July 22.

Kurtz, J.L., and Lyubomirsky, S. 2008. Toward a durable happiness. In S.J. Lopez and J.G. Rettew (eds.), *The Positive Psychology Perspective Series*, vol. 4. Westport, CT: Greenwood.

LaBarre, P. 2002. Weird ideas that work. *Fast Company* 54:68–73.

Lachman, V. 2001. Personality disorders in the workplace: identification and intervention. Presentation for the Forum on Healthcare Leadership, Philadelphia, August 19.

Lancaster, L., and Stillman, D. 2002. *When Generations Collide: How to Solve the Generational Puzzle at Work*. New York: HarperCollins.

Lanser, E.G. 2001. Leveraging your nursing resources. *Healthcare Executive* 16(4): 50–51.

Larkin, H. 2008. Your future chief of staff? *Hospitals & Health Networks* 82(3):30–34.

Larson, C.E., and LaFasta, F. 1989. *Team Work: What Must Go Right/What Can Go Wrong*. Newport Park, CA: Sage.

Larson, M. 2007. Florida hospitals find wealth of talent among people over 50. *Workforce Management Online*. [Online information; retrieved November 27, 2008.] http://www.workforce.com/section/06/feature/we/16/53/index.html.

Lauter, V.Z. 2006. The many ways to hold onto good employees. *H&HN OnLine*. [Online information; retrieved August 31, 2006.] www.hhnmag.com.

Lauter, V.Z. 2007 Better recruiting tactics. *H&HN OnLine*. [Online information; retrieved February 2, 2007.] www.hhnmag.com.

Lazoritz, S., and Carlson, P. 2008. Don't tolerate disruptive physician behavior. *American Nurse* 3(3):20–22.

Leander, W., Shortridge, D., and Watson, P. 1996. *Patients First*. Chicago: Health Administration Press.

Lee, C. 1999. Mean streets and rude workplaces: the death of civility. *Training* 36(7):24–30.

Lee, F. 2004. *If Disney Ran Your Hospital: 9½ Things You Would Do Differently*. Bozeman, MT: Second River Healthcare Press.

Leebov, W. 2006. Healthy respect. *H&HN OnLine*. [Online information; retrieved December 19, 2006.] www.hhnmag.com.

Leebov, W. 2007. A five-point plan for breakthroughs. *H&HN OnLine*. [Online information; retrieved October 16, 2007.] www.hhnmag.com.

Lencioni, P. 2002. *The Five Dysfunctions of a Team: A Leadership Fable*. San Francisco: Jossey-Bass.

Lima, T.H. 2007. Attracting and retaining your nursing staff. *Voice of Nursing Leadership* (3):6–7.

Loehr, J., and Schwartz, T. 2003. *The Power of Full Engagement: Managing Energy, Not Time, Is the Key to High Performance and Personal Renewal*. New York: Free Press.

Longo, J., and Sherman, R.O. 2007. Leveling horizontal violence. *Nursing Management* (March):34–51.

Lorimer, W., and Manion, J. 1996. Team-based organizations: leading the essential transformation. *Patient-Focused Care Association Review* (Summer):15–19.

Losada, M. 1999. The complex dynamics of high performance teams. *Mathematical and Computer Modeling* 30:179–92.

Ludema, J.D., Cooperrider, D.L., and Barrett, F.J. 2000. Appreciative inquiry: the power of the unconditional positive question. In P. Reason and H. Bradbury (eds.), *Handbook of Action Research*. London: Sage.

Lydon, J.E., and Zanna, M.P. 1990. Commitment in the face of adversity: a value-affirmation approach. *Journal of Personality and Social Psychology* 58(6):1040–47.

Lykken, D. 1999. *Happiness: What Studies on Twins Show Us about Nature, Nurture, and the Happiness Set Point*. New York: Golden.

Lyubomirsky, S. 2006. Is it possible to become lastingly happier? Answers from the modern science of well-being. In *Vancouver Dialogues*. Vancouver, BC: Truffle Tree.

Lyubomirsky, S., King, L.A., and Diener, E. 2005. The benefits of frequent positive affect: does happiness lead to success? *Psychological Bulletin* 131(6):803–55.

Mackoff, B.L., and Triolo, P.K. 2008a. Why do nurse managers stay? Building a model of engagement: part 1, dimensions of engagement. *Journal of Nursing Administration* 38(3):118–24.

Mackoff, B.L., and Triolo, P.K. 2008b. Why do nurse managers stay? Building a model of engagement: Part 2, Cultures of engagement. *Journal of Nursing Administration* 38(4):166–71.

Mackoff, B.L., and Triolo, P.K. 2008c. Line of sight: the crucible in nurse manager engagement. *Nurse Leader* 6(4):21–26.

Makin, P.J., Cooper, C.L., and Cox, C.J. 1996. *Organizations and the Psychological Contract: Managing People at Work*. Westport, CT: Quorum.

Manion, J. 1989. Professional collaboration: more than a committee structure. *Nursing Options* 1(4):9–12.

Manion, J. 1990. *Change from Within: Nurse Intrapreneurs as Health Care Innovators*. Washington, DC: American Nurses Association.

Manion, J. 1993. Chaos or transformation? *Journal of Nursing Administration* 23(5): 41–48.

Manion, J. 1997. Teams 101: the manager's role. *Seminars for Nurse Managers* 5(1): 31–38.

Manion, J. 1998. *From Management to Leadership: Interpersonal Skills for Success in Health Care*. Chicago: AHA Press.

Manion, J. 2000. Retaining current leaders: a gold mine in your back yard. *Health Forum Journal* 43(5):24–27.

Manion, J. 2002a. *Joy at Work: As Experienced, As Expressed*. Unpublished doctoral dissertation. Fielding Graduate Institute, Santa Barbara, CA.

Manion, J. 2002b. Life at the crossroads. *American Journal of Nursing Career Guide* (January):20–23.

Manion, J. 2003. Joy at work: creating a positive workplace. *Journal of Nursing Administration* 33(12):652–59.

Manion, J. 2004a. Community in the workplace. *Journal of Nursing Administration* 34(1):46–53.

Manion, J. 2004b. Nurture a culture of retention: front-line nurse leaders share perceptions regarding what makes—or breaks—a flourishing nursing environment. *Nursing Management* 35(4):28–39.

Manion, J. 2004c. Strengthening organizational commitment: understanding the concept as a basis for creating effective workforce retention strategies. *The Health Care Manager* 23(2):167–76.

Manion, J. 2005. *From Management to Leadership: Practical Strategies for Health Care Leaders*, second edition. San Francisco: Jossey-Bass.

Manion, J. 2008. Does your job make you happy? How to decide whether it's time to move on. *American Journal of Nursing Career Guide* (January):11–12.

Manion, J., and Bartholomew, K. 2004. Community in the workplace. *Journal of Nursing Administration* 34(1):46–53.

Manion, J., Lorimer, W., and Leander, W. 1996. *Team-Based Health Care Organizations: Blueprint for Success*. Gaithersburg, MD: Aspen.

Manion, J., Sieg, M.J., and Watson, P.W. 1998. Managerial partnerships: the wave of the future? *Journal of Nursing Administration* 28(4):47–55.

Manion, J., and Watson, P.W. 1995. Developing team-based patient care through reengineering. In S.S. Blancett and D. Flarey (eds.), *Reengineering Nursing and Health Care*. Gaithersburg, MD: Aspen.

Marsh, A. 2005. The art of work. *Fast Company* 78(8):77–79

Martin, R. 2007. How successful leaders think. *Harvard Business Review* 85(6):1–9.

Maxwell, J. 2003. Inspiration point. *Nurse Leader* (September/October):8.

Mayer, J.D., Salovey, P., and Caruso, D.R. 2000. Models of human intelligence. In R.J. Sternberg (ed.), *Handbook of Human Intelligence*, second edition. New York: Cambridge University Press.

Mayer, R., and Schoorman, D. 1998. Differentiating antecedents of organizational commitment. *Journal of Organizational Behavior* 19(1):15–28.

Maymin, S. 2007. What is positive psychology? *Positive Psychology News Daily*, January 1. [Online information; retrieved June 28, 2008.] http://pos-psych.com/news/senia-maymin/2007010115.

McCarthy, D. 1997. *The Loyalty Link*. New York: John Wiley & Sons.

McConnell, C.R. 2006. Succession planning: valuable process or pointless exercise? *The Health Care Manager* 25(1):91–98.

McIntosh, B., Palumbo, M., and Rambar, B. 2002. *The Older Nurse: Clues for Retention*. Burlington: Office of Nursing, Workforce, Research, Planning and Development, University of Vermont.

McKenna, E.P. 1997. *When Work Doesn't Work Anymore: Women, Work, and Identity*. New York: Delacorte Press.

McNeese-Smith, D.K. 2001. Building organizational commitment among nurses. *Journal of Healthcare Management* 46(3):173–87.

McNeese-Smith, D.K., and Crook, M. 2003. Nursing values and a changing nurse workforce: values, age, and job stages. *Journal of Nursing Administration* 33(5): 260–70.

Meilaender, G.C. (ed.) 2000. *Working: Its Meaning and Its Limits*. Lafayette, IN: University of Notre Dame Press.

Melrose, K. 1996. Leader as servant. *Executive Excellence* 13(4):20.

Menninger, B. 2001. The sad state of healthcare staffing. *Health Leaders* (August): 42–50.

Meyer, J., and Allen, N.J. 1984. Testing the 'side-bet theory' of organizational commitment: some methodological considerations. *Journal of Applied Psychology* 69(3):372–78.

Meyer, J., Allen, N.J., and Smith, C.A. 1993. Commitment to organizations and occupations: extensions and test of a three-component conceptualization. *Journal of Applied Psychology* 78(4):538–51.

Meyer, J., Paunonen, S., Gellatly, I., Goffin, R., and Jackson, D. 1989. Organizational commitment and job performance: it's the nature of the commitment that counts. *Journal of Applied Psychology* 74(1):152–56.

Michalopoulos, A., and Michalopoulos, H. 2006. Management's possible benefits from teamwork and the nursing process. *Nurse Leader* 4(6):52–55.

Miller, J.B. 1976. *Toward a New Psychology of Women*. Boston: Beacon Press.

Moore, T. 1994. *Care of the Soul*. New York: Harper Perennial.

Moran, J. 2008. Assistant director of Magnet Operations, American Nurses Association. Personal e-mail communication, July 16.

Morgan, C. 2005. Growing our own: A model of encouraging and nurturing aspiring leaders. *Nursing Management* 11(9):27–30.

Morgan, G. 1998. *Images of Organization: The Executive Edition*. San Francisco: Berrett-Koehler.

Morissette, R., Schellenberg, G., and Silver, C. 2004. Retaining older workers. *Perspectives on Labour and Income* 5(10). [Online information; retrieved November 27, 2007.] http://www.statcan.ca/english/freepub/75-001XIE/11004/art-2.html.

Murphy, M., Burgio-Murphy, A., and Young, J. 2007. Building trust in the workplace. *Leadership IQ*, pp. 1–8.

Murray, B. 2003. Positive discipline reaps retention. *Nursing Management* 34(6):19–22.

Mycek, S. 1998. Leadership for a healthy 21st century. *Healthcare Forum Journal* 41(4):26–30.

Myers, D.G. 1992. *The Pursuit of Happiness: Discovering the Pathway to Fulfillment, Well-being, and Enduring Personal Joy*. New York: Avon.

Myers, D.G., and Diener, E. 1995. Who is happy? *Psychological Science* 6(1):10–19.

Nadler, D.A., and Tushman, M.L. 1997. *Competing by Design: The Power of Organizational Architecture*. New York: Oxford University Press.

Natale, P. 2008. Chief nursing officer at Detroit Medical Center. Personal communication, July 14.

Naylor, T.H. 1996. The search for community in the workplace. *Business and Society Review* 97:42–48.

Naylor, T.H., Willimon, W.H., and Osterberg, R. 1996. *The Search for Meaning in the Workplace*. Nashville, TN: Abingdon Press.

Needleman, J., Buerhaus, P., Mattke, S., Stewart, M., and Zelevinsky, K. 2002. Nurse-staffing levels and the quality of care in hospitals. *New England Journal of Medicine* 346(22):1715–22.

Noer, D.M. 1993. *Healing the Wounds: Overcoming the Trauma of Layoffs and Revitalizing Downsized Organizations*. San Francisco: Jossey-Bass.

Nohria, N., Groysberg, B. and Lee, L.E. 2008. Employee motivation: a powerful new model. *Harvard Business Review* 86(July/August):78–84.

Norman, L. 2005. The older nurse in the workplace: does age matter? *Nursing Economics* 23(6):282–88.

O'Brien-Pallas, L., Duffield, C., and Alksnis, C. 2004. Who will be there to nurse? Retention of nurses nearing retirement. *Journal of Nursing Administration* 34(6):298–302.

O'Brien-Pallas, L., Duffield, C., Murphy, G.T., Birch, S., and Meyer, R. 2005. *Nursing Workforce Planning: Mapping the Policy Trail*. Geneva, Switzerland: International Council of Nurses.

Oster, C. 2004. Director of organizational development for General Motors. Personal conversation, Pontiac, MI, June.

Ott, W., and Abrams, M.N. 2008. Retention and the value of work. *H&HN OnLine*. [Online information; retrieved March 9, 2008.] www.hhnmag.com.

Palese, A., Pantali, G., and Saiani, L. 2006. The management of a multigenerational nursing team with differing qualifications: a qualitative study. *The Health Care Manager* 25(2):173–93.

Parker, M., and Kupperschmidt, B.R. 2002. Connection failure. *Nursing Spectrum Career Management*. [Online information; retrieved November 27, 2008.] http://www.NursingSpectrum.com/CareerFitnessOnline.

Parker, P. 1997. Teamwork and team players. *Team Management Briefings* 5(5):8.

Parsons, M.L., Cornett, P.A., and Golightly-Jenkins, C. 2006. Laying the groundwork by listening to nurse managers. *Nurse Leader* 4(6):34–39.

Patterson, L., and Deblieux, M. 1993. *Supervisor's Guide to Documenting Employee Discipline*. Carlsbad, CA: Parker & Sons.

Peck, M.S. 1987. *The Different Drum: Community Making and Peace*. New York: Simon & Schuster.

Peters, T., and Austin, N. 1985. *A Passion for Excellence*. New York: Random House.

Peterson, C., and Seligman, M.E.P. 2004. *Character Strengths and Virtues: A Classification Handbook*. Washington, DC: American Psychological Association.

Pfeffer, J. 1999. Practices of successful organizations. *Health Forum Journal* 42(2): 55–58.

Phillips, D. 1992. *Lincoln on Leadership: Executive Strategies for Tough Times*. New York: Warner.

Pinchot, G., and Pinchot, E. 1994. *The Intelligent Organization: Engaging the Talent and Initiative of Everyone in the Workplace*. San Francisco: Berrett-Koehler.

Pittman, A. 2007. Nursing and football: a team analogy. *Nurse Leader* 5(12): 42–44, 53.

Pittman, M.A., and Svensson, P. 2008. Ensuring global human resources for health. *H&HN OnLine*. [Online information; retrieved April 15, 2008.] www.hhnmag.com.

Plotkin, H. 1999. Six Sigma: what it is and how to use it. *Harvard Management Update* 4(6):6–7.

Ponte, P.R., Kruger, N., DeMarco, R., Hanley, D., and Conlin, G. 2004. Reshaping the practice environment: the importance of coherence. *Journal of Nursing Administration* 34(4):173–79.

Porter-O'Grady, T. 1992. *Implementing Shared Governance: Creating a Professional Organization*. St. Louis: Mosby.

Porter-O'Grady, T. 2001. Is shared governance still relevant? *Journal of Nursing Administration* 31(10):468–73.

Porter-O'Grady, T. 2003. Creators and dreamweavers: building conspiracies for innovation. *Nurse Leader* 1(1):30–32.

Porter-O'Grady, T., Alexander, D.K., and Minkara, N. 2006. Constructing a team model: creating a foundation for evidence-based teams. *Nursing Administration Quarterly* 30(3):211–20.

Post, N. 1989. Managing human energy: an ancient tool of change experts. *OD Practitioner* 6:14–16.

Post, N. 1993. Presentation on systems energetics, Philadelphia.

Powell, D.H. 1999. Retaining third-seasoners: the time is ripe. *Healthcare Executive* (November/December):4–10.

Powell, J.M., Kanny, E.M., and Ciol, M.A. 2008. State of the occupational therapy workforce: results of a national study. *American Journal of Occupational Therapy* 62(1):97–105.

Putnam, R. 2000. *Bowling Alone*. New York: Simon & Schuster.

Raines, C. 2002. *Managing Millenials*. [Online information; retrieved November 24, 2007.] http://www.generationsatwork.com/articles/millenials.html.

Rath, T. 2007. *StrengthsFinder 2.0*. New York: Gallup Press.

Raudsepp, E. 1981. *How Creative Are You?* New York: Putnam.

Reed, S. 2007. Tapping into discretionary effort: the grail of hospital leadership. *Nurse Leader* 5(10):51–54.

Reina, D., and Reina, M.L. 1999. *Trust and Betrayal in the Workplace: Building Effective Relationships in Your Organization.* San Francisco: Berrett-Koehler.

Reiners, G. 2008. Staff nurses' perceptions of supervisory leadership styles. Personal communication, July 12.

Reivich, K., and Shatte, A. 2002. *The Resilience Factor: Seven Essential Skills for Overcoming Life's Inevitable Obstacles.* New York: Broadway.

Richards, D. 1995a. *Artful Work: Awakening Joy, Meaning, and Commitment in the Workplace.* New York: Berkley.

Richards, D. 1995b. Artistry and the experience of joy. *Journal for Quality and Participation* 18(7):6–9.

Riggs, C.J., and Rantz, M.J. 2001. A model of staff support to improve retention in long-term care. *Nursing Administration Quarterly* 25(2):43–54.

Rogers, L.G. 2005. Why trust matters. *Journal of Nursing Administration* 35(10): 421–23.

Rogers, R. 1994. The psychological contract of trust. *Executive Excellence* 11(7):6.

Rosenfield, P. 2007. Workplace practices for retaining older hospital nurses: implications from a study of nurses with eldercare. *Policy, Politics, & Nursing Practice* 8(2):120–29.

Rousseau, M.F. 1991. *Community: The Tie That Binds.* New York: University Press of America.

Royal College of Nursing, Australia 2004. *The Treasury's Discussion Paper: Australia's Demographic Challenges.* [Online information; retrieved December 29, 2007.] http:www.demographics.treasury.gov.au/content/_download/subs/Royal_College_of_Nursing.pdf.

Ruggiero, J.S. 2005. Health, work variables, and job satisfaction among nurses. *Journal of Nursing Administration* 35(5):254–70.

Runy, L.A. 2003. How committed are health care employees? *Hospitals & Healthcare Networks* 77(11):28.

Runy, L.A. 2008. High-performing executive teams. *Hospitals & Health Networks* 82(4):59–66.

Ryan, K.D., and Oestreich, D.K. 1991. *Driving Fear out of the Workplace: How to Overcome the Invisible Barriers to Quality, Productivity and Innovation.* San Francisco: Jossey-Bass.

Sánchez, M., Pardo, A.P., Sánchez, D.C., Gelado, Y.N., and Garcia, M. 2008. Nurses' perception of noise levels in hospitals in Spain. *Journal of Nursing Administration* 38(5):220–22.

Santamour, B. 2004. Staffing watch. *Hospitals & Health Networks* 78(8):24.

Santos, S.R., Carroll, C.A., Cox, K.S., Teasley, S.L., Simon, S.D., Bainbridge, L., Cunningham, M., and Ott, L. 2003. Baby Boomer nurses bearing the burden of care: a four-site study of stress, strain, and coping for inpatient registered nurses. *Journal of Nursing Administration* 33(4):243–50.

Santos, S., and Cox, K. 2000. Workplace adjustment and intergenerational differences between Matures, Boomers, and Xers. *Nursing Economics* 18(1): 7–13.

Scalise, D. 2004. Shhh, quiet please! *Hospitals & Health Networks* 78(5): 16–17.

Schofield, D.J., and Beard, J.R. 2005. Baby Boomer doctors and nurses: demographic change and transitions to retirement. *Medical Journal of Australia* 183(2):80–83.

Scholtes, P. 1998. *The Leader's Handbook.* New York: McGraw-Hill.

Schuster, D.T. 1990. Work, relationships, and balance in the lives of gifted women. In H. Y. Grossman and N. L. Chester (eds.), *The Experience and Meaning of Work in Women's Lives*, pp. 189–211. Hillsdale, NJ: Lawrence Erlbaum Associates.

Schutz, W.C. 1989. *Joy: 20 Years Later*, revised edition. Berkeley, CA: Ten Speed Press.

Schwartz, B. 2004. *The Paradox of Choice: Why More Is Less*. New York: Harper-Collins.

Schwartz, T. 2007. Manage your energy, not your time. *Harvard Business Review* 85 (October):63–73.

Scott, E.S., and Cleary, B.L. 2007. Professional polarities in nursing. *Nursing Outlook* 55(5):250–55.

Searcy, B. 2003. Director of employee and labor relations for Genesys Regional Medical Center, Grand Blanc, MI. Personal conversation.

Seashore, C.N., Seashore, E.W., and Weinberg, G.M. 1999. *What Did You Say? The Art of Giving and Receiving Feedback*. Columbia, MD: Bingham House.

Seiling, J.G. 1997. *The Membership Organization: Achieving Top Performance through the New Workplace Community*. Palo Alto, CA: Davies-Black.

Seligman, M.E.P. 1998. *Learned Optimism: How to Change Your Mind and Your Life*. New York: Pocket.

Seligman, M.E.P. 2002. *Authentic Happiness: Using the New Positive Psychology to Realize Your Potential for Lasting Fulfillment*. New York: Free Press.

Seligman, M.E.P., Steen, T.A., Park, N., and Peterson, C. 2005. Positive psychology progress: empirical validation of interventions. *American Psychologist* 60(5): 410–21.

Senge, P.M. 1990. *The Fifth Discipline: The Art and Practice of the Learning Organization*. New York: Doubleday/Currency.

Sengupta, K., Abdel-Hamid, T.K., and Van Wassenhove, L.N. 2008. The experience trap. *Harvard Business Review* 86(2):94–109.

Shaffer, C.R., and Anundsen, K. 1993. *Creating Community Anywhere: Finding Support and Connection in a Fragmented World*. New York: Jeremy P. Tarcher/Putnam.

Sheehan, M. 2008. Understanding opposition. *Harvard Business Review* 86(2):21.

Shendell-Falik, N. 2008. A positive approach to safer handoffs: using AI to improve patient care outcomes. Presentation at the NRC Picker annual symposium, Palm Springs, CA, September 28.

Sherman, R.O. 2006. Leading a multigenerational nursing workforce: issues, challenges, and strategies. *Home ANA Periodicals* 11(2).

Sherwood, G. 2003. Leadership for a healthy work environment: caring for the human spirit. *Nurse Leader* 1(5):36–40.

Silberstang, J. 1995. Does joy in work have a place on your balance sheet? *Journal for Quality and Participation* 18(7):20–23.

Smith, H.L., Hood, J.N., Waldman, J.D., and Smith, V.L. 2005. Create a favorable practice environment for nurses. *Journal of Nursing Administration* 35(12): 525–32.

Snow, C.C., Lipnack, J., and Stamps, J. 1999. The virtual organization: promises and payoffs, large and small. In C.L. Cooper and D.M. Rousseau (eds.), *Trends in Organizational Behavior: The Virtual Organization*, pp. 15–30. New York: John Wiley & Sons.

Spencer, A.L. 1982. *Seasons: Women's Search for Self through Life's Stages*. New York: Paulist Press.

Spiegelman, P. 2007. Brand loyalty from the inside out. *H&HN OnLine*. [Online information; retrieved November 6, 2007.] www.hhnmag.com.

Spinks, N., and Moore, C. 2007. The changing workforce, workplace, and nature of work: implications for health human resource management. *Nursing Leadership* 20(3):26–41.

Spitzer, R. 2007. Commitment goes both ways. *Nurse Leader* 5(10):4.

Stacey, R.D. 1992. *Managing the Unknowable: Strategic Boundaries between Order and Chaos in Organizations*. San Francisco: Jossey-Bass.

Stanton, M.W. 2004. Hospital nurse staffing and quality of care. Agency for Healthcare Research and Quality. AHRQ Publ. 04-0029. [Online information; retrieved 12/19/08.] http://www.ahrq.gov/research/nursestaffing/nursestaff.htm.

Stefaniak, K. 2007. Discovering nursing excellence through appreciative inquiry. *Nurse Leader* 5(4):42–46.

Strachota, E., Normandin, P., O'Brien, N., Clary, M., and Krukow, B. 2003. Reasons registered nurses leave or change employment status. *Journal of Nursing Administration* 33(2):111–17.

Strack, R., Baier, J., and Fahlander, A. 2008. Managing demographic risk. *Harvard Business Review* 86(2):119–28.

Stuenkel, D.L., and Cohen, J. 2005. The multigenerational workforce: essential differences in perception of work environment. *Journal of Nursing Administration* 35(6):283–85.

Sull, D.N., and Houlder, D. 2005 Do your commitments match your convictions? *Harvard Business Review* 83(1):82–91.

Sutton, R. 2002. *Weird Ideas That Work: 11½ Practices for Promoting, Managing, and Sustaining Innovation*. New York: Free Press.

Swearingen, S., and Liberman, A. 2004. Nursing generations: an expanded look at the emergence of conflict and its resolution. *The Health Care Manager* 23(1):54–64.

Taylor, B.J. 2004. Improving communication through practical reflection. *Reflections on Nursing Leadership* (second quarter):28–38.

Terez, T. 1999. Meaningful work. *Executive Excellence* 16(2):19.

Terkel, S. 1972. *Working*. New York: Pantheon.

Thomas, K.W. 2000. *Intrinsic Motivation at Work: Building Energy and Commitment*. San Francisco: Berrett-Koehler.

Thomas, S.P. 2004. *Transforming Nurses' Stress and Anger: Steps toward Healing*, second edition. New York: Springer-Verlag.

Thompson, D.N., Wolf, G.A., and Spear, S.J. 2003. Driving improvement in patient care: lessons from Toyota. *Journal of Nursing Administration* 33(11):585–95.

Thrall, T.H. 2005. Retirement boom? *Hospitals & Health Networks* 79(11):30–38.

Thrall, T.H. 2006. Staffing watch. *Hospitals & Health Networks* 80(4):24.

Thrall, T.H. 2007. Residency program helps rural hospitals attract, keep nurses. *Hospitals & Health Networks* 81(12):24–25.

Tichy, N., and Cardwell, N. 2002. *The Cycle of Leadership: How Great Leaders Teach Their Companies to Win*. New York: HarperBusiness.

Thompson, J., Wieck, K.L., and Warner, A. 2003. What perioperative and emerging workforce nurses want in a manager. *AORN Journal* 78(2):246–49, 252–56, 258, 261.

Totterdell, P. 2000. Catching moods and hitting runs: mood linkage and subjective performance in professional sport teams. *Journal of Applied Psychology* 85(6):848–59.

Totterdell, P., Kellett, S., Teuchmann, K., and Briner, R.B. 1998. Evidence of mood linkage in work groups. *Journal of Personality and Social Psychology* 74(6):1504–15.

Tourigny, L., and Pulich, M. 2008. Improving retention of older employees through training and development. *The Health Care Manager* 25(1):43–52.

Trigg, R. 1973. *Reason and Commitment*. Cambridge, UK: Cambridge University Press.

Tubbs, W. 1993. Karoushi: stress-death and the meaning of work. *Journal of Business Ethics* 12:869–77.

Tucker, A.L., and Edmondson, A.C. 2003. Why hospitals don't learn from failures: organizational and psychological dynamics that inhibit system change. *California Management Review* 45(2):55–72.

Tucker, A.L., and Spear, S.J. 2006. Operational failures and interruptions in hospital nursing. *Health Services Research* 41(3):643–62.

Tushman, M.L., and O'Reilly, C.A. 1999. Building ambidextrous organizations: forming your own "skunk works." *Health Forum Journal* 42(2):20–23, 64.

Vance, M. 1982. *Creative Thinking*. Chicago: Nightingale-Conant.

Vestal, K. 2006. Ex-employees: can they come back? *Nurse Leader* 4(10):6, 14.

Vestal, K. 2007. The one thing you need to know. *Nurse Leader* 5(10):6–8.

Vestal, K. 2008. Managing interruptions. *Nurse Leader* 6(6):8–9.

Vogl, A.J. 1997. Soul searching: looking for meaning in the workplace. *Across the Board* 34(9):16–24.

Wall, B. 2007. Being smart only takes you so far. *Training & Development* 61(1):64–68.

Walker D.M. 2007. Older Workers: Some Best Practices and Strategies for Engaging and Retaining Older Workers. Testimony before the U.S. Senate Special Committee on Aging, February 28. [Online information; retrieved November 27, 2007.] http://www.gao.gov/cgi-bin/getrpt?GAO-07-433T.

Waterman, R.H. 1992. *Adhocracy: The Power to Change*. New York: W.W. Norton.

Watson, N. 2008. Director of human resources at Mercy Hospital/Allina Hospitals & Clinics, Minneapolis, MN. Personal conversation, July 15.

Watson, R., Manthorpe, C., and Andrews, J. 2003a. *Nurses over 50: Options, Decisions and Outcomes*, Bristol, UK: University of Hull.

Watson, R., Manthorpe, C., and Andrews, J. 2003b. Older nurses and employment decisions. *Nursing Standard* 18(7):35–40.

Weaver, T. 2008. Enhancing multiple disciplinary teamwork. *Nursing Outlook* 56(3):108–14.

Webber, A.M. 1998. Danger: toxic company. *Fast Company* 19:152–61.

Weber, D.O. 2003. Ideology. *Health Forum Journal* 47(3):21–24.

Weber, D.O. 2005. The toll on hospital workers, part 2. *H&HN OnLine*. [Online information; retrieved August 25, 2005.] www.hhnmag.com.

Wedman, D. 2008. Personal conversation, July 7.

Wesorick, B. 2002. 21st century leadership challenge: creating and sustaining healthy healing work cultures and integrated service at the point of care. *Nursing Administration Quarterly* 26(5):18–32.

Wheatley, M.J. 1999. *Leadership and the New Science: Learning about Organizations from an Orderly Universe*, second edition. San Francisco: Berrett-Koehler.

Whiley, K. 2001. The nurse manager's role in creating a healthy work environment. *AACN Clinical Issues* 12(3):356–65.

Whyte, D. 2001. *Crossing the Unknown Sea: Work as a Pilgrimage of Identity*. New York: Riverhead.

Wieck, K.L. 2000. Tomorrow's nurses: are we ready for them? *Texas Nursing* (June/ July):1-4.

Wieck, K.L. 2003. Faculty for the millennium: changes needed to attract the emerging workforce into nursing. *Journal of Nursing Education* 42(4):151–58.

Wieck, K.L., Prydun, M., and Walsh, T. 2003. What the emerging workforce wants in its leaders. *Journal of Nursing Scholarship* 34(3):283–88.

Wiener, Y. 1982. Commitment in organizations. *Academy of Management Review* 7(3):418–28.

Wiggins, M. 2001. Personal communication.

Williams, E.S., Manwell, L.B., Konrad, T.R., and Linzer, M. 2007. The relationship of organizational culture, stress, satisfaction, and burnout with physician-reported error and suboptimal patient care: results from the MEMO study. *Health Care Management Review* 32(3):203–12.

Wolf, E. 2001. Defying age bias in the workplace. *Healthcare Executive* (November/ December):5–10.

Wolf, G., Triolo, P., and Ponte, P.R. 2008. Magnet recognition program: the next generation. *Journal of Nursing Administration* 38(4):200–204.

Wolff, S.B. 1998. *The Role of Caring Behavior and Peer Feedback in Creating Team Effectiveness.* Unpublished thesis, Boston University.

Womack, J.P., and Jones, D. 1996. *Lean Thinking: Banish Waste and Create Wealth within Your Organization.* New York: Simon & Schuster.

World Health Organization (WHO). 2006. *Working Together for Health: The World Health Report 2006.* Geneva, Switzerland: WHO.

Worthington, C.H. 1994. *Beyond Job Satisfaction: The Phenomenon of Joy in Work.* Unpublished doctoral dissertation, Georgia State University, Atlanta.

Wycoff, J. 1991. *Mindmapping: Your Personal Guide to Exploring Creativity and Problem-Solving.* New York: Berkley.

Zander, R.S., and Zander, B. 2000. *The Art of Possibility: Transforming Professional and Personal Life.* Boston: Harvard Business School Press.

Zemke, R. 1996. The call of community. *Training* 33(3):24–30.

Zemke, R. 1999. Problem-solving is the problem: don't fix that company. *Training* 36(6):26–33.

Zemke, R. 2002. Generational diversity in health care: the management challenge. Seminar at VHA Leadership Conference, Chicago.

Zemke R., Raines, C., and Filipczak, B. 2000. *Generations at Work: Managing the Clash of Veterans, Boomers, Xers, and Nexters in Your Workplace.* New York: AMACOM.

Index